3D Printing in Orthopaedic Surgery

3D Printing in Orthopaedic Surgery

EDITED BY

MATTHEW DIPAOLA, MD
Clinical Assistant Professor of Orthopaedics
  and Sports Medicine
Jacobs School of Medicine
University at Buffalo
Buffalo, NY, United States

FELASFA M. WODAJO, MD
Virginia Cancer Specialists
Associate Professor Orthopedic Surgery
VCU School of Medicine
Assistant Professor Orthopedic Surgery
Georgetown University Hospital
Fairfax, VA, United States

ELSEVIER

ELSEVIER

3251 Riverport Lane
St. Louis, Missouri 63043

3D Printing in Orthopaedic Surgery   ISBN: 978-0-323-66211-6

Notices

Publisher: Mica Haley
Acquisition Editor: Kayla Wolfe
Editorial Project Manager: Jennifer Horigan
Project Manager: Poulouse Joseph
Designer: Alan Studholme

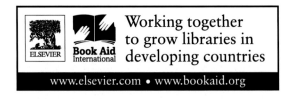

Working together
to grow libraries in
developing countries

www.elsevier.com • www.bookaid.org

List of Contributors

Adam E. Jakus, PhD
Chief Technology Officer
Dimension Inx LLC
Chicago, IL, USA

Sourabh Manoj Saptarshi, MS
Digital Manufacturing Laboratory
University at Buffalo
Buffalo, NY, USA

Chi Zhou, PhD
Assistant Professor
Industrial and Systems Engineering
University at Buffalo
Buffalo, NY, USA

Sanjay P. Prabhu, MBBS, DCH, FRCR, DABR
Staff Pediatric Neuroradiologist
Director, Advanced Image Analysis Lab
Clinical Director, SIMPeds3D Print Service
Medical Director, Imaging Informatics
Boston Children's Hospital
Assistant Professor of Radiology
Harvard Medical School
Boston, MA, USA

Gilbert G. Berdine, MD
Associate Professor of Medicine
Internal Medicine
Texas Tech University Health Sciences Center
Lubbock, TX, USA

Faculty Affiliate
Free Market Institute
Lubbock, TX, USA

Michael Weinberg, JD
New York, NY, USA

Matthew DiPaola, MD
Clinical Assistant Professor of Orthopaedics and
Sports Medicine
Jacobs School of Medicine
University of Buffalo
Buffalo, NY, USA

William M. Mihalko, MD, PhD
J. R. Hyde Professor
Campbell Clinic Department of Orthopaedic Surgery &
Biomedical Engineering
Univ. of Tennessee-Campbell Clinic
Memphis, TN, USA

Paul A. Anderson, MD
Professor
Orthopedic Surgery and Rehabilitation
University of Wisconsin
Madison, WI, USA

Jerry D'Alesio, PHD
VP Research and Advanced Engineering
R&D
Onkos Surgical
Parsipanny, NJ, USA

Andy Christensen, BS
Somaden LLC
Littleton, Colorado, USA

Division of Medical Physics
Department of Radiology
University of Ottawa
Ottawa, Ontario, Canada

H. Brent Bamberger, DO
Program Director
Kettering Health Network
Orthopedic Surgery Department at Grandview
Dayton, OH, USA

James R. Jastifer, MD
Orthopaedic Surgery
Borgess Medical Center

Clinical Assistant Professor
Department of Orthopaedic Surgery
Western Michigan University Homer Stryker M.D.
   School of Medicine
Kalamazoo, MI, USA

Christian DiPaola, MD
Associate Professor
Dept. of Orthopaedics and Rehabilitation
UMass Memorial Medical Center
Worcester, MA, USA

Associate Professor
Radiation Oncology
UMass Memorial Medical Center
Worcester, MA, USA

John R. Burleson, MD
Dept. of Orthopedic Surgery
UMass Memorial Medical Center
Worcester, MA, USA

Brian M. Haus, MD
Chief, Pediatric Orthopaedic Surgery
Orthopaedic Surgery
UC Davis Children's Hospital
Sacramento, CA, USA

Lawrence I. Karlin, MD
Assistant Professor of Orthopaedic Surgery
Harvard Medical School
Associate Attending
Department of Orthopaedic Surgery
Boston Children's Hospital
Boston, MA, USA

Eric T. Ricchetti, MD
Department of Orthopedic Surgery
Orthopedic and Rheumatologic Institute
Cleveland Clinic
Cleveland, Ohio, USA

Deepak M. Cheriachan, MD
Department of Orthopedic Surgery
Orthopedic and Rheumatologic Institute
Cleveland Clinic
Cleveland, Ohio, USA

Sridhar R. Rachala, MD
Clinical Assistant Professor
Orthopaedic Surgery
University at Buffalo
SUNY
Buffalo General Hospital
Buffalo, NY, USA

Amir Sternheim, MD
Joint Head 3D Surgical Lab
National Unit of Orthopaedic Oncology
Tel-Aviv Medical Center
Tel-Aviv
Israel

Sakler School of Medicine
Faculty of Medicine
Tel-Aviv University
Tel-Aviv
Israel

Bruno Borralho Gobbato, MD
Chief Division Shoulder Surgery
Orthopedic Surgery
Hospital São José
Jaraguá do Sul
Santa Catarina
Brazil

Chief Division Shoulder Surgery
Orthopedic Surgery
IOT Jaraguá
Jaraguá do Sul
Santa Catarina
Brazil

Felasfa M. Wodajo, MD
Virginia Cancer Specialists
Associate Professor Orthopedic Surgery
VCU School of Medicine
Assistant Professor Orthopedic Surgery
Georgetown University Hospital
Fairfax, VA, United States

Sean Gao, DO
Kettering Health Network
Orthopedic Surgery Department at Grandview
Dayton, OH, USA

Joseph Dallis Stephens, DO
Kettering Health Network
Orthopedic Surgery Department at Grandview
Dayton, OH, USA

Caleb Piatt, DO
Kettering Health Network
Orthopedic Surgery Department at Grandview
Dayton, OH, USA

Taylor Hockman, DO
Heritage College of Osteopathic Medicine
Athens, OH, USA

Andrew Hills, DO
Lake Erie College of Osteopathic Medicine
Erie, PA, USA

Jay Thompson, DO
Rocky Vista Universty College of Osteopathic Medicine
Parker, CO, USA

Morgan Smith, DO
Texas College of Osteopathic Medicine
Forth Worth, Texas, USA

David Martineau, MD
Research Director
Kettering Health Network
Orthopedic Surgery Department at Grandview
Dayton, OH, USA

Peter A. Gustafson, PhD
Associate Professor of Mechanical and Aerospace
    Engineering
Western Michigan University
Michigan, USA

Associate Professor of Medical Engineering
Western Michigan University
Homer Stryker M.D. School of Medicine
Michigan, USA

Andrea S. Bauer, MD
Assistant Professor of Orthopaedic Surgery
Harvard Medical School
Associate Attending
Department of Orthopaedic Surgery
Boston Children's Hospital
Boston, MA, USA

Joseph P. Iannotti, MD
Department of Orthopedic Surgery
Orthopedic and Rheumatologic Institute
Cleveland Clinic
Cleveland, Ohio, USA

Muhammad Nadeem, MBBS
Research Scholar
University at Buffalo
SUNY
Buffalo, NY, USA

Eric Jackson, DO
Fellow
Adult Reconstructive Orthopaedic Surgery
University at Buffalo
SUNY
Buffalo, NY, USA

Yair Gortzak, MD
National Unit of Orthopaedic Oncology
Tel-Aviv Medical Center
Tel-Aviv, Israel

Sakler School of Medicine
Faculty of Medicine
Tel-Aviv University
Tel-Aviv, Israel

Yehuda Kolander, MD
National Unit of Orthopaedic Oncology
Tel-Aviv Medical Center
Tel-Aviv, Israel

Sakler School of Medicine
Faculty of Medicine
Tel-Aviv University
Tel-Aviv, Israel

Solomon Dadai, MD
Joint Head 3D Surgical Lab
National Unit of Orthopaedic Oncology
Tel-Aviv Medical Center
Tel-Aviv, Israel

Sakler School of Medicine
Faculty of Medicine
Tel-Aviv University
Tel-Aviv, Israel

Building the Future of Orthopedics: One Layer at a Time

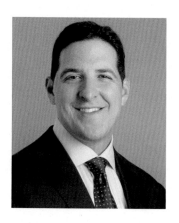

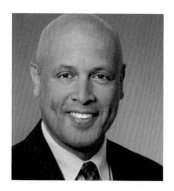

Although additive manufacturing and 3D printing technologies have been in existence since the 1980s, their adoption in orthopedics has begun to reach an inflection point. A combination of factors has opened a fascinating new era in manufacturing, one that puts more power in the hands of the inventor and more personalization for the end user.

Orthopedics has always been a very tangible field. As surgeons, our charge is often to reimagine and reshape anatomy. In this respect, the advancements in 3D printing technologies may have met their ideal medical specialty in orthopedics.

In this volume, we will explore the history of additive manufacturing in general and orthopedics more specifically. There are chapters dedicated to the engineering aspects of 3D printing and to the software tools used to create print-ready models from CT scans. A thought-provoking chapter explores the possible economic and regulatory repercussions of democratized 3D printing. Other chapters provide an overview of 3D printing in arthroplasty, in orthopedic resident education and on how to set up an inexpensive home/office 3D print "shop" for printing your own bone models.

The largest portion of this volume consists of orthopedic surgeon authors delving into the uses of 3D printing in their respective subspecialties. We found many of these case examples both eye opening and inspiring.

As orthopedic surgeons, we feel we are witnessing the beginning of a more personalized approach to understanding and reconstructing musculoskeletal anatomy. We hope you enjoy your journey through this text as much as we have in putting it together.

Matthew DiPaola, MD
*Clinical Assistant Professor Orthopaedics
and Sports Medicine
Jacobs School of Medicine University
at Buffalo
UBMD Orthopedics and Sports Medicine
Buffalo, NY*

Felasfa M. Wodajo, MD
*Virginia Cancer Specialists
Associate Professor, Orthopedic Surgery,
VCU School of Medicine
Assistant Professor, Orthopedic Surgery,
Georgetown University Hospital
Fairfax VA*

Contents

SECTION I
3D PRINTING PRINCIPLES

1 **An Introduction to 3D Printing—Past, Present, and Future Promise**, *1*
   Adam E. Jakus, PhD

2 **Basics of 3D Printing: Engineering Aspects**, *17*
   Sourabh Manoj Saptarshi, MS and Dr. Chi Zhou, PhD

3 **From CT and MR Images to 3D Printed Models—Software Basics for the Surgeon**, *31*
   Sanjay P. Prabhu, MBBS, DCH, FRCR, DABR

4 **Economic and Regulatory Perspectives on Additive Manufacturing**, *41*
   Gilbert G. Berdine, MD, Matthew DiPaola, MD, and Michael Weinberg, JD

SECTION II
OVERVIEW OF 3D PRINTING IN ORTHOPEDICS

5 **Additive Manufacturing of Arthroplasty Implants**, *49*
   William M. Mihalko, MD, PhD

6 **3D Printing for Education and Surgical Planning in Orthopedic Surgery**, *55*
   Paul A. Anderson, MD

7 **3D Printing for Commercial Orthopedic Applications: Advances and Challenges**, *65*
   Jerry D'Alessio, PhD, and Andy Christensen, BS

SECTION III
3D PRINTING IN ORTHOPEDICS: SUBSPECIALTIES

8 **3D Printing in Orthopedics: Upper Extremity Trauma and Deformity**, *85*
   Sean Gao, DO, Joseph Dallis Stephens, DO, Caleb Piatt, DO, Taylor Hockman, DO, Andrew Hills, DO, Jay Thompson, DO, Morgan Smith, DO, David Martineau, MD, and H. Brent Bamberger, DO

9 **Three-Dimensional Printing Technology in Foot and Ankle Surgery**, *95*
   James R. Jastifer, MD and Peter A. Gustafson, PhD

10 **3D Printing in Spine Surgery**, *105*
   John Burleson, MD and Christian DiPaola, MD

11 **Pediatric Hip and Acetabulum**, *123*
   Brian M. Haus, MD

12 **Pediatric Spine and Extremity**, *137*
   Lawrence I. Karlin, MD and Andrea S. Bauer, MD

13 **3D Printing in Orthopedics—Upper Extremity Arthroplasty**, *151*
   Deepak M. Cheriachan, MD, Matthew DiPaola, MD, Joseph P. Iannotti, MD, PhD, and Eric T. Ricchetti, MD

14 **3D Printing in Hip and Knee Arthroplasty**, 171
Muhammad Nadeem, MBBS, Eric Jackson, DO and Sridhar R. Rachala, MD

15 **3D Printing in Orthopedic Oncology**, 179
Amir Sternheim, MD, Yair Gortzak, MD, Yehuda Kolander, MD, and Solomon Dadia, MD

SECTION IV
FUTURE OF 3D PRINTING

16 **Setting Up Your Own Home 3D Printing "Plant"**, 195
Bruno Borralho Gobbato, MD

INDEX, 209

CHAPTER 1

An Introduction to 3D Printing—Past, Present, and Future Promise

ADAM E. JAKUS, PHD

INTRODUCTION

The progress of human civilization is commonly defined by material-named ages—stone, bronze, iron, steel, silicon/computer, etc. However, the onset of these ages do not denote when these materials were first discovered, but rather, when humanity began to master their isolation and ability to manufacture with them, creating useful devices and objects that ultimately propelled technology and civilization to achieve its present form. Until very recently, manufacturing, regardless of the materials being utilized, has been primarily "subtractive" in nature—raw materials are isolated, collected, transformed into bulk forms, which are in turn manipulated, machined, and reduced to create the final objects. These processes have been effectively utilized to shape our world and produce nearly every single device in use today, including for medicine—from the simplest plastic disposables to the most advanced metallic and ceramic surgical tools and implants and many human- and animal-derived biologics. Despite the enormous progress that has been made, the subtractive nature of traditional manufacturing processes has numerous limitations that have ultimately driven a new paradigm in manufacturing—additive manufacturing (AM), now commonly, and collectively referred to as "3D printing."

"3D printing" has become the common term that refers to a broad collection of additive-based technologies—technologies that operate on the principal of creating objects from the bottom-up, bit-by-bit or layer-by-layer, rather than top-down, removing excess bulk material until the final object is revealed (subtractive manufacturing). A simplified representation of these distinct additive and subtractive processes is illustrated in Fig. 1.1. The term "3D printing"

technically refers to additive technologies based on the deposition of materials. Another technique is selective delivery of energy to a material, resulting in selective curing or sintering to create a three-dimensional object. However, despite the technical differentiation between the terms, "3D printing" has become colloquially dominant and is utilized to refer to the collection of AM technologies that will be discussed in this and proceeding chapters. These technologies range from simple room temperature nozzle extrusion of pastes and "3D inks" to high-energy electron beam selective sintering/melting of metallic powder beds and everything in between—all of which have applications in orthopedics and the broader fields of surgery and medicine, including use for modeling, surgical guides, training devices, orthotics, prosthetics, permeant implants, and tissue regenerative implants. For additional specifics on the continuously evolving definitions and standards related to additive manufacturing, the reader can refer to ASTM International document F42 and ISO TC 261.

At present, 3D printing is being utilized in nearly every single industry, trade, and field for innumerable applications, ranging from production of simple models, toys, food, and high art and fashion items to advanced parts for aircraft and orbital transportation. However, 3D printing is perhaps most at home and has the longest history within the medical fields—where enabling the creation of distinct objects that represent or can replace varied, anatomic parts of individuals, of which no two are exactly alike, is perfectly suited. In this case, "history" refers to only the past 30—35 years, beginning in the mid-1980s with the introduction of the first additive technologies for modeling and rapid prototyping, up to the present day, where both one-off, patient-matched devices as well as

3D Printing in Orthopaedic Surgery. https://doi.org/10.1016/B978-0-323-58118-9.00001-4

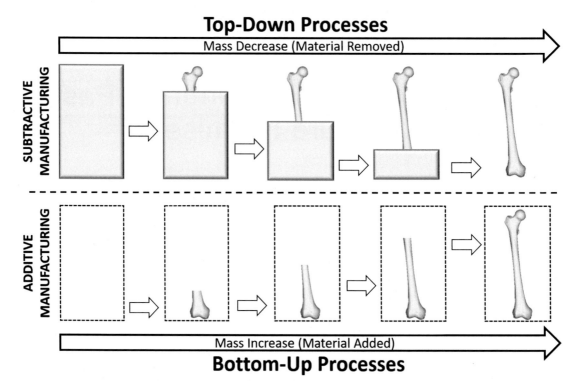

Top-Down Processes
Mass Decrease (Material Removed)

SUBTRACTIVE MANUFACTURING

ADDITIVE MANUFACTURING

Mass Increase (Material Added)
Bottom-Up Processes

FIG. 1.1 A simplified schematic illustration highlighting the general distinction between subtractive and additive manufacturing ("3D printing") processes.

mass-produced, regulatory-approved, 3D printed medical products have become increasingly ubiquitous. At the same time, the development of new and advanced biomaterials and biologics, along with live cell and tissue bioprinting and related biofabrication technologies are beginning to be clinically introduced, foreshadowing a future where 3D printing is not only commonly utilized to create models, guides, and inert implants, but also highly bioactive, tissue regenerative devices that promise to transform orthopedic medicine and healthcare at large. This chapter gives a brief overview of the history, present state, and projected future of 3D printing in medicine and orthopedics, along with a brief introduction and discussion to the basic premises, technologies, materials, and processes that collectively underlie 3D printing.

3D PRINTING: FROM PAST TO PRESENT
To fully appreciate the current state, as well as the future of 3D printing in orthopedics, it is important to understand the technologies' collective history and rapid progression. This not only places the current state of 3D printing in perspective but will enable the reader to

appreciate how quickly the field is moving and where it might be in 5, 10, or 15 years from the present. The following section describes the broader history of AM, not specifically focusing on orthopedics, or even the broader fields of medicine. Nevertheless, it should be noted that surgery and medicine were at the forefront of every single major progression in the technology.

The history of AM, or 3D printing, can be distinguished into five, or possibly six, distinct eras. The first era began in the late 1970s and continued through the early 1980s and is defined by isolated examples of what could be considered the forerunners of AM technologies ("Proto Additive Manufacturing"). The second era began in the mid-1980s and continued to approximately 1990 and denotes the development and initial introduction of three of major, foundational 3D printing technologies, as well as the founding of the first 3D printing companies, two of which remain major industry players to this day. The third era, from 1990 to approximately 2005, denotes an extended period of 3D printing technology maturation within the original private companies, the introduction of additional, major 3D printing technologies, as well as the tandem development and advancement of computational and

3D imaging capabilities. The fourth era, from 2005 to 2012, which noncoincidentally aligns with the expiration of the original 3D printing patents, mainstream adoption of social media, as well as the start of the "maker movement," represents the period in which 3D printing begins to be widely introduced to and adopted by audiences beyond the original big industry players. The fifth era, beginning in 2012/2013 and continuing into 2017, or the present day depending on opinion, represents what could be described as an awakening of 3D printing. New additive technologies, 3D printable materials, and even bioprinting began to be widely adopted, going mainstream, and being substantially funded and supported by major federal government efforts and entities. These five/six eras and associated, select major events within and related to AM and 3D printing are illustrated in the timeline in Fig. 1.2 and further expanded upon later, with additional attention given to the medical fields.

First Era (Late 1970s to Early 1980s)—Proto Additive Manufacturing

Publicly available knowledge and sources related to the first successful examples of AM are limited. However, anecdotally, technologies related to contemporary, advanced aerospace manufacturing were believed to have been applied in isolated instances to create minimal fidelity structures based on low resolution imaging data. However, the first public article, specifically on the

subject of AM, "Automatic method for fabricating three-dimensional plastic model with photo-hardening polymer," was published in the first half of 1981 and authored by Hideo Kodama[1] of the Nagoya Municipal Industrial Research Institute in Japan. This paper first described what is known as today as the stereolithography (SLA) process.

Second Era (Mid-1980s to 1990)— Introduction of Additive Manufacturing

The mid- to late 1980s saw the first commercially viable examples of multiple 3D printing technologies be developed and begin to take off. Chuck Hull is often credited with being the inventor of 3D printing. He was granted a patent related to the stereolithographic process in 1986, but was not the first creator of the process as can be seen from Hideo Kodama's earlier work, as well as an earlier French patent application filed by Alain Le Mèhautè, Jean-Claude Andrè, and Olivier de Witt. Despite this, Chuck Hull did develop the SLA file format, .STL, which remains the predominant file type used for 3D printing across a range of stereolithographic and nonstereolithographic processes. Chuck Hull went on to cofound 3D Systems, which remains a major industry player in both medical and nonmedical markets. The 1986 patent was followed closely by patents for powder bed–based selective laser sintering (SLS; 1989) by Carl Deckard (cofounder of Desk Top

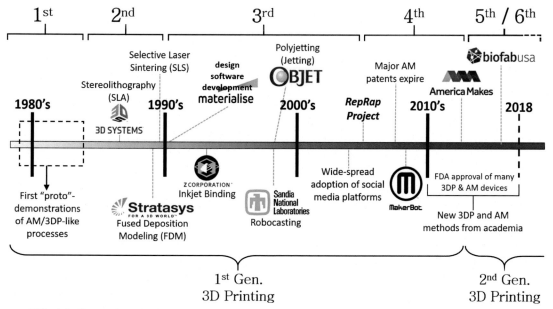

FIG. 1.2 Summarized timeline with major eras and select events in the history of additive manufacturing (AM) and 3D printing (3DP).

Manufacturing; later acquired by 3D Systems) and material deposition–based fused deposition modeling (FDM; 1989) by Scott Crump, cofounder of Stratasys, which also remains one of the largest players in the industry. These three original AM and 3D printing technologies, SLA, SLS, and FDM, remain in frequent use today and provided the technologic foundation for the emergence of many additional resin bath–, powder bed–, material deposition–based, and hybrid 3D printing technologies (described later) that are utilized today. During this period, and continuing through the 1990s and early 2000s, AM and 3D printing processes were not commonly referred to as such; "rapid prototyping" was the preferred terminology, as the processes were predominantly utilized for creating models and prototypes of products to be fabricated and produced using traditional manufacturing methods.

Third Era (1990–2005)—Computational Capabilities Increase and Industrial 3D Printing Matures

One of the major limitations of early 3D printing, or rapid prototyping, technologies was the inability to efficiently generate, store, and translate complex three-dimensional digital data into 3D printable files. Whether that data was made from scratch, via early computer-aided design software, or was generated via serial three-dimensional imaging processes such as magnetic resonance imaging or computer-aided tomography, the process was cumbersome and required computational skills as well as computational power. The hardware (3D printer) was not yet effectively matched with the software. During this period, desktop computation and data storage capabilities began to exponentially increase. In tandem, numerous three-dimensional software and modeling companies were founded, including Materialise, which remains a major global player in three-dimensional software development, data acquisition, refinement, modeling, and 3D printing, consulting in medical and nonmedical fields. This period also witnessed the maturation of the original SLA, SLS, and FDM prototyping technologies as well as the first examples of new processes, such as ink-jet binding (1993, Z Corporation—merged with 3D Systems in 2012), polyjetting (1998, Objet—merged with Stratasys in 2011), and robocasting (extrusion-based 3D printing).

Contemporaneously with the advancements being made in computing power and imaging software, maturation of original and introduction of new 3D printing technologies, and establishment of imaging and 3D printing service and consulting companies, select clinicians began to utilize the process to aid in complex surgical cases. At the time, these efforts were primarily focused on hard tissue, complex, craniomaxillofacial (CMF) pediatric abnormalities and traumatic injuries. With the ability to work with physical, life-size representations of a specific patient's anatomic defects, complex tasks and operations could be planned prior to surgery, and the models could even be utilized intraoperatively as guides as well as used outside the operating room as tools and aids for physician-physician and physician-patient communications. Although there are several isolated examples of 3D printing being used for orthopedic surgical planning and modeling during the 1990s, 3D printing in medicine during this era was primarily driven by the needs of and challenges faced by CMF and oral surgeons. It would not be until the fourth and fifth eras that 3D printing, both for individual patients as well as mass-produced products, became more widespread within the field of orthopedics.

Fourth Era (2005–2012)—Rapid Expansion and Increased Awareness of 3D Printing

From an anthropologic perspective on technology evolution and development, the fourth era of 3D printing is rather fascinating. Rather than any major technologic breakthrough, it was primarily the alignment of major legal and social events/groups that resulted in the rapid expansion and mass awareness of 3D printing. These events were the expiration of the original 3D printing–related patents from the 1980s, emergence and widespread adoption of social media, and the founding of the RepRap Project at the University of Bath in the United Kingdom, which became a major part of the young "maker movement," and ultimately the company MakerBot, arguably the first major consumer-focused 3D printing company. These efforts not only resulted in an explosion of media and mass public awareness of 3D printing technology, particularly SLA and FDM, but also resulted in the development of consumer-scale and priced 3D printers (or build-your-own 3D printer kits) that soon became widely available in conjunction with open-source software and file sharing community sites. It is because of the sudden and rapid increase in awareness of 3D printing during this period, and lack of awareness of its prior history, that 3D printing is often viewed as a very new technology, despite it having been in use for more than three decades.

Perhaps as a result of the increased global awareness of the technology as well as what could be considered inaccurate exaggerations about being able to make anything, 3D printing technology began to be rapidly adopted by academic and clinical research institutions, subsequently becoming not only a vital tool to aid in existing research but becoming the subject of research itself. During this time, the use of 3D printed surgical models, guides, basic prosthetics and orthotics, and other simple polymeric and metallic devices become increasingly commonplace in orthopedics and the broader medical fields. At the same time, the US government, still recovering from the major economic collapse of 2008, saw 3D printing and advanced manufacturing technologies (a term that encompasses additive technologies and other new manufacturing processes) as an opportunity to rebuild the United States' manufacturing prowess. With this in mind, the National Network for Manufacturing Innovation (NNMI; also known as Manufacturing USA) was launched in 2012, with the National Additive Manufacturing Innovation Institute (NAMII; also known as America Makes) being the first institute established as part of the network. With these series of events, 3D printing had come to the forefront of industry, the maker movement, academia, medicine, and US (and subsequently international) government; setting the stage for an explosion in hardware, software, materials, and application research, development, and adoption.

Fifth Era (2012—2017/Present)— New Materials and Technologies and Second-Generation 3D Printing

Prior to 2012, the majority of major advancements in the field of 3D printing was due to advances in hardware and software, as well as increased social awareness and technology sharing. Now, with the technology beginning to receive the full attention of industry, academia, government, and medicine, major developments, primarily led by the creation of new, advanced, highly functional, and 3D printable materials, were beginning to lead the technology away from one-off prototypes, models, guides, etc. made of simple plastics and metals, to being suitable for mass production of complex products, as well as products that could potentially repair or regenerate biologic tissues, such as bone, cartilage, muscle, and more.

In addition to the new continued focus on technology and material development for 3D printing, this period has seen the introduction of many regulatory-approved 3D printed devices. As of the time of this writing, the US Food and Drug Administration (FDA) has approved more than 100 3D printed medical devices—ranging from simple surgical tools to complex implantables such as mass-produced, off-the-shelf vertebral interbody cages and patient-matched cranial implant devices—with many more products approved for use in Europe and Asia. During this period,

additional US government organizations, including the National Institutes of Health (NIH), Department of Defense (DoD), Department of Veteran Affairs (VA), and the FDA began targeted research, development, and public-private funding initiatives in the fields of medical 3D printing, with the FDA releasing its first complete guidance document on AM and 3D printing of medical devices in December 2017 and additional statements enforcing their commitment to progressing advanced regenerative medicine technologies in November 2017. And in July 2017, the Advanced Regenerative Manufacturing Institute (ARMI), or Bio-FabUSA, a US government public-private partnership and part of NNMI was launched with the goal of "…mak[ing] practical the large-scale manufacturing of engineered tissues and tissue-related technologies, to benefit existing industries and grow new ones." (www.armiusa.org)

Because of the societal and technologic distinctions that have resulted in this, the fifth era, relative to previous eras, it would be appropriate to say that we are in the second generation of 3D printing, as opposed to the first generation that defined eras 1—4. As first-generation technologies (SLA, SLS, FDM, inkjet binding, polyjetting) continue to mature and take hold in orthopedics as means for surgical training, modeling, and planning, as well as for producing orthotics and permanent polymeric or metallic implants, second-generation AM and 3D printing technologies are beginning to emerge.

Sixth Era (Present)—New Materials and Advanced Biomedical 3D Printing

The continuation of the fifth era, or arguably the start of the sixth, is focused on the development of new advanced materials. Unlike the first-generation technologies, which have been improved primarily through advances and refinement in hardware and utilize well-established, inert materials, second-generation 3D printing technologies are being enabled by rapid improvements in three-dimensional imaging and advanced robotics as well as the development and introduction of new, highly biofunctional materials (Biomaterial 3D printing), including hydrogel and live cell/tissue fabrication, permitting partial or even whole tissue and organs to be created. These emerging 3D printing processes, including, but not limited to *3D painting* and bioprinting, combined with the ubiquity of first-generational technologies, ensure that AM and 3D printing will continue to play a vital role in orthopedic practice in the coming years; from training and education all the way to permanent, integrative implants and even tissue engineering, regeneration, and replacement.

UNDERSTANDING THE COMPONENTS, PROCESSES, MATERIALS, AND CLASSIFICATIONS OF 3D PRINTING

With the overall history of 3D printing established and placed in perspective of present and upcoming technologies, it is important to understand the vital elements that make up 3D printing as well as the common and emerging 3D printing process used in medicine and orthopedics. These topics will be expanded upon in later chapters but are introduced here to give the reader a foundational and functional understanding of the processes and the vocabulary necessary to understand the deeper technologic and application concepts.

3D Printing Technologies and Processes

AM refers to fabrication methods that create objects from the bottom-up, piece-wise or continuously, as opposed to top-down, or subtractive (traditional), manufacturing which can be divided into three major categories: energy-based, materials deposition–based,

and combination. Six of the core technologies and their functional processes are outlined in Fig. 1.3, with specific technologies mentioned and very briefly discussed later.

ENERGY-BASED TECHNOLOGIES

Energy-based AM approaches require the directed, controlled application of energy to a resting material to transform it into a solid structure. These processes can be further divided into two major categories: those that utilize liquid resin (monomers mixed with a photo-reactive reagent) baths, in conjunction with selective application of noncoherent light (resin bath–based lithography), and those that utilize solid, packed powder (metal, alloy, or thermoplastic) beds, in conjunction with a coherent energy beam (laser or electron). Energy-based technologies are currently the most commonly utilized, industrial AM techniques and include SLA, SLS, and direct laser melting (DLM).

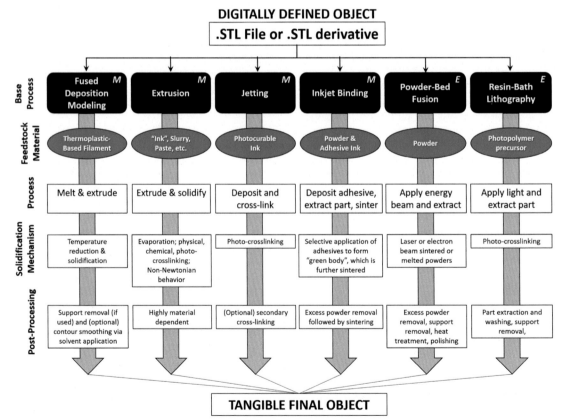

FIG. 1.3 Generalized processes and defining features of the six major families of AM technologies. Subfamilies and hybrid technologies exist for each category, but are not included in the figure. "*M*" or "*E*" refers to "materials deposition–based" or "energy-based" technology, respectively.

Despite their differences, resin bath and powder bed–based technologies share several major similarities. First, they both require excess starting material (aka feedstock), in the form of liquid resin or solid powders, to fill the volume of the bath or bed, respectively. Owing to the selective application of energy, the majority of original feedstock is not utilized during the fabrication process. Second, excess liquid/powder residue must be removed from the fabricated part. Third, tight porosity or completely enclosed (solid wall) architectural features cannot be practically fabricated due to the need to remove unreacted or unsintered/melted resin or powder, respectively. Fourth, postprocessing is often required, which is often referred to as "secondary curing" in the case of resin-based materials, or thermal homogenization and/or densification in the case of metals. Finally, these processes are currently not compatible with multiple materials.

Resin bath–based lithographic (light-based polymerization) processes—This subfamily of energy-based AM includes SLA, direct light projection, continuous liquid interface polymerization (CLIP), and two-photon polymerization. Feedstock resins are primarily comprised of carbon-based monomeric units and photoinitiator molecules. Generally, upon exposure to specific wavelengths of light, polymerization leads to observable solidification of the exposed region of the resin bath. This process can be discrete, layer-by-layer, or in the case of the newer CLIP processes, continuous. Because this process is high resolution, but primarily restricted to photocurable plastics, the resulting objects are primarily used as visual prototypes, models, and guides, as opposed to functional implants and load-bearing structures. Additionally, due to the current inability to remove all toxic monomeric units and photoinitiator, parts created using resin bath–based lithographic processes are not utilized or currently recommended for implantation.

Powder bed–based selective sintering and melting processes—This subfamily of energy-based AM and 3D printing processes includes SLS, DLM, and electron beam melting. Feedstock powders can be thermoplastics, such as polycaprolactone (PCL), acrylonitrile butadiene styrene, polylactic acid (PLA), and polyether ether ketone, as well as prealloyed metals, such as 300 series stainless steels, Ti64 (titanium-6 aluminum-4 vanadium), or cobalt-chromes. The powders must be of specific size and shape to attain optimal packing necessary for successful sintering. Once packed and level, a high-energy laser or electron beam sinters or melts powder particles together in the outline of that particular layer/cross-section of the object being built. The application of high-energy laser or electron beams, combined with the small size and environmental reactivity of dry powder materials, requires extensive safety precautions to be taken before, during, and after processing. This also requires that powder beds be fully enclosed, and the chambers purged and often filled with inert gas (argon, nitrogen, helium, depending on the material) prior to beginning fabrication. Finished objects must be carefully extracted from the powder beds and physically cleaned to remove unsintered or partially sintered powders. Metallic parts must often undergo additional mechanical (surface smoothing or roughening) or thermal (microstructural homogenization or precipitation) treatments prior to use.

MATERIAL DEPOSITION–BASED TECHNOLOGIES

Material deposition AM technologies utilize the ejection or laminar extrusion of materials in a layer-by-layer process to create solid, three-dimensional structures without the need for powder beds or resin baths. These processes include FDM, inkjetting and polyjetting, direct ink writing (DIW)/robocasting, 3D painting, and bioprinting. The deposited material must be self-supporting shortly after deposition to maintain architectural fidelity and allow for additional layers of material to be deposited, as well as bond with subsequently deposited layers of material. This requirement has historically restricted utilized materials to thermopolymers, photopolymers, low particle-content composite polymers, and thick gels. However, recent developments have enabled an extensive variety of materials to be compatible with materials deposition–based AM processes such as plastics, composites, metals and alloys, ceramics, acellular biologics, and living cells.

Inkjetting/Polyjetting—Unlike the other technologies in this category, inkjetting and polyjetting (tradename) do not extrude, but instead thermally or piezoelectrically eject material out of a cartridge in a process very similar to common inkjet 2D printing. This deposited material is then solidified via some mechanism prior to jetting additional material onto the previously deposited layer. This mechanism is highly material dependent and can be anything from thermal, photochemical, or chemical/ionic.

Fused deposition modeling—Perhaps the most widely known 3D printing process is simply the extrusion of melted or softened thermoplastics (fed from a spool or from powder reservoir) out of a nozzle. The material solidifies as a result of cooling to ambient temperature upon extrusion. This process is restricted to select thermoplastics and lightly loaded thermoplastic composites.

Extrusion 3D Printing (i.e., *robocasting, DIW*)—This broad process is similar to FDM, but does not melt the feedstock materials prior to deposition, and usually occurs at or near room temperature. These processes utilize a liquid "ink" or thick paste/slurry extruded out of a syringe/nozzle. Inks are usually comprised of a powder, organic or nonorganic solvent(s), and binder material (usually a polymer soluble in selected solvent(s)). In some instances, a powder may not be present, in which case the resulting solid material is comprised only of polymer. Resulting DIW and robocast structures are generally quite fragile or difficult to handle and are thus often restricted to several layers. However, objects can be postprocessed, via chemical reaction or thermal sintering, in the case of metals and alloys, to attain structurally stable objects. These processes can be utilized for additively manufacturing a variety of materials, including polymers, metals, ceramics, and electronics. However, due to the difficulty in obtaining quality, larger 3D parts, the processes have been primarily adopted for creating electronics (primarily planar) within other 3D printed materials.

3D painting—3D paints are liquids comprised of a powder, polymer binder, solvents and are 3D printed via extrusion at or near room temperature. Although the polymer binder and solvents remain the same among distinct 3D paints, it is the type of powder that defines the 3D paint, much in the same way pigment powders define the color of traditional patients. In the case of 3D paints, however, the comprising powder defines whether it is particular biomaterial, metal, alloy, ceramic, or electronic material. 3D paints deviate from DIW inks in multiple ways. Perhaps the most significant difference is that 3D paints, unlike DIW inks, do not rely on material-specific chemistries or electrostatic stabilization (positive-negative material interactions) to produce 3D printable formulations. This means that 3D paints' ability to be 3D printed is primarily independent of the composing, defining, powder material, enabling the creation, development, and utilization of a wide variety of 3D printable materials. Their material-agnostic nature also allows for 3D paints to be mixed prior to 3D printing, without significantly compromising 3D printing parameters. An analogy would be that one does not change the way they paint a wall just because they decide to change the color of paint they are using. Similarly, in 3D paint, one does not need to change the way they 3D print simply because they are changing materials. Finally, they can be 3D printed at much faster rates than robocasting, DIW, or FDM processes and result in solid structures that are mainly powder (the functional material), yet

remain mechanically stable and even flexible and elastic in many cases. Although 3D painting is a new process, it has already been applied to 3D printing a wide variety of materials, including highly bioactive, cell-free, osteogenic[2,3] and neurogenic materials,[3,4] bioelectronics,[4] tissue-specific decellularized extracellular matrices,[5] metals and alloys,[6,7] and more.[8]

Bioprinting—Bioprinting actively utilizes living cells and tissues in the feedstock material.[9] Note, based on this definition, "medical 3D printing" is not synonymous with "bioprinting," nor is it synonymous with adding cells to a 3D printed structure post printing and prior to use.[10] Because living cells need to survive throughout the AM process while still maintaining 3D printability (ability to be extruded and maintain shape upon deposition), bioprinting mediums frequently take the form of polysaccharide or natural or synthetic-based proteinaceous hydrogels. Additional information regarding bioprinting can be found in the following section.

Combination Energy-Material Deposition Technologies

Inkjet binding—With this technology, an inkjet head selectively jets adhesive binder onto the surface of a powder bed, selectively gluing particles together. The resulting solid part, known as a green body, is extracted from the bed, and postprocessed via sintering, to yield a final part. This process is frequently used to create ceramic models and molds.

Laser metal/Wire deposition processes—A complex additive process that requires the tandem operation and movement of a high-powered laser and powder spray or metal wire deposition. The laser continuously sinters the sprayed metal powder or wire as it is being deposited in place. This process can create complex 3D parts and is primarily utilized to repair or refurbish already existing metal parts.

Laminated object manufacturing—Laminated object manufacturing (LOM) is the collective name given to additive processes that utilize precisely cut, individual sheets of material, which are positioned, layered, and fused, or laminated, together to create three-dimensional objects. LOM is one of the oldest additive techniques, originally utilized to create architectural models from layers of cut paper, but is now frequently utilized in conjunction with advanced composite, sheet feedstocks. The process used to cut individual layers from sheets of material is material dependent, but includes physical cutting with blades as well as energy beams (laser, electron, or ion beams). Fusing the individually cut and stacked layers together is also highly material dependent, but can include liquid or gelled adhesives, thermal welding, mechanical/ultrasonic welding, among others.

THE 3D PRINTING TRIAD: THE HARDWARE, SOFTWARE, AND MATERIAL

Regardless of the 3D printing process being utilized, the end result will depend on the application and interaction of three major components: hardware, software, and material (Fig. 1.4). Attention is most frequently given to the hardware (the 3D printer itself), which creates the object. However, it is the software—which defines the shape of the object and the manner in which the hardware builds the object—and the material—which defines the functionality of the object—that are absolutely vital to the successful application of 3D printing in any given scenario. The triad is enclosed within "user training, skill, and experience" because 3D printing is not (yet) an automatic process; it requires user training, skill, and experience just like any other manufacturing process.

Software utilized for creating and preparing a digital file for 3D printing encompasses everything from 3D imaging acquisition, computer-aided design, and .STL transformation programs. Similar to the extensive range of 3D printer hardware and types, there are a wide variety of individual software programs as well as software suites, ranging from low to high end, that are available for generating a digital representation of the desired object, which can be subsequently converted into a 3D printable file type (usually a .STL) of that object, and translated such that the 3D printer hardware can determine appropriate three-dimensional motion paths. Even the most advanced piece of hardware will be ill-suited to create the user-designed objects if paired with inappropriate software or poor input data. Conversely, a low-end 3D printer paired with the right type of design, visualization, and conversion (to .STL) software along with good inputs, such as a digitally defect-free designs or clean three-dimensional imaging data, will likely be able to produce objects adequate for many applications. It should be noted that many lower end and consumer 3D printers can utilize open-source, free software. However, despite being readily available and free, open-source software is typically less user-friendly than programs intentionally engineered for a specific piece of 3D printing hardware and require the user to know or develop coding knowledge. On the higher end of medical 3D printing software are program suites such as Materialise's *Mimics*, which has been at the forefront of medical three-

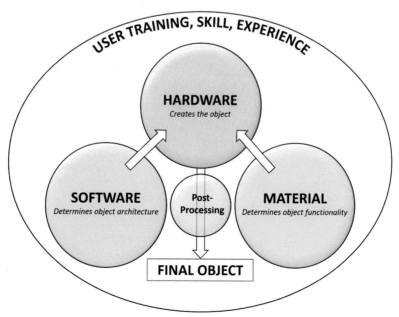

FIG. 1.4 3D printing is dependent on the input materials, which determine the functionality of the final object; the software, which defines the architecture of the final object; and the hardware, or the 3D printer itself, which creates the physical object. Depending on the process and materials being used, postprocessing after 3D printing may be required to yield the final object.

dimensional, digital modeling technology since the early 1990s. Thus, it is important for a potential purchaser or user of a 3D printer to consider software just as carefully as hardware.

Perhaps the most import component of the 3D printing triad is the material. As discussed at the beginning of this chapter, historic ages have been defined by the types of materials humans have been able to manufacture (stone, bronze, iron, steel, silicon, etc.)—not necessarily how those materials are manufactured or what final objects are produced. Analogously, 3D printing, as a field, is advancing in large part due to the increased availability and compatibility of various materials with existing and emerging hardware. As mentioned earlier, the first published paper on the subject of AM was "Automatic method for fabricating three-dimensional plastic model with photo-hardening **polymer**"[1] (emphasis added). Thus, simple plastics were the first materials made compatible with 3D printing hardware (original SLA processes). This was followed by thermoplastics and lightly loaded **thermoplastic composites** (FDM) in the late 1980s and early 1990s, simple **metals, alloys, and ceramics** throughout the 1990s (SLS, Inkjet Binding, and related processes), and eventually "functional" medical and nonmedical materials (robocasting, other extrusion-based processes, and 3D painting), including **advanced hydrogels, acellular biomaterials, and live cells and simple biologic**

tissues in the 2000s and 2010s. Indeed, the importance of the material cannot be overstated, as material developments in 3D printing have transformed a field once referred to as *rapid prototyping* to a field that 30 years later includes *bioprinting*, or the ability to 3D print live cells and functional biologic tissues. Present and emerging materials compatible with the various hardware platforms are illustrated in Fig. 1.5.

While the hardware (3D printer) creates the physical product, characterized by an architecture that has been previously, digitally defined in the software (.STL), it is the material, its chemistry, microstructure, surface properties, etc. that impart functionality, or biofunctionality, in the case of implantables, to the final product. Even with the best raw data, software, and hardware, if the appropriate material is not selected or compatible with the manufacturing process, the resulting end object will not have the necessary functionality or applicability. An extreme example that illustrates this point is 3D printing a kidney (or any organ or anatomic part). An object shaped like a kidney but 3D printed using plastic will have very different properties and applicability than one 3D printed from kidney-specific bioactive materials or even live kidney-related cells and tissue fragments. Even though these two "kidneys" may look and feel similar, they could not be more different—with one potentially being useful as a medical model for teaching and the other being potentially

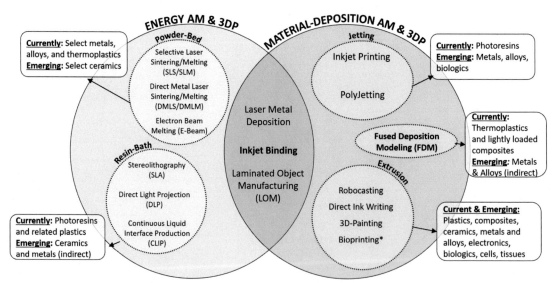

FIG. 1.5 Generalized description of major subprocesses within the six primary additive manufacturing (AM) technologies and corresponding current and emerging material compatibilities. Bioprinting is denoted with an "*" because bioprinting itself is not a specific process, but refers to any 3D printing (3DP) process that makes use of live cells or tissue. Bioprinting is also not entirely restricted to extrusion-based processes, although extrusion represents the majority of process used in conjunction with cell or tissue 3DP.

useful for restoring biologic kidney functions. Although this is an extreme example, it can be translated to any other medical 3D printing scenario. Thus, a 3D printer user should be ever aware of the importance of materials and material selection when producing objects for particular applications.

Beyond the triad, Fig. 1.4 also highlights "postprocessing," which will not be comprehensively discussed in this chapter. However, it is important to keep in mind that, depending on the hardware and material type utilized to create an object, that object may require additional postprinting processing before it can be effectively utilized. Postprocessing can include everything from 3D printed support material removal, chemical smoothing of plastic parts, homogenization heat treatments and secondary machining and polishing of metal parts, or even biologic culture and mechanical, electrical, and or chemical stimulation and conditioning of bioprinted objects. Clearly, postprocessing is highly material dependent, and depending on the material being utilized or intended object application, postprocessing can be relatively quick and easy (i.e., support removal) or require an extended period of time and skill (tissue and organ maturation and conditioning).

MEDICAL 3D PRINTING

Up until this point, this chapter has served as an introduction to 3D printing as a whole—not giving much additional attention to 3D printing in medicine or specifically to orthopedics. This is because the 3D printing processes and underlying technologies, except for perhaps bioprinting, are not particular to specific industries, fields, or applications. Proceeding chapters will discuss orthopedic 3D printing topics in detail, but to place past, present, and emerging 3D printing medical technologies in context, it is important to have a cursory understanding of the three major categories of medical 3D printing: traditional, advanced biomaterials, and bioprinting (Fig. 1.6). These categories are primarily distinguished by material, and thus functionality. Both advanced biomaterials and materials for bioprinting (bioinks) draw from the same base biomaterial palette (Fig. 1.7). However, the distinguishing feature is that bioinks contain live cells, whereas the remaining biomaterial inks do not. The following section gives a brief overview of the three main categories of medical 3D printing and the corresponding subcategories.

1. Traditional medical 3D printing

Traditional medical 3D printing, arbitrarily named because it has been in use for several decades, has become increasingly commonplace across surgical disciplines, including orthopedics, with many FDA-approved off-the-shelf and patient-matched products on the market. Orthopedic application of traditional 3D printing includes surgical planning and/or training models, cutting and placement guides, custom tooling, orthotics, and permanent implantable products. Generally, these objects are comprised of established polymers or medically relevant metals and alloys, such as Ti64, and are primarily utilized for visualization purposes (nonimplantable) or structural purposes (implantables). For the purposes of this definition, and to further separate from new, advanced biomaterials, common biodegradable polymers, and related composites, are also included in this category. Traditional biodegradable polymers, primarily 3D printed via FDM approaches, include but are not limited to PLA, polyglycolic acid, polylactic-co-glycolic acid, and PCL.[11] Although biodegradable, resorbable, and relatively biocompatible depending on application, these polymers do not have strong, intrinsic bioactivity and are thus more similar to permanent structural polymers and alloys than tissue regenerative or biofunctional materials. However, these polymeric materials can be postprocessed with bioactive particles and biologics to impart limited degrees of tissue specific biofunctionality and tissue regeneration potential.[12,13]

2. Advanced biomaterials (includes acellular biologics) medical 3D printing

Advanced biomaterials encompass a range of acellular materials derived from 3D printable "inks" and are defined by the following characteristics. First, the resulting printed material is comprised entirely or primarily (>50% by volume) of the bioactive component, rather than a bioinert or low bioactivity binder. Second, temperatures greater than those commonly observed in biologic environments ($37°C$) are not required at any stage of the manufacturing or preparation process. This characteristic precludes materials 3D printed via FDM and powder bed processes. Third, the resulting 3D printed materials induce tissue-specific responses and desired regenerative behavior. Again, this precludes generic biodegradable polymers that do not exhibit tissue-specific behavior. Fourth, the biomaterial ink is co-3D printing compatible with other biomaterial inks, allowing for fabrication of multimaterial, multifunctionality objects. Finally, the manufactured material exhibits mechanical properties and handling characteristics that make them highly amenable to the surgical procedures and

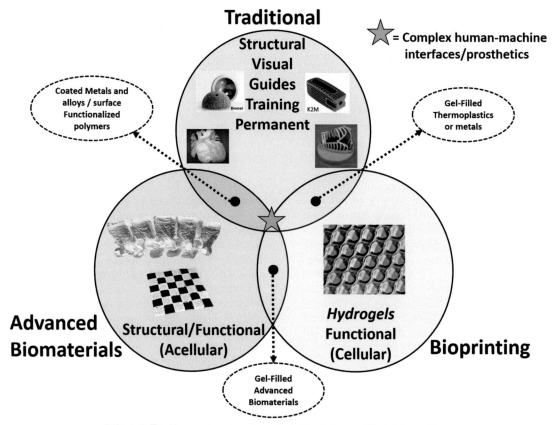

FIG. 1.6 The three categories of medical 3D printing and their intersections.

applications for which they are intended.[10] The US FDA has yet to approve a 3D printed advanced biomaterial for orthopedic applications, but it is likely that numerous musculoskeletal-focused, advanced biomaterials will be approved and on the by the early 2020s. If current trends hold, these will primarily be orthopedic-focused biomaterials that can be applied to existing, established orthopedic indications, for example, 3D printed biologic versions of existing orthopedic products used to treat common, existing orthopedic indications. These will hit the market before more advanced/exotic products that will likely require PMA approvals.

3D painting is an example of a new process compatible with 3D printing of a variety of materials,[2,3,5−7,9] including advanced biomaterials, such as *"Hyperelastic Bone(TM)"* (HB)[2,3] and *3D-Graphene* (3DG).[2,9] Such materials exhibit high, tissue-specific bioactivity and are 3D printed and processed under room temperature conditions. They are mechanically robust and have excellent handling characteristics despite being comprised of upwards of 75% brittle materials. The processing at ambient temperatures allows for incorporation of organic molecules and factors directly into the ink prior to 3D printing, permitting the user to augment the materials without compromising printability. 3D painted materials are generally not as mechanically rigid as traditionally 3D printed medical materials, nor are they necessarily as bioactive as bioprinted structures containing living cells; however, their handling characteristic, bioactivity, and stability (shelf-life, shipping, and packaging) offer a valuable compromise between the two classes of medical 3D printing and may make them ideal for near future orthopedic use in a variety of musculoskeletal indications.

3. Bioprinting (includes cellular biologics)
   Although frequently used interchangeably with all forms of medical 3D printing, the term

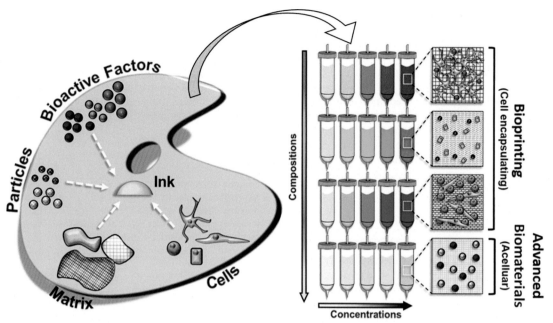

FIG. 1.7 The biomaterial ink palette and its components and resulting types of 3D printable materials. (Modified from Jakus AE, Rutz AL, Shah RN. Advancing the field of 3D biomaterial printing. *Biomed Mater*. 2016;11(1) with permission.)

"bioprinting" specifically refers to the process of 3D printing using cell encapsulating materials, called bioinks. In its simplest form, a bioink is comprised of a matrix material, usually a hydrogel (>90% water by weight) containing live cells of at least one type. The matrix material comprising the hydrogel can be synthetic, such as polyethylene glycol; naturally derived (protein or polysaccharide), such as gelatin; or a synthetic-natural hybrid.[9] Cell types can include but are not limited to cell lines, primary cells, adult stem cells, and induced pluripotent stem cells.[10]

Because bioinks contain living cells, bioprinting faces numerous additional challenges beyond those common to all extrusion-based 3D printing methods. These can be categorized as 3D printing, structure, and cell encapsulation. The first two include such requirements as the ability for the material to be laminarly extruded, self-supporting upon deposition, biocompatible, and mechanically robust enough to be handled and clinically applied without failure. The third category, cell encapsulation, requires that the bioink itself be short-term (hours) and long-term (days to weeks) cytocompatible and support the viability and function of the

encapsulated cells. Cytocompatibility of the biomaterial is often inversely proportional to the weight percent solids content of the encapsulating gel matrix. However, mechanical properties and capacity to be self-supporting upon deposition, and thus 3D printable, are most often proportional to the weight percent solids content. These two competing criteria, among others, related to 3D printability and cytocompatibility present a significant obstacle to the technical and clinical advancement of bioprinting technologies.[14] However, new approaches, such as partial gel cross-linking are being developed to permit bioinks to be both highly cytocompatible and 3D printable. An additional major challenge to bioprinting is that temperature (~37°C) and sterility must be maintained during the entire process, from cell acquisition and bioink synthesis through final application. Unlike traditional and advanced biomaterials, which can be sterilized using existing, approved methodologies, there are no currently established methods for sterilizing bioprinted structures. Finally, the impact of the shear forces on the cells during extrusion as well as the tendency for the cells to settle in the bioink prior to printing must be considered.

Being able to 3D print live, functional cells within a bioactive matrix in a structurally organized and predetermined fashion is the first step toward direct complex tissue and organ fabrication. With the cells already present, bioprinted structures have the potential to create their own vasculature, produce growth factors and additional biologic species, and rapidly integrate with surrounding tissues upon implantation. Although no bioprinted structures have yet been FDA approved for specific indications, the rapid, continuing advances in laboratory research have already yielded functional examples of bioprinted living cartilage,[15] tendons,[16] and muscle.[17]

THE FUTURE OF MEDICAL 3D PRINTING

The previous sections describe the collective history and give a broad overview of the current state of 3D printing. In only a few decades, the technology has moved from niche, plastic rapid prototyping and model making to the first demonstrations of viable, bioprinted tissues and the introduction of new advanced, acellular biomaterials, such as *HB*. Much of this progress has occurred only over the past decade, with 3D printing becoming mainstream in a wide variety of industries, including healthcare and medicine, where more than 100 3D printed products have been FDA approved for use. As traditional medical 3D printing becomes the new standard of care, with physicians frequently using 3D printed surgical models for planning and training, guides for cutting, external orthotics and prosthetics, and patient-matched and off-the-shelf parts, we have seen the rapid emergence of new materials and technologies, along with official acknowledgments by major standards and regulatory agencies that a major shift in healthcare technology is imminent, if not already underway.

Owing to the rapid rate in which the field has developed, especially over the past decade, it is difficult to make accurate predictions about the future of medical 3D printing. However, using history as a guide, in conjunction with emerging, wide-scale efforts, such as BioFabUSA, it is safe to predict that the coming decade will witness the introduction of many new traditionally 3D printed medical products, as well as acellular 3D printed and cellular, bioprinted tissue regenerative biologics for existing and de novo musculoskeletal, orthopedic indications. Beyond new products and technologies being introduced in the near future, it is

likely that 3D printing methods and technologies will likely become common educational subjects for physicians and surgeons during medical training, along with the establishment of specifically qualified and regulated, medical 3D printing vocations and professions. Regardless of the specifics, 3D printing will play increasingly common, integral roles in orthopedic education, training, and surgical practice.

REFERENCES

1. Kodama H. Automatic method for fabricating a three-dimensional plastic model with photo-hardening polymer. *Rev Sci Instr.* 1981;52(11):1770–1773.
2. Jakus AE, Rutz AL, Jordan SW, et al. Hyperelastic "bone": a highly versatile, growth factor-free, osteoregenerative, scalable, and surgically friendly biomaterial. *Sci Transl Med.* 2016;8(358):358ra127.
3. Jakus AE, Shah RN. Multi- and mixed 3D-printing of graphene-hydroxyapatite hybrid materials for complex tissue engineering. *J Biomed Mater Res A.* 2017;105A(1).
4. Jakus AE, Secor EB, Rutz AL, Jordan SW, Hersam MC, Shah RN. Three-dimensional printing of high-content graphene scaffolds for electronic and biomedical applications. *ACS Nano.* 2015;9(4):4636–4648.
5. Jakus AE, Laronda MM, Rashedi AS, et al. "Tissue papers" from organ-specific decellularized extracellular matrices. *Adv Funct Mater.* 2017;27(34):1700992-n/a.
6. Jakus AE, Taylor SL, Geisendorfer NR, Dunand DC, Shah RN. Metallic architectures from 3D-printed powder-based liquid inks. *Adv Funct Mater.* 2015;25(45):6985–6995.
7. Taylor SL, Jakus AE, Shah RN, Dunand DC. Iron and nickel cellular structures by sintering of 3D-printed oxide or metallic particle inks. *Adv Eng Mater.* 2017;19(10).
8. Jakus AE, Koube KD, Geisendorfer NR, Shah RN. Robust and elastic lunar and martian structures from 3D-printed Regolith ink. *Sci Rep.* 2017;7.
9. Rutz AL, Hyland KE, Jakus AE, Burghardt WR, Shah RN. A multimaterial bioink method for 3D printing tunable, cell-compatible hydrogels. *Adv Mater.* 2015;27(9):1607.
10. Jakus AE, Rutz AL, Shah RN. Advancing the field of 3D biomaterial printing. *Biomed Mater.* 2016;11(1).
11. Woodruff MA, Hutmacher DW. The return of a forgotten polymer-Polycaprolactone in the 21st century. *Prog Polym Sci.* 2010;35(10):1217–1256.
12. Lee CH, Cook JL, Mendelson A, Moioli EK, Yao H, Mao JJ. Regeneration of the articular surface of the rabbit synovial joint by cell homing: a proof of concept study. *Lancet.* 2010;376(9739):440–448.
13. Serra T, Mateos-Timoneda MA, Planell JA, Navarro M. 3D printed PLA-based scaffolds: a versatile tool in regenerative medicine. *Organogenesis.* 2013;9(4):239–244.

14. Malda J, Visser J, Melchels FP, et al. 25th anniversary article: engineering hydrogels for biofabrication. *Adv Materials (Deerf Beach FLA)*. 2013;25(36):5011−5028.

15. O'Connell G, Garcia J, Amir J. 3D bioprinting: new directions in articular cartilage tissue engineering. *ACS Biomater Sci Eng*. 2017.

16. Rimann M, Laternser S, Keller H, Leupin O, Graf-Hausner U. 3D bioprinted muscle and tendon tissues for Drug development. *Chimia*. 2015;69(1):65−67.

17. Merceron TK, Burt M, Seol Y-J, et al. A 3D bioprinted complex structure for engineering the muscle−tendon unit. *Biofabrication*. 2015;7(3):035003.

CHAPTER 2

Basics of 3D Printing: Engineering Aspects

SOURABH MANOJ SAPTARSHI, MS • DR. CHI ZHOU, PHD

INTRODUCTION TO 3D PRINTING

3D printing also referred to as *rapid prototyping* or *additive manufacturing* is a method of manufacturing objects layer by layer using three-dimensional software planning and material deposition techniques. In contrast, many traditional manufacturing techniques such as grinding or milling are *subtractive* in nature; that is, they rely on removing material to shape a finished object.

The process involves a series of operations from Computer Aided Design (CAD) conceptualization to setting the right parameters and finally to produce the final three-dimensional model of the virtual design. 3D printing has impacted almost all industries including food, automobile, defense, art, aerospace, construction, medicine, dentistry, prosthetics, and beyond.

In this chapter we will briefly outline some of the technologic and engineering underpinnings of 3D printing. The intended audience is the clinician or technician who has a cursory understanding of the field. It is intended to give a better technical understanding and overview of the processes, technologies, and design steps involved in 3D printing in general. It is by no means a comprehensive review of the subject matter. The field has grown too large and technically complex to cover all of the technical facets of the 3D printing process in such a small space. For a very detailed review of 3D printing, especially as it relates to bioengineering subject matter, we refer you to the comprehensive text Essentials of 3D Biofabrications and Translation by Atala and Yoo. It is an extraordinarily detailed and well-referenced text on the subject matter.

HISTORY OF 3D PRINTING

The 3D printing technologies first became available in the late 1980s. The very first patent was filed by Dr. Hideo Kodama, in Japan, in 1980. The patent was rejected as Dr. Kodama missed the 1-year deadline to file the patent. It was not until 1986 that the first patent was awarded in the field of 3D printing to Charles(Chuck) Hull for his Stereolithography apparatus(SLA). Chuck Hull cofounded 3D Systems, which is one of the largest organizations in the 3D printing world today.[1,2] Fast forward to the 21st century, today's printers boast the ability to create objects in different materials, including plastic, metal powders, metal alloy powder, concrete cement, composites, polymers, and bioinks, each having its own advantages and limitations. The technologies also let users decide part properties such as density, strength, and stiffness.

Since its inception in the 1980s, the 3D printing life cycle can be broadly classified into three prominent eras based on the technologic advancement that were observed:[2,3]

1. **Early years: 1981 to 1999**

   It was during this stage that most of the technologies were being invented and companies were filing patents to safeguard their work. 3D Systems, cofounded by Chuck Hull, introduced the first SLA-1 printer in 1987. In 1988, DTM Inc. made the first SLS printer, and in 1992, Stratasys secured the patent rights for its Fused Deposition Modeling (FDM) procedure.[1–3] This was an era of innovation and many technologies were invented during this early phase.

2. **1999 to 2010**

   By the start of the millennium, 3D printing had observed technologic advancements and an increase in usage and applications. 3D printing saw use in the fields of medicine and biology, aerospace, automotive, and construction industries. Some of the biggest breakthroughs in the medical field happened when scientists at Wake Forest Institute for Regenerative Medicine successfully 3D printed a working human bladder.[2,3] They printed a synthetic scaffold of the bladder and coated it with the host's cells.[2,3] This ensured that the body would accept the organ without any complications. The scientists were successfully able to implant the bladder in human patients. Even though there were such major breakthroughs, the general public was still not completely aware and well informed about the technology partly because of multiple factors including cost of printing, ease of operation, part accuracy, and printer/material availability. Commercially available 3D printers were expensive and desktop printers were not common. Only major corporations and research institutes were able to afford a 3D printer.

Until 2009, inventors of most of the technologies held the patents to their work and a monopoly over their manufacture and distribution. The expirations of these patents paved the way for many start-ups to manufacture affordable and reliable open-sourced 3D printers. In 2004, engineers from the British University started the open design RepRap project, which allowed users to freely download printer software and designs. The project was started with the concept of self-replication.[4] As affordable and highly accurate 3D printers became readily available, many new businesses and service bureaus started to emerge, which provided entrepreneurs and designers the ability to invest less capital and print multiple iterations of their part to test their ideas.

3. **2011 to the present day**

3D printing technology has advanced at a rapid rate over the last few years. The market now offers many affordable and reliable desktop 3D printers that can be purchased for under $500. Tremendous advancement has been made in other sectors as well. 3D printed parts are now being used in commercial airplanes, 3D printed food is now a reality and bioprinting has seen an increase in its application in the development of bioengineered tissues.

3D printing techniques are heavily reliant on software applications. The rapid increase in processing power and speed from improvements in chip technology (Moore's Law) has led to decreases in the overall cost of operation, increased accuracy of printers, and improved ease of operation. As costs have plummeted, 3D printers have moved out of solely the realm of industry and into the hands of hobbyists and tinkerers, making printing supplies more plentiful and opening up new use cases for printing.

APPLICATIONS OF 3D PRINTING
Below is a list of a few examples of the sectors that benefitted due to 3D printing and continue to make advances.

Food
Natural Machines has created a 3D printer called Foodini (Fig. 2.1), which is capable of 3D printing food from freshly prepared ingredients (Fig. 2.2).[5] An exciting possibility is using this method for manned space travel missions.

Construction
San Francisco–based start-up Apis Cor 3D printed a 400 sq. foot house for about $10,000 in a Russian town within 24 h.[6] The 3D printer used concrete as raw material to build.

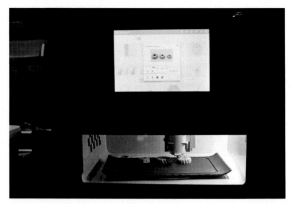

FIG. 2.1 Corn cob dish being printed by Foodini using all natural components. (Natural Machines: https://www.naturalmachines.com/.)

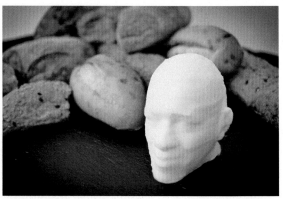

FIG. 2.2 Miniature 3D printed head made out of butter by Foodini. (Natural Machines: https://www.naturalmachines.com/.)

Art

In 2014, the Smithsonian Institution added the first ever 3D printed sculpture, a portrait of President Obama, to its presidential collection.[7] The face was scanned using more than 50 high-resolution 3D scanners and then accurately 3D printed.

Automobile

The 1360 HP Koenigsegg One:1 supercar has a variable turbo which has intricate designs and assemblies which cannot be achieved by regular casting process. The entire turbo is printed as one single piece instead of assemblies.[8]

Aviation

General Electric uses a 3D printed fuel nozzle in its LEAP engines which are fitted on the A320neo, Boeing 737 MAX, and COMAC C919. Before 3D printing, the fuel nozzle was made up of 20 parts assembled together, but now it is just one single part. The design also reduces the carbon deposits, which contributes to clean fuel burn.[9]

Medical Applications

Scientists and medical practitioners have 3D printed orthopedic implants, jaws, ear molds, customizable hearing aids, and other devices for patients.[10]

Archeology

3D printing and 3D scanning are being used by archaeologists to capture and remake ancient artifacts or art pieces that were destroyed due to various reasons. These tools can also be used to scan and print missing fossil bones for researchers to study or be used in museums in lieu of the real fossil.[11]

TYPES OF TECHNOLOGY

3D printing has advanced significantly in technologic sophistication since its inception in the 1980s. Early platforms were SLA-based printers that used liquid polymers as raw material, but printing techniques have expanded to multiple different platforms and now a wide variety of techniques are employed.[12]

For legal reasons, various manufactures used different acronyms for describing the same process. The term Fused Deposition Modeling and its abbreviation FDM are trademarked by Stratasys.[13] Other manufacturers with similar technology have come up with their own abbreviations; for example, RepRap project named it fused filament fabrication (FFF), whereas Markforged calls it CFF.[14] To avoid confusion caused by having multiple names for the same technique, the American Society of Testing and Materials (ASTM) decided to group similar processes together and categorized the technologies under seven headings (ASTM F2792 − 12a) as follows:[12,15]

1. Vat photopolymerization
2. Material extrusion
3. Directed energy deposition (DED)
4. Powder bed fusion (PBF)
5. Binder jetting (BJ)
6. Material jetting (MJ)
7. Sheet lamination (SL)

These are described briefly in the following sections. A summary of their minimum design features is seen in Table 2.1.

TABLE 2.1
Table shows the minimum design values to be considered while designing parts for a particular technology[16,17,21,34]

Type of Technology	MINIMUM DESIGN DIMENSIONAL CONSIDERATION (IN MM)[a]			
	Minimum Feature	Wall Thickness	Hole Diameter	Assembly Spacing
Vat photopolymerization	0.2	0.4	0.5	0.5
Extrusion	2	1	2	0.3
Powder-based fusion				
Thermoplastic powder	0.8	0.7	1.5	0.3
Metal parts	0.6[b]	0.5[b]	1.5[b]	–[b]
Binder jetting	2	2	1.5	0.2
Material jetting	0.5	1	1.5	0.2
Sheet lamination	2–3	0.5	–	–

[a] Minimum dimensional thickness can depend heavily on the structure and design of the 3D model.
[b] The values mentioned are general guidelines for designing metal printed parts. The values can differ for different metal powder and also on the structure to be built.

Vat Photopolymerization

3D printing parts using liquid photopolymer (liquid resin) is one of the oldest technologies developed and enjoys widespread applications to this date. Photopolymerization processes use liquid photopolymers as the building material. Upon contact with UV light, the resin undergoes curing because of chemical reactions (Fig. 2.3). The UV light bonds the polymer molecules to each other, thus forming a continuous chain. In desktop styled printers, the printer prints the part hanging upside down (or inverted) from the build plate. Instead of the build plate going down after each layer as with most other technologies, the build plate in a photopolymerization-based printer goes up. This is because these printers have a light source in the bottom section of the printer. This directs an image on the build platform using mirrors attached to galvanometers of the part in the X and Y direction along the build plate. After each layer is printed, fresh resin is redistributed for the process to continue. Because of this inverted styled printing, in most cases, the parts do need supports to hold them in place. As the raw material is liquid resin, this opens the door for creating and customizing various types of resins for different engineering and prototyping applications. Parts printed out of this process have a superior surface finish, are capable of high accuracy and resolution, and can be used for a wide variety of applications.

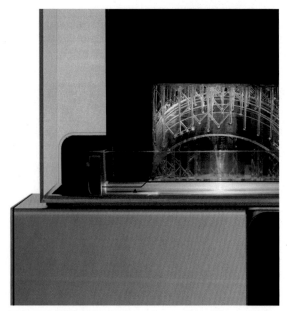

FIG. 2.3 UV light traces the cross-section of the part being printed and in the process builds the part layer by layer. (Formlabs: https://formlabs.com/3d-printers/form-2/.)

While printing using vat photopolymerization techniques, few design considerations such as a minimum wall thickness of 0.4 mm, a minimum hole diameter of 0.5 mm, a minimum part clearance of 0.5 mm for assemblies must be kept in mind for a successful print.[16,17]

Two primary configurations were developed for photopolymerization precess based on their exposure strategy

- Stereolithography
- Digital Light Processing

Vat Photopolymerization is the main technology and stereolithography and DLP are two types of processes under it.

Stereolithography (SLA)

SLA uses UV light and a photo-curable resin to 3D print the part layer by layer. It contains a vat or tray filled with photopolymerizable resin. The platform (build plate) lowers into the resin vat and UV light traces out the shape of the first cross-section on the build plate, thus curing the resin. The build plate then moves up and a sweeper (or a tilt motion in some printers) redistributes fresh resin in the vat. The process then repeats itself. Subsequent layers adhere to the previous layer, thus the part builds layer by layer. 3D Systems is one of first and remains a major manufacturer of SLA-based machines. Several companies such as the Massachusetts-based company Formlabs is also leading the race to provide quality and affordable desktop-based SLA 3D printers to users (Fig. 2.4). They offer a variety of materials including but not limited to standard colored resins, engineering resins (flexible, tough, high temp, durable), dentistry resins (for making dental products such as retainers and aligners), and castable resins (for making custom jewelry).[18]

Digital Light Processing

Digital light processing (DLP) is similar to SLA in the sense that both the processes use photopolymerizable resin and a sweeper to redistribute resin. However, in this process, a DLP projector projects the entire image of the cross-section of the part at once. Because the projector is a digital screen, the image of each layer is composed of square pixels, resulting in a layer formed from small rectangular bricks called voxels.[19] Accuracy of the parts depend on the projector's resolution. The higher the projector resolution, the crisper the voxels and hence a higher resolution part.

After printing a part using the photopolymerization technique, the part needs to be dipped in an isopropyl alcohol (IPA) bath for a few minutes to remove the excess resin stuck to the part. Supports are then clipped off using a pair of clippers (Fig. 2.5). After cleaning, parts are usually baked in a UV light box to stabilize their physical properties.[20]

Material Extrusion

Material extrusion is a process in which semisolid material is extruded from a nozzle and deposited layer by

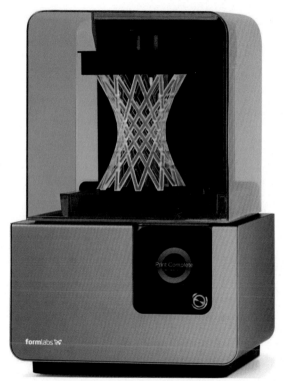

FIG. 2.4 Formlabs form 2. (Formlabs: https://formlabs.com/media/upload/_thumbs/Form-2-printer-three-quarters-Hart_q7J639F.jpg.960x0_q80.jpg.)

layer on the build plate. The nozzle heats the filament and extrudes it. The basic idea remains the same, depositing or stacking layers of material one above the other to create a three-dimensional model. The extruder houses the nozzle and moves in X and Y direction to deposit material, while the build platform moves up or down in the Z direction (Fig. 2.6).

Extruding thermoplastic material can also be referred to as FFF or FDM.[13] The filament passes through a set of rollers that control the feed rate of the material. Unlike the photopolymerization process where the model and supports are made of the same material, extrusion technique offers the flexibility to incorporate an additional nozzle which can be used to extrude soluble support material which can be dissolved in a solvent bath (Fig. 2.7). This reduces the painful clipping and sanding process. Stratasys's Idea series printers Mojo and uPrint (Figs. 2.8 and 2.9) are two of the many printers that have dual nozzle configurations to extrude support and model material. Not all extrusion-based printers provide the flexibility of incorporating an additional nozzle to extrude support material.

The two most widely used thermoplastic materials are acrylonitrile butadiene styrene (ABS) and polylactic acid (PLA). They come in the form of spool, and both

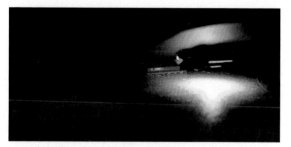

FIG. 2.6 Extruder is melting plastic and depositing it layer by layer thus creating a 3D object. (Stratasys, Ltd.)

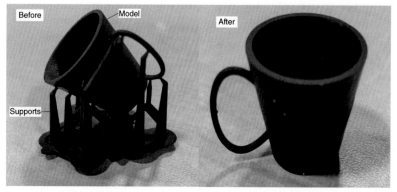

FIG. 2.5 Before and after clipping the supports off the part.

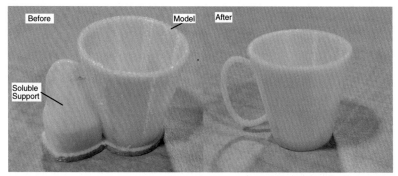

FIG. 2.7 Before and after dissolving the supports by immersing the 3D printed part in a solvent bath.

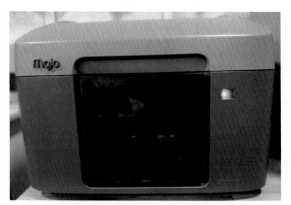

FIG. 2.8 Stratasys Mojo is part of the Idea series printers. (Stratasys, Ltd.)

ABS and PLA are safe to work with as they do not emit any toxic smoke when heated. ABS has a tendency to warp. To prevent warping, the parts are printed in a heated environment either on a heated build plate or in a heated chamber. Stratasys, 3D systems, Ultimaker, LulzBot, Markforged, Hyrel, etc. are some of the leading manufacturers that offer extrusion-based 3D printers. Along with ABS and PLA, many printers can also print using nylon, composites, clay, etc. depending on the printer and the nozzle specification.

There are various applications of extrusion technique in fields such as construction, food, prototyping, automobile, etc., but one of the most exciting applications is in the medical field. Also known as extrusion-based bioprinting (EBB), EBB has made substantial progress during the last decade. EBB uses extrusion principles and creates 3D tissues from bioinks using a layer-by-layer deposition process.[21,22] 3D tissues can be printed using scanned CT or MRI images.[22,23] Using a computer program, the printer lays

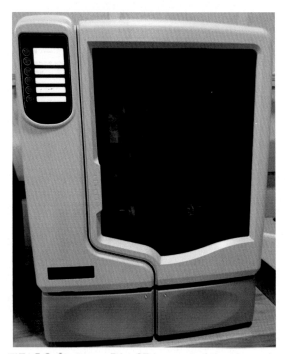

FIG. 2.9 Stratasys uPrint SE is a part of the Idea series printers. (Stratasys, Ltd.)

down precise layers of bioinks either by a pneumatic or piston-driven deposition system.[24]

While printing thermoplastic parts using extrusion techniques, few design considerations such as a minimum wall thickness of 1 mm, a minimum hole diameter of 2 mm, a minimum part clearance of 0.3 mm for assemblies must be kept in mind for a successful print.[16,25] Furthermore, if the angle of the overhang is less than 45 degrees, then the feature does not need supports.

Thermoplastic material extrusion–based printers offer an affordable and viable option for prototyping. There are plenty of printers available starting from just $200 (e.g., XYZprinting da Vinci mini, Prusa i3, RepRap Guru, etc.) which can print parts using ABS, Nylon, PLA, high-impact polystyrene (HIPS), etc. and provide good part accuracy and a decent build volume, enabling the user to print a small- to medium-sized part. This breakthrough has enabled people to have a 3D printer at home to experiment with their designs. Another advantage of extrusion printers is the ready availability of raw materials. The material spools are easily available and are affordable (anywhere between $20-$50 per kilogram).

Powder Bed Fusion (PBF)

PBF is a process in which powdered material is sintered or melted to form a part by using either laser, electron beam, or thermal heat as the power source. There are three vital components to all PBF systems—a nozzle which houses the energy source necessary to combine the material, a modeling chamber where the part is built, and a feedstock to replenish material in the modeling chamber. Irrespective of the power source, all the techniques maintain a constant build chamber temperature just below the melting point of the powdered material (different for different powdered materials).[26] This is essential to minimize the power requirement, to reduce overall build time, and to prevent the part from warping because of accumulated stress due to nonuniform thermal expansion and contraction.[27] Warping due to nonuniform thermal expansion and contraction is a major issue while printing metal parts.

For the first layer, the modeling chamber is lowered to the appropriated depth and filled with the powdered material. Depending on the technology, either laser, electron beam, or thermal heat is directed onto the powdered material to sinter or melt the powder together tracing the first cross-section of the part. Once the first layer is printed, the build chamber is slightly lowered and a roller or blade restocks fresh powder from the feed and the process is repeated.

As the raw material is in the powdered form while printing with thermoplastic powders such as plastic, nylon, polyamide, etc., there is no need to add an additional support structure to support overhangs or the part as the unused powder acts as a cushion and provides support to the part. However,

this is not the case while printing with metal powder such as nickel alloy, stainless steel, cobalt, titanium alloy, etc. Because metal powder has higher density than thermoplastic powders, there is a need to add support structures to prevent the part being printed from warping or buckling under its own weight and also to support overhangs.

There are five distinct PBF methods based on the type of power source.[26,27] They are as follows:
1. Selective laser sintering (SLS)
2. Direct metal laser sintering (DMLS)
3. Selective heat sintering (SHS)
4. Selective laser melting (SLM)
5. Electron beam melting (EBM)

Laser Sintering

- SLS is one of the most common laser sintering (LS) processes. It is most commonly used for producing thermoplastic parts and uses a laser beam to sinter the material together. The modeling chamber is filled with nitrogen gas to minimize oxidation of the powdered material.[27] Parts printed out of this method have high strength and are cost effective. Medical and healthcare, military, and automobile are a few of the industries that use this process to build functional parts and prototypes for testing.

- DMLS is the same as SLS, but instead of printing plastic parts, metal parts are printed using powdered metal as the feed. Support structures are needed to print metal parts. DMLS offers an affordable and reliable source for producing custom-made prosthetics or implants for patients. DMLS is also used for toolmaking.

- SHS fuses the powdered thermoplastic material by using a thermal print head. Blueprinter, a Danish company, invented and patented SHS technology in the early 2000s.[28] Because SHS uses a thermal print head instead of a complex laser system to print parts; the parts made are affordable, thus offering a cost-effective method for manufacturing prototype parts.

German companies EOS and SLM, Swiss company Sintratec, Polish company Sinterit, and US-based companies 3D Systems and Formlabs are few of the manufacturers that supply desktop- and industrial-grade LS 3D printers. These printers can print dimensionally accurate parts using thermoplastic powders and metal powders such as stainless steel, titanium, and nickel alloys.

Melting

- **In SLM**, the metal powder is fully melted instead of being sintered. A high-powered fiber laser is used to melt the powder and print it layer by layer. As the powder is melted rather than being sintered, the laser can be used to control the physical properties of the part by altering the lattice formation as per requirement.[26] Similar to its sintering siblings, in SLM, the print chamber is filled with an inert gas to slow down the oxidation of powdered material. This technology is widely used in the aerospace and medical industry.
- **EBM** uses a high-energy electron beam to melt the metal powder. EBM method operates in a vacuum chamber.[27] The electron beam is moved in the X and Y axes via electromagnet deflection.[26] Complete dense metal parts can be accurately made with EBM method. Arcam, a Swedish company is currently the only manufacturer that provides EBM 3D printers.

Once printing is completed, all of the unused powder is sucked out of the modeling chamber to reveal the final part. This unused powder can be recycled and reused for the next build. This ability to recycle and reuse unused powder further helps to reduce the overall operation cost. Stratasys Direct Manufacturing did a study to understand whether the mechanical properties of parts made out of reused powder in a DMLS printer degrades over time, and found that reusing the powder did not affect the mechanical properties and that the parts had the same mechanical properties after multiple reuse. They also proved that mixing old powder with new powder did not affect the mechanical properties.[29]

General postprocess includes removing unused powder from the part using an air gun in case of plastic parts or grinding the part down in case of metal parts. The metal parts are subjected to heat treatment (annealing) by baking them in an oven to enhance mechanical properties. Complete and utmost importance must be given to personnel safety. Proper personal protective equipment (PPE) such as face mask, goggles, laboratory coat, etc. must be worn all the time while dealing with loose powder.

Directed Energy Deposition (DED)

In directed energy deposition, metal powder or metal wire is fused together and deposited on a build plate by either an electron or high-power laser beam.[27] The deposition and melting of metal powder happens simultaneously. The nozzle and the power source setup are typically mounted on a multiaxis arm. Because the material deposition and fusion process happens simultaneously, DED printers are faster than their powder bed cousins. Optomec Inc., Trumpf, Sciaky Inc., BeAM are a few of the companies that manufacture printers that use high-power laser beams to fuse the metal together.

Because the arm can move in various axes, the nozzle can deposit material at any angle to the build plate. The reverse is also possible, as in the arm and the power source are fixed while the build plate is mounted on a multiaxis platform. This unique ability to have multiple axes of movement makes it ideal to be used for repairing and maintaining structural parts.[27] DED method can also be used to repair turbine blades and other high-end equipment.[30] Sciaky's Electron Beam Additive Manufacturing process is capable of printing very large parts (larger than 19 ft.) in one go.[31]

Postprocessing involves machining the supports off and also surface machining to achieve the desired tolerance. Heat treatment might be needed to enhance mechanical properties of the part.

Binder Jetting (BJ)

BJ is a 3D printing process in which liquid binding agent is carefully sprayed to bind powder particles together to produce a 3D part. Just like PBF, BJ unit consists of a feedstock with the powdered material, a roller or blade to restock the powder in the chamber, and a nozzle to selectively spray the binding agent across a thin cross-section of powder. Once a layer is completed, the build platform lowers down and a roller or blade refills the chamber with fresh powder. Over time, the part develops through the layering of powder and binder agent. BJ is capable of printing a variety of materials including nylon, thermoplastics, and ceramics. Parts made out of BJ do not need additional supports as the parts are supported by the loose powder. This enables parts to be stacked over one another to increase the number of parts printed at once. Complete assemblies can be printed using this method, thus avoiding the need for tedious and challenging assemblies. Another advantage of this technology is that parts can be printed in full color and in multiple color combinations. 3D Systems's ProJet CJP ×60 printer series can print parts in full CMYK color.

While printing using BJ techniques, few design considerations such as a minimum feature thickness of 2 mm, a minimum hole diameter of 1.5 mm, a minimum thickness of 3 mm for unsupported walls etc. must be kept in mind for a successful print.[16]

Similar to PBF, the powdered material used in a BJ printer can also be recycled and reused. Proper PPE such as face mask, goggles, laboratory coat etc. must be worn all the time while dealing with loose powder. Post-process cleaning such as blowing excess powder off the part must be done inside a closed chamber. As the parts are held together by the epoxy binding agent, parts directly out of the build platform tend to be brittle, fragile, and have limited mechanical characteristics. Postprocessing involves infiltrating the part with either resin, epoxy, or saltwater to make it stronger and durable.

Material Jetting (MJ)

MJ (also known as inkjet printing) jets fine drops of liquid photopolymer on the build tray either in a continuous or drop-on-demand approach.[27] The process is similar to an inkjet printer that sprays ink on paper to print. Multiple print heads jet material simultaneously to create layers, which is instantly cured by UV light bulb which is attached to the extruder along with the nozzles. MJ is considered to be a very accurate form of 3D printing. Once done, the parts can be used without additional postcuring. MJ process always uses support material to completely surround and support the part. The support material like the model material is jetted onto the build tray by multiple nozzles. In 2011, Stratasys bought Objet Geometrics Ltd, an Israel-based company which had multiple patents for its PolyJet technology[13] (Fig. 2.10). ProJet MJP series by 3D Systems works on the same principle. One key difference being that the MJP series uses a waxlike support material.

While printing using MJ techniques, few design considerations such as a minimum feature thickness of 0.5 mm, a minimum hole diameter of 0.5 mm, a minimum thickness of 1 mm for unsupported walls etc. must be kept in mind for a successful print[16] (Table 2.1).

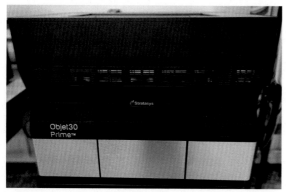

FIG. 2.10 Stratasys Objet30 Prime is part of the Design series printers. (Stratasys, Ltd.)

As MJ uses liquid polymer as material, it is possible to combine multiple different polymers within the same 3D printed part to create parts with different physical properties and have multicolored parts. Additionally, entire assemblies can be printed at once using the MJ printing process, reducing the need for multiple printing and combining multiple parts. Parts printed out of MJ have a very smooth surface finish.

Postprocessing in the case of the Objet series printers is done by removing the support material by using a high-powered waterjet system. This is at a disadvantage when the wall thickness is too thin. The water pressure might cause some features to break, hence special care must be taken while removing supports off thin-walled parts. The Projet MJP series uses a waxlike support material which can be easily melted away after printing, thus avoiding the need for a power wash to remove supports. The only disadvantage to this method is that if the wall thickness is too thin, the parts can warp while melting.

Sheet Lamination (SL)

SL uses sheets of paper as raw material to build the part. Most lamination printers use A4 size paper as the feed material. The paper is coated with a heat-sensitive adhesive. To build an object, layers of paper are stacked on top of each other and a heated roller or press is used to melt the adhesive, which forces the layers to stick to each other.[32] A blade then cuts the material as per the cross-section of the part. After a layer of the object is cut, the build platform lowers down and fresh set of paper is pulled from the feedstock and the heated roller or press is again used to bind the new layer to the ones under it. This process is repeated until the entire object has been printed. The blade cross-hatches the excess material, making it easier to remove the waste once the part is fully printed.[33] Typical layer resolution depends on the material feedstock and usually ranges from one to a few sheets of paper. For a successful print, the minimum wall thickness must be 0.5 mm.[34] At CES 2016, Ireland-based Mcor introduced Arke, which is a successor to its industrial-grade SL printer Iris. Arke uses regular paper as feed. Parts made out of this process can be printed in full CMYK color.

The advantage of this technology is that, as it uses regular printing paper as raw material, the parts can be printed at a fraction of the cost compared with other technologies. The downside to this technology is that there is a lot of wastepaper generated.

Once an object is done printing, it is removed from the build tray, and excess paper is removed to reveal the final part. The final part can be treated with epoxy to improve the strength of the part and to give it a nice shiny appearance.

3D PRINTING WORKFLOW

While in some ways 3D printing simplifies the manufacturing process by integrating the assembly of a given product layer by layer, it is still quite a complex undertaking that requires multiple well-orchestrated steps to materialize a CAD concept to a physical part.

We will take you through a basic workflow that one must traverse in order to produce any 3D printed part.

The process can be broadly broken down into three major areas as follows:[12,35]

- Preprocessing—preparing the model
- Processing—preparing to 3D print the model
- Postprocessing—removing and cleaning the model

Preprocessing
Step 1: Preparing the CAD model

The first and foremost element of 3D printing is the CAD model (Fig. 2.11). This is the visualization phase. There are various CAD packages available in the market such as Solidworks and CATIA developed by Dassault Systèmes, Fusion 360 and Inventor developed by Autodesk, Creo developed by PTC as well as free, open-source options such as FreeCAD, Rhino, and OpenSCAD. All of these software products give the user freedom and the power to model a creative or functional part. CATIA is used mostly for surface modeling and is a popular CAD package in the automobile and aircraft industry. Solidworks and Creo are mid-level user-friendly CAD packages. Solidworks has great product-rendering features, whereas Creo has great assembly features.

While designing a model for 3D printing, the designer must take into consideration various factors which affect the final outcome of the part. Each technology has different capabilities and limitations. Depending on the printing technology to be used, the designer may need to minimize the angle of overhangs to avoid the need for supports and pay extra attention to unsupported walls, engraved details, holes, connecting parts, tolerance, etc. as discussed earlier. These constraints must be considered while designing parts.

Step 2: STL conversion

Once the part has been modeled, the next step is to convert the CAD model into an STL file. STL is a neutral file format recognized, and read by every printer and is the standard file format. STL uses triangles (polygons) (Fig. 2.12) to describe the surfaces of an object.[33] STL has several acronyms such as Standard Triangle Language and Stereolithography Tessellation Language.

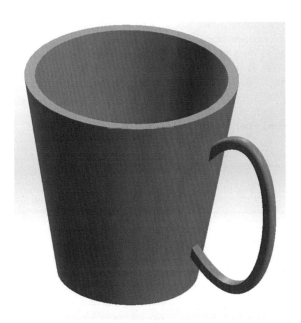

FIG. 2.11 CAD model of the part that being printed.

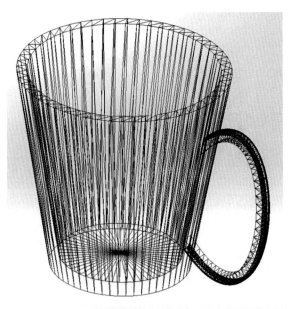

FIG. 2.12 STL triangles (polygons).

OBJ format is an alternative to STL file, which is gaining popularity. OBJ files are capable of storing extra information such as texture maps, color, and other details of the CAD model that the STL file does not save. If a user wants to print a multicolor part, the file should be saved as .OBJ rather than as .STL file format. Although, STL files are still widely used and every printer accepts STL files, OBJ file format can be easily exported from most CAD tools and is supported by almost all new 3D printers.

Step 3: Uploading the part to the printer

Once an STL file has been generated, the file is imported into a slicer program. This program takes the STL file, slices it in horizontal layers, calculates the time needed to print the part and amount of material used, and then converts the instructions into G-code. This is a set of computer codes which holds instructions for movement of the 3D printer.[36] Slicer settings have a huge impact on the final outcome and quality of the part and can be the difference between a successful and a failed print. The optimal slicer settings depend on the design, the material being used, and the type of printer being used. Open-sourced printers generally do not have an associated custom slicer. This gives the user the freedom and flexibility to use different slicing software. Autodesk Netfabb is one of the most popular and widely used slicing software as it has features that help to repair STL files. Others such as Slic3r, Cura, IceSL, and Z-Suit are also available for use. In case of closed sourced desktop printers, the manufacturer provides custom slicing software package which does all the abovementioned steps without the need for the user to separately create the G-codes. Refer to Chapter 3 "From CT and MR images to 3D printing - Software Basics for the Surgeon" for more information.

Processing

Step 4: Printer setup

Before beginning the printing process, one must ensure that the printer has enough raw material. Each printing technology has its unique setup requirements. Few of the most popular materials are spools of PLA or ABS thermoplastic, nylon, photocurable liquid resin, powdered metal such as titanium, nickel, or cobalt alloy, and thermoplastic powdered material. There are few uncommon materials such as flexible material NinjaFlex, wood-textured material, clay, HIPS plastic, etc. which are used for specific purposes and require different print settings and specialized equipment to print.

Step 5: Part manipulation and build

Once the printer is ready for printing, the next step is to manually import the sliced STL part into the printer by opening the file in the printer software. In case of closed sourced printers, the software lets the user perform various operations to the STL file such as duplicating, orienting, and positioning the parts. Once the desired parameters are set, the slicer will generate the G-code and the support structures for the part (if needed) and send the codes to the printer. In case of open-sourced printers, the user can import the sliced part generated by the slicer software. The printer will then start the printing process and build the part layer by layer. Very minimum supervision is needed at this stage unless the print fails due to conditions such as not enough material, temperature error, power outages, etc.

Postprocessing

Step 6: Remove the part

After the part has been printed, it needs to be taken out of the 3D printer. Printers with closed chambers may require some added time to make sure that it is safe to take the part out. For others, the build plate can be immediately taken out. The build plate, chamber, or the part may be hot, so necessary precautions must be followed while removing the part. For some machines, it might be as simple as twisting or plucking the part out of the build plate, whereas for some, you may need to use a joint knife to remove the part from the build plate.

Step 7: Cleaning/Final touchups

The final stage of 3D printing is cleaning the part. Because of structural constraints, a part might need support structures to print overhangs and once printed, the supports need to be removed from the part. Few technologies such as SLS, BJ, SL, etc. do not need additional supports as the raw material provides support to the structure. Supports can be clipped and sanded in case of photopolymerization printers, dipped in a solvent bath to be dissolved or clipped and sanded in case of extrusion printers, removed using a waterjet in case of MJ printers, or ground down in case of metal printers. After cleaning, the part is ready to be used as per desired.

3D SCANNING

A 3D scanner is a device that scans an object and collects data on its shape and appearance. The data are then used to construct digital models. 3D scanning has opened up new possibilities for reverse engineering. Designers could modify an existing object without having to remake the whole CAD model of the part. They could make the necessary alterations to the scanned model and 3D print it to verify the part. In addition to automobile and aerospace, 3D scanning can be used in biology and archeology. There are various types of 3D scanners available now. It is important to note that the accuracy and amount of details captured depends on the resolution of the scanner.

ADVANTAGES OF 3D PRINTING

Understanding the different advantages of 3D printing allows a user to make sound decisions when selecting a type of printing process to print a part. Even though the technology is still developing, there are various advantages and compelling reasons to incorporate the technology in our day-to-day activities.

- Traditional manufacturing process requires the use of warehouses to meet ever-growing and changing demands. With 3D printing, this is not necessary anymore. Parts can be manufactured on-site, which reduces the problem of storage and supply chain.
- 3D printing helps to minimize the number of intermediary steps involved to manufacture a part. Unlike the conventional subtractive process, where a part might have to go through repetitive operations such as milling, drill, lathe, etc. to be finished, 3D printing needs only a handful of operations. The ability to produce a part in one step greatly reduces the dependence on different manufacturing processes.
- 3D printing also reduces the amount of waste material generated. Waste scrap is a huge problem in industries. Companies generate tons of scrap during the intermediary processes and most of it is either recycled or dumped. As 3D printing uses a fixed amount of material, the amount of waste generated is minimized, thus saving costs.
- 3D printing allows the user to be as creative as possible. If one can model it, the 3D printer can print it. This flexibility allows artists to be creative in their work by creating unique designs for concept manufacturing. Conventional manufacturing has limited creativity and a fixed scope of use.
- 3D printing can be used to reduce the amount of moving parts. The entire assembly can be manufactured at once using 3D printing techniques. This reduces the effort to assemble the part (Fig. 2.13).

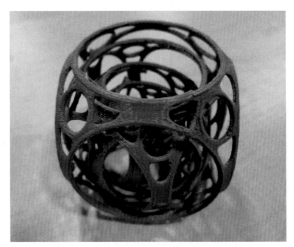

FIG. 2.13 Gyro Air. It is a multiassembly model and was printed as a single piece. (Gyro Air by Dalpek. File downloaded from: https://www.thingiverse.com/thing: 653085.)

- Parts made up of multiple materials are possible with 3D printing. As discussed in the previous section, various technologies offer the benefit of manufacturing a part using different materials at once. This opens door for customization.

LIMITATIONS OF 3D PRINTING

Although 3D printing has many applications, it is still unlikely to replace many traditional manufacturing methods. It has plenty of limitations and has a long way to go before it is truly user-friendly and can be used by any one from a beginner to an expert in 3D printing.

- Time: Even though there has been a remarkable breakthrough in the technology, the process is still slow and takes a while to print a medium to a large part. This limits the number of parts one can print at a time.
- New materials are being developed every day to provide better choices to the user. The issue is the cost of these materials. Material development plays a huge part in the progress of 3D printing. The commonly used materials such as ABS and PLA are affordable and readily available, but other specialty materials (such as polymers, metals, etc.) are still expensive and further add to the operations cost. A 1 kg spool of PLA costs anywhere between $20–$50, whereas a 1 L bottle of photocurable polymer can cost anywhere between $100–$500.

- Cost is a major roadblock of this technology. Even though there are hundreds of affordable and reliable printers in the market, they all have a small build volume and cannot build a large functioning part. Higher end printers are big and expensive to buy and to operate. This limits the market, which is ready to welcome 3D printing into its operations.

- Another limitation is the material characteristics. Materials such as ABS and PLA used in extrusion printers have very high melting points and have a rough finish. To get a smooth surface finish, additional postprocessing is required such as sanding or in case of ABS, acetone vapor can be used to smooth the surface. The fumes might be harmful if inhaled directly. Material such as nylon is highly susceptible to absorbing moisture. This causes the part to fail as the moisture in the material prevents the material from retaining its extruded shape. Thermoplastic powders for BJ and PBF too need to be stored in a moisture-free environment. In case of vat photopolymerization and MJ printers, the liquid resin has a shelf life and if not used regularly can go bad and not print a successful part.

- Size is another restriction. It is difficult to manufacture a very large part with 3D printing techniques.

- The main reason why 3D printing took a while to kick off is because of patent restrictions. Companies that filed for the patents held on to their intellectual properties and had monopoly over the technology for many years. It was not until the early 2000s that the patent started to expire, thus paving the way for start-ups and other companies to explore the field.

- There are many sites such as GrabCAD and Thingiverse that provide platform for designers to upload their files for others to view and download. This causes concerns over intellectual properties. Anyone can use the files made by others without any prior permission. It is especially challenging to control the content available through these websites. It is absolutely possible for designers to upload the CAD model of a weapon which can be freely circulated and downloaded by many and can be misused.

SUMMARY

Today, 3D printing is becoming increasingly popular among the public. Many of the big manufacturers are teaming up with schools to educate children on the technology and provide them with hands-on experience. This evolution has changed the way we look at conventional manufacturing. We encounter multiple parts that are 3D printed without even noticing. Leading airlines such as Etihad and Emirates are using 3D printed panels in many of their newer planes, automobile manufacturers are substituting conventional manufacturing process with 3D printing for producing various functional and esthetic parts, personalized jewelry can be manufactured without any restriction, custom shoes based on one's feet can be 3D printed. With the invention of 3D printers such as Foodini[5] that can print delicious-looking food, we can already start to see how 3D printing might enter the home. A lot can be attributed to the fact that the overall cost of owning, operating, and maintaining a 3D printer has decreased by thousands of dollars, while the technology keeps improving. We can imagine a day when every household will have a 3D printer to prepare food, repair broken parts, make jewelry, and create shoes. With the rate of improvement seen over just a few years, the future of this technology is bright.

REFERENCES

1. The Free Beginner's Guide: 3Dprintingindustry.com. https://3dprintingindustry.com/3d-printing-basics-free-beginners-guide#02-history.
2. Flynt J. A Detailed History of 3D Printing: 3Dinsider.com. http://3dinsider.com/3d-printing-history.
3. Goldberg D. *History of 3D Printing: It's Older than You Are.* Redshift by Autodesk; 2014. https://www.autodesk.com/redshift/history-of-3d-printing/.
4. *The Official History of the RepRap Project.* All3DP.com; April 8, 2016. https://all3dp.com/history-of-the-reprap-project/.
5. Natural Machines. www.naturalmachines.com/press-kit/.
6. Koslow T. *3D Printed House — World's 35 Greatest 3D Printed Structures.* All3dp; 2017. https://all3dp.com/1/3d-printed-house-homes-buildings-3d-printing-construction/.
7. Brooks K. *14 Ways 3D Printing Has Changed the Art World.* Updated December 6, 2017. Huffpost; 2014. https://www.huffingtonpost.com/2014/06/30/3d-printing-art_n_5534459.html.
8. One:1; koenigsegg. https://www.koenigsegg.com/one1/.
9. Keller T. *An Epiphany of Disruption: GE Additive Chief Explains How 3D Printing Will Upend Manufacturing.* GE Reports; 2017. https://www.ge.com/reports/epiphany-disruption-ge-additive-chief-explains-3d-printing-will-upend-manufacturing/.
10. Birrell I. *3D-Printed Prosthetic Limbs: The Next Revolution in Medicine.* The Guard; 2017. https://www.theguardian.com/technology/2017/feb/19/3d-printed-prosthetic-limbs-revolution-in-medicine.

11. *3D Scanning and 3D Printing for Museums and Archeology Aniwaa*. https://www.aniwaa.com/3d-printing-for-archeology-and-museology/.

12. Gibson I, Rosen D, Stucker B. Introduction and basic principles. In: *Additive Manufacturing Technologies*. New York, NY: Springer; 2010. https://doi.org/10.1007/978-1-4419-1120-9. e-ISBN: 978-1-4419-1120-9.

13. *Legal Information*. http://www.stratasys.com/legal/legal-information.

14. *Terms of Condition Markforged*. https://markforged.com/terms-conditions/.

15. Barnatt C. *3D Printing*. 2nd ed. ExplainingTheFuture.com; November 7, 2014. ISBN-13: 978−1502879790.

16. Brpckotter R. *Key Design Considerations for 3D Printing*: 3D Hubs. https://www.3dhubs.com/knowledge-base/key-design-considerations-3d-printing.

17. *Formlabs Design Guide*: Formlabs.com. https://formlabs.com/media/upload/formlabs-design-guide.pdf.

18. *Resources*: Formlabs.com. https://formlabs.com/resources/.

19. *3D Printing Technology Comparison: SLA Vs DLP*. Formlabs; November 16, 2016. https://formlabs.com/blog/3d-printing-technology-comparison-sla-dlp/.

20. *The Ultimate Guide to Stereolithography (SLA) 3D Printing in Tutorials*: Formlabs.com. https://formlabs.com/blog/ultimate-guide-to-stereolithography-sla-3d-printing/.

21. Falguni P, Jinah J, Jin Woo L, Dong-Woo C. Essentials of 3D biofabrication and translation. In: *Extrusion Bioprinting*. 2015.

22. Vijayavenkataraman S, Fuh JYH, Lu WF. *3D Printing and 3D Bioprinting in Pediatrics*. 2017. https://doi.org/10.3390/bioengineering4030063. PMCID: PMC5615309.

23. You F, Eames BF, Chen X. *Application of Extrusion-Based Hydrogel Bioprinting for Cartilage Tissue Engineering*. ISSN: 1422−0067.

24. Ozbolat IT, Hospodiuk M. Current advances and future perspectives in extrusion-based Bioprinting. In: *Biomaterials*. vol. 76. 2016:321−343. ISSN: 1878−5905.

25. *Design Guide I Materialize*. https://i.materialise.com/3d-printing-materials/abs/design-guide.

26. Gibson I, Rosen D, Stucker B. Powder bed fusion processes. In: *Additive Manufacturing Technologies*. New York, NY: Springer; 2010. https://doi.org/10.1007/978-1-4419-1120-9. e-ISBN: 978-1-4419-1120-9.

27. Loughborough University. *About Additive Manufacturing*: Additive Manufacturing Research Group. http://www.lboro.ac.uk/research/amrg/about/the7categoriesofadditive-manufacturing/.

28. Jakk. *What Is Selective Heat Sintering (SHS), and How Does it Work?* GoPrint3D; April 6, 2016. https://www.goprint3d.co.uk/blog/selective-heat-sintering-shs-work/.

29. Mutchler E, Carter A. *Additive Metals: Achieving Process Repeatability*: Stratasys Direct Manufacturing Webinar. https://www.stratasysdirect.com/resources/webinars/additive-manufacturing-metal-achieving-process-repeatability.

30. Peels J. *Comparison of Metal 3D Printing − Part Two: Directed Energy Deposition*. July 28, 2017.

31. *Electron Beam Additive Manufacturing (EBAM)*: Sciaky Inc. http://www.sciaky.com/additive-manufacturing/wire-am-vs-powder-am; https://3dprint.com/182367/directed-energy-deposition/ .

32. Gibson I, Rosen D, Stucker B. Sheet lamination processes. In: *Additive Manufacturing Technologies*. New York, NY: Springer; 2010. https://doi.org/10.1007/978-1-4419-1120-9. e-ISBN: 978-1-4419-1120-9.

33. Palermo E. *What Is Laminated Object Manufacturing?* Livescience; October 9, 2013. https://www.livescience.com/40310-laminated-object-manufacturing.html.

34. *Matrix 300+/IRIS Training & Set-Up Manual*: Mcor Technologies. https://www.pfsgraphics.com/new-equipment/3dprinters/mcor/technical/Mcor_Iris_Matrix300A_OperationalManual.pdf.

35. Crawford S. *How 3-D Printing Works*. HowStuffWorks; March 1, 2011. https://computer.howstuffworks.com/3-d-printing.htm.

36. Redwood B, *The Additive Manufacturing Process*: 3D Hubs. https://www.3dhubs.com/knowledge-base/additive-manufacturing-process.

CHAPTER 3

From CT and MR Images to 3D Printed Models—Software Basics for the Surgeon

SANJAY P. PRABHU, MBBS, DCH, FRCR, DABR

INTRODUCTION

Advanced image visualization techniques have been used widely by clinicians in all the surgical specialties including orthopedics to display and visualize complex pathologies. Clinicians rely on these images to understand relationships between anatomic structures, a key step in planning a surgical procedure. These images are also used to communicate findings to other members of the clinical team involved in care of the patient and convey the details of the technique to trainees and patients.

More recently, three-dimensional (3D) visualization has extended beyond display on a screen to include 3D printed models that are capable of providing tangible depth information about anatomic and pathologic states. Surgical benefits of 3D printed models include improved surgical planning via rehearsal of procedures using bespoke patient-specific models, enhanced diagnostic quality, decreased patient exposure time to general anesthesia, decreased patient blood loss, and smaller wound exposure needs.[1–3] 3D printed models also enable better communication between clinical teams and facilitate more meaningful patient and trainee education.[4]

Improvements in medical imaging modalities, such as computed tomography (CT) and magnetic resonance imaging (MRI), have enabled capture of anatomic data with submillimeter resolution. Added to this, modern segmentation techniques are constantly being improved to display anatomic structures in high detail, and modern 3D printers can create models with layer thicknesses on the order of microns. As the use of 3D printed models generated from Digital Imaging and Communications in Medicine (DICOM) images for planning interventions and fabricating implants becomes more prevalent and considered part of routine clinical care, clinicians should become well versed in various 3D printing technologies, software programs and materials used to create 3D printed anatomic models, and latest guidelines being developed to ensure optimal and accurate prints.

Creating a 3D printed model of an anatomic structure seen on imaging studies entails converting and manipulating imaging data stored in the DICOM format into a file format that can be handled by 3D printers. In this chapter, we will discuss steps involved in creating a 3D printed model, with emphasis on the step of image acquisition and ways to convert DICOM images into a file that can be converted to an accurate print. We will also discuss common challenges and pitfalls in the process and ways to overcome them.

STEPS IN WORKFLOW CREATING A MEDICAL 3D MODEL[5] (FIG. 3.1)

Step 1: Ideation

The first step in the process of a creating a 3D printed model is to ascertain whether 3D printing will add value over and above conventional imaging studies and other techniques that allow manipulation of patient images on a screen in two-dimensional (2D) or 3D space.[6–8] The decision to 3D print may be informed by reading about the experience of other surgeons who have operated on similar cases, review of peer-reviewed literature, or one's own prior experience. In many cases, surgeons decide to use 3D printing for the first time to help with procedures that they have found challenging or complex, cases with large number of possible variations to the approach or in rare cases that have no clearly defined solution. Occasionally, the decision to create a 3D printed model arises from a clinical conference where there is

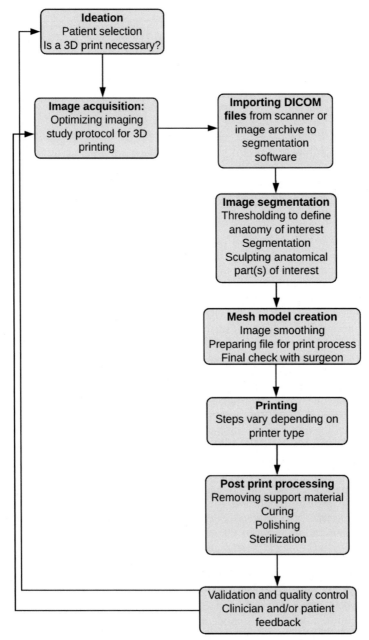

FIG. 3.1 Workflow for printing patient-specific models for surgical planning. *DICOM*, digital imaging and communications in medicine.

difference of opinion between members of the surgical team on how to treat a particular condition, or where the radiologist suggests a print might be helpful in clarifying the anatomy or where the anatomy is too complex to be understood from conventional imaging studies and visualization methods or where the surgical team thinks an innovative approach might provide a better solution to the clinical problem.

Once the decision to get a 3D printed model has been made, it is important to clearly define the purpose of the model, as this will inform subsequent steps in the process. These steps include deciding which structures should be included in the print, specifications of whether the material needs to be easily cut and manipulated, and whether the printed model will be taken into the surgical field, thereby requiring sterilization. It is important for the entire team (orthopedic surgeon, radiologist, and engineers) to clearly understand these requirements at the outset. While specific details might change during the process, the ultimate aim of the model should be kept in mind throughout the process.

Step 2: Image Acquisition

The next step is to acquire images of the structure/s that have to be included in the 3D printed model. 3D models can be printed using the data from a wide variety of cross-sectional imaging studies including CT, MRI, ultrasound studies, and conventional angiography studies.

If a 3D printed model is anticipated prior to image acquisition, the imaging study should be tailored to acquire high-quality images to show the anatomic structure that is the focus of the print.[9] In orthopedics, the bones are the most common structures of interest and therefore CT is the imaging modality of choice most often. However, in our pediatric-focused practice, we print a majority of our osseous models for surgical planning of upper and lower limb procedures from MRI acquisitions. While segmentation of MRI images to parse out osseous structures is relatively more time consuming using existing software tools, this method avoids radiation and also provides a "one-stop shop" enabling visualization of cartilage, muscles, vascular anatomy, and other soft tissues on a single study.[10,11]

Most orthopedic surgeons rely on models created using a single modality (typically CT for osseous models and MRI for soft tissue lesions such as tumors). However, in some cases, prints based on multiple modalities can be created using a combination of contemporaneously obtained CT and MRI. This step is facilitated by overlaying the two DICOM data sets and coregistering them using various open source or commercially available applications such as 3D Slicer prior to segmentation to extract the soft tissue information from MRI and the bone and/or vascular information from CT. Alternatively, coregistration can be carried out after creation of the printable STL files in 3D space using specific landmarks on the images.[12] For example, in some prints, it may be important to also visualize surrounding vascular structures, bowel, cartilage, or ligaments in addition to the bones. In these cases, care should be taken to ensure optimal CT contrast bolus timing and acquire the most appropriate MR sequences to visualize the soft tissue and vascular structures of interest, as described in more detail in following sections.

In addition to anatomic data, some models allow incorporation of other data into the model utilizing functional studies such as radionuclide studies, called by some authors as five-dimensional printing, as time and physiologic activity are added to the 3D model.[13]

A dialog between the surgeon and the radiologist is key to ensuring that the imaging study is performed optimally both to answer the clinical question and provide images that can be used to create a 3D printed model. The bottom line is that if a structure is not imaged optimally or not imaged at all due to inadequate coverage in field of view of the scan, then it is not possible to accurately segment that structure and visualize it in the printed model.

It is extremely important to understand that a "diagnostic" imaging study is not necessarily an optimal study for optimal 3D print generation. In particular, studies that a radiologist or surgeon considers adequate for diagnosis may be too noisy (low signal to noise), have low spatial resolution, or not include the thinnest image sets to enable creation of a usable and accurate 3D printed model. As a rule of thumb, scan parameters used to generate a 3D printed model of a structure will be the same as those that allow optimal visualization of the targeted anatomic structure. Volumetric images acquired with a slice thickness of 1−2 mm in thickness (or lower) in case of CT and 1−2 mm on MRI are ideal for creation of 3D printed models. Most importantly, gaps between slices should be avoided. While it is still possible to create a 3D model from images acquired with a slice thickness greater than 2−3 mm, or even with images containing gaps between slices, the resulting prints are not accurate enough to help with precise surgical planning. Careful attention to scan parameters may assist in the process of mesh generation (discussed later) and create higher quality models.[14]

With regard to scan acquisition settings for CT, it is better to err on the side of higher tube currents (mA), or higher tube potential (kV) depending on body habitus, to ensure noise is minimized in cases where high-quality 3D printing is required. Other important factors that influence spatial resolution and image noise in CT are slice thickness and reconstruction kernels. Thicker images can result in discontinuous, stair-step-like boundaries on the segmented model. The reconstruction kernel defines the filter used to reject noise on a CT scan. We choose different kernels based on the type of image that we are trying to create. For imaging the bones or lungs, we choose a sharp kernel as we want to accentuate small, discrete features such as fractures, nodules, fine reticulation. Conversely, a softer kernel is used to visualize soft tissues such as the brain or abdominal organs such as the liver or kidneys, as these structures have larger features with mild differences in attenuation. These reconstruction kernels used to create different sets of images should be distinguished from the different window settings used to view the images at the workstation that depend upon the underlying attenuation values of these tissues. Another way to look at reconstruction kernels is that we have to use softer kernels where there is less contrast and a higher priority in removing noise. On a practical note, reconstruction kernels affect the spatial resolution and image noise, which need to be balanced based on the type of 3D model. For example, for models requiring fine detail, such as sharp delineation of fracture lines and bone fragments, a sharp kernel is more appropriate to get the best spatial resolution. On the other hand, for models that require moderate to large size, low contrast objects, such as the vascular structures, pelvis, or dysplastic hips, a smooth kernel is more appropriate to control image noise.

Timing of contrast bolus is also very important to maximize visualization and ensure accurate segmentation of vascular and soft tissue structures. If a print request calls for inclusion of the femoral artery, for example, the contrast injection and bolus timing for a CT angiogram of the lower limb vasculature can be adjusted to enable optimal delineation of the femoral artery and its branches while excluding the venous structures. A lower tube potential (kV) can help increase the relative enhancement of iodinated contrast medium in vascular models.

Finally, it is important to remember that artifacts on the acquired imaging data sets, including streak artifacts, blooming, or beam hardening, will also be represented in the 3D mesh generated from it and in turn will be seen in the 3D printed object. Beam hardening is an artifact on CT that is characterized by dark streaks along the long axis of a single high attenuation object and bright streaks adjacent to the dark streaks. This is particularly a problem with metal implants and in areas where there are sharp outlines of bone like the posterior fossa in the brain. Blooming refers to foci of calcification or heterotopic bone appearing larger than they actually are due to partial volume artifact, particularly when combined with motion artifact and when a low-density structure is located close to the higher density focus.

In pediatric patients, the need to minimize dose per the "as low as reasonably achievable (ALARA)" principle results in noisier images. In these cases, iterative reconstruction and denoising techniques such as isotropic total variation and four-dimensional noise reduction can be helpful to reduce noise while preserving image features, allowing for faster and more automated segmentation.

Another useful technique to consider is application of metal artifact reduction algorithm to scans acquired with dual energy technique available on some modern CT scanners to reduce artifacts from metallic hardware, which can be particularly problematic in orthopedic cases with prior instrumentation.

To summarize, higher mA, smaller voxel sizes, lower slice thickness, and sharp kernel settings are appropriate for capturing fine image detail but may necessitate more manual segmentation and postprocessing to smooth the model due to image noise.[14] Conversely, larger voxel size and "soft" reconstruction kernels facilitate more automated segmentation and produce smoother 3D models, albeit at the cost of loss of model detail. For example, in order to print a long bone from a CT, the axial images created with a soft tissue algorithm are ideal—as long as demonstrating fine bone detail such as a subtle fracture line is not the object of the study.

Step 3: Image Segmentation

The next step is to import the images from the hospital picture archiving and communication system (PACS) system into a segmentation software package. Some segmentation software programs include a converter that handles the conversion from the DICOM format, whereas others require conversion to a format readable by segmentation programs.

Segmentation refers to the process of isolating the structure of interest from the rest of the imaged anatomy and defining boundaries between various structures in images to create patient-specific, highly accurate computer models of organs and tissue. Basic segmentation approaches rely on the differences in pixel density (on CT) or signal intensity (on MRI) of each tissue type on imaging studies. As long as the imaging study has been optimized to visualize these differences between tissue types, it is possible to distinguish between tissues and identify boundaries. For instance, CT is the modality of choice for segmenting and printing osseous structures due to the inherent higher contrast between the bone and surrounding soft tissues. Enhancement with iodinated contrast enables delineation of enhancing tumors and vascular structures on contrast-enhanced CT studies. MRI scans can differentiate between various types of soft tissues based on differences in signal intensities of tissues including water, fat, calcium, and protein on various sequences. Also, certain MRI techniques can delineate vascular structures without addition of contrast medium based on the movement of blood.

In some cases, combined use of CT and MRI can help create accurate models for surgical planning by coregistration scans. For example, in cases of a pelvic or long bone tumor, the bony margins can be defined on CT, whereas the soft tissue component of the tumor and sites of tumor invasion, periosteal elevation, and/or edema within the bone is best defined on MRI. A single model created using the information from both modalities allows the surgeon to plan resection and reconstruction utilizing all available information.

There are a number of commercial and open source image segmentation tools with their own advantages and disadvantages Table 3.1. We can summarize this topic by saying that there is no single segmentation technique, which is suitable for all images and applications, and almost all the tools have a learning curve. As the segmentation packages are constantly undergoing changes, we will not elaborate on individual software tools in this chapter. The key points to note when choosing a software tool for image segmentation are ease of use, ability of the tool to segment the structures that are most commonly printed in one's practice, availability of training or help with challenging segmentations, and the cost of the tool.

Newer and faster segmentation techniques that are based on nonlinear filtering, active contour modeling, statistical thresholding, and morphologic postprocessing are currently being developed. Fully automatic segmentation of arbitrary anatomic structures from 3D medical image data is an unsolved problem to date. This means that the surgeon, radiologist, or engineer will have to manually identify, at least in part, the various anatomic structures so they can be printed as separate objects. The degree of manual segmentation depends upon several factors including the degree to which contrast and spatial resolution between structures is optimized on the imaging study and the software used to segment the data. Although fully automatic segmentation would be ideal for clinical analysis and 3D printing, the complexity of anatomic structures across populations and the variability of different imaging modalities have hitherto hindered development of a general-purpose fully automatic 3D segmentation framework. Work in this area is currently

ongoing with new computer vision (machine learning) approaches being developed.[15]

Segmented images designated for printing patient-specific models for surgical planning should be carefully reviewed for anatomic accuracy irrespective of the software tool or underlying segmentation technique used. This check should preferably be assigned to a physician, either the surgeon or a radiologist familiar with the anatomy and the surgical procedure being planned.[3] Also, it should be pointed out that one of

TABLE 3.1
Examples of Segmentation Software

Software	Features	Comments
Osirix MD/ Osirix Lite[a]	• MacOS only • Manual editing • Segmentation by region growing	• $/Free (OsiriX Lite) • Osirix MD FDA cleared
3D Slicer[a]	• Cross platform (Windows, MacOS, Linux) • Manual editing • Thresholding • Variety of filters tailored for segmentation of specific anatomy • Allows image registration and fusion	• Open source • Online training resources (e.g., Wiki and tutorials) • Challenging with low contrast studies
Mimics inPrint (Materialise)	• Windows only • Thresholding • Manual editing • Anatomy-specific modules	• Customer support • Training part of setup costs • FDA approved (501K clearance) • $$$
InVesalius[a]	• Cross platform (Windows, MacOS, Linux) • Manual editing • Thresholding • Volume rendering using ray casting technique	• Free, open source • Detailed manuals in multiple languages

[a] Free and Open Source software.

the largest sources of error in a 3D model is at this step of tissue segmentation. Even when an expert checks segmentation, there is an inherent variation in the degree of accuracy of the printed models due to over- or underestimation of small nonuniform structures, particularly soft tissues, irrespective of the segmentation tool used.[16] Ways to mitigate or minimize this is to employ frequent quality checks on the scanner and have calibration tools that allow for quality checks on printed models at regular intervals.

Step 4: Mesh Model Creation, Smoothing, and Preparing for Print Process

The segmented anatomy is converted into a special file format called .STL using a wide array of computer-aided design (CAD) tools. STL Table 3.2 was originally derived from the word stereolithography, and now stands for Standard Tessellation Language, a term that refers to the tiling or layering of geometric shapes and patterns. The simplest explanation of an STL file is that it represents the surface geometry of a 3D object as a series of connected polygons without any representation of color, texture, or other common model attributes. Triangles are the most frequently used shape and will be referred to as such in the following discussion.[9] This 3D mesh of triangles defines the object that is being printed, and the term "mesh" refers to the fact that the model is not solid, but has a mesh or netlike appearance. Postprocessing of the mesh enables correcting of errors and discontinuities that arise during the segmentation and exporting process, making the mesh "watertight." It is important to carefully choose the number of triangles that represents the model; if too many triangles are created, the .STL file size can become unmanageable, and if too few triangles are created, curved areas are not properly defined, resulting in creation of false edges in smoothly curved parts of the model.

Further manipulation involves fixing flaws in the segmented model in preparation for 3D printing. The precise steps to clean the model differ with each commercially and open source software program and is beyond the scope of this chapter. However, irrespective of which software tool is used, the common principles include fixing holes in the segmented model to make it watertight, hollowing the model by defining a thickness between the inner and outer walls to reduce costs (as a solid model requires more material than a hollow one), removing discontinuous portions of the mesh that are not required to be part of the model, and joining up elements that are artificially separated

TABLE 3.2
Examples of Mesh Manipulation/Cleaning Software

Software	Features	Comments
Meshmixer*	• Cross platform (Windows and MacOS) • Drag and drop mesh mixing • 3D sculpting • Hollowing, hole filling, and auto-repair • Automatic surface alignment	• Free • Clean, simple interface • Easy to learn
Blender*	• Cross platform (Windows, MacOS, Linux) • Versatile 3D sculpting tools • Mesh analysis • Curve displays • Multiresolution mesh modeling	• Free and open source • Steep learning curve • Detailed website with step-by-step instructions • Powerful and freely customizable
3-Matic (Materialise)	• Windows only • Excellent meshing capabilities and repair tools • Allows mesh preparation for finite element simulations • Integrated full suite solution with other Materialise products	• $$$ • Various modules tailored to need • Excellent training and customer support

*Free and open source software

from the model during segmentation. Finally, additional elements such as segmented anatomic structures from another imaging study (e.g., MRI) or hardware components may also be added at this stage.

Step 5: Printing

The refined mesh model is then sent to the printer in a variety of file formats. The most common and universal file formats for 3D printing are STL, VRML (also called WRL), and the .OBJ format.

As mentioned, the STL file format carries the surface geometry of the object without any specific color representation. This is typically the file format for use with desktop 3D printers. VRML ("vermal," .WRL file extension) stands for "Virtual Reality Modeling Language" is a newer digital 3D file type that also includes color, so it can be used on desktop 3D printers with more than one extruder (i.e., two or more nozzles that each can print with a different color plastic) or with full-color binder jetting technology. The OBJ file format can encode both color and texture information and is gaining more traction in the 3D printing world with the advent of full color printing. This format supports both approximate and precise encoding of surface geometry. When using the approximate encoding, it allows the surface mesh to be created using polygons such as quadrilaterals in addition to triangular facets. When using precise encoding, it uses smooth curves and surfaces such as NURBS (nonuniform rational basis spline, a mathematical model commonly used in computer graphics for generating and representing curves and surfaces that offers flexibility and precision for handling both analytic [surfaces defined by common mathematical formulas] and modeled shapes).

In addition, many 3D printer manufacturers have their own proprietary input file formats that contain instructions specific to the methodology for that make or model and that are compatible only with that manufacturer's software. Examples of such proprietary file formats include the .form file, used with the PreForm software for Form1 or Form2 printers, or the .zpr format, proprietary to the ZPrint and ZEdit software used with ZCorp binder jet printers. This does not constitute a barrier to print as the printer software allows the user to generate the proprietary file format from the base STL or WRL file.

There is a newer file format being developed called the 3D Manufacturing Format (3 MF) which allows design applications to send full-fidelity 3D models to a mix of applications, platforms, services, and printers. This newer 3 MF is a universal specification engineered to avoid the problems associated with other 3D file formats. It is currently being worked upon and refined by a large consortium of industry partners and has the potential to be a file format for use in medical 3D printing in the near future.

A description of types of printers and printing techniques can be found in Chapters 1 and 2.

Step 6: Postprint Processing/Polishing

After the object is printed, it is often necessary to remove the residual material or supporting structures. The time required for this step depends on the type of printer and the type of model being printed. In addition to clearing the support material, polishing, coloring, reconstruction, or material hardening (infiltration) may also be necessary depending on the proposed use of the model. It is important not to lose important details such as the contours of bones or smooth out subtle fractures during this stage. Also, the time required for this step should be considered when determining the time required to print a model, particularly in an emergency situation (see Table 3.2).

Step 7. Validation and Quality Control

A key factor in ensuring the 3D printed models can be used in surgical planning is the accuracy of the model.[16] The accuracy of the model can be affected by errors that can occur during each of the steps described previously. Errors can become cumulative and significantly affect the model accuracy and utility.[14] There are no clear guidelines for quality control processes, and they are still a "work in progress." Most 3D printing laboratories with sufficient volumes, particularly laboratories that undertake additive manufacturing of implantable devices, have developed internal measures to minimize and mitigate errors when they do occur.

Potential validation steps include comparison of the final mesh model resulting after postprocessing and smoothing with the initial imaging study prior to sending the file to the printer.[14] Second, the measurements of the 3D printed object are compared with intraoperative measurements to assess accuracy. Finally, the 3D printed object can be scanned using a high-resolution technique (like a micro-CT scanner), and the resulting images are compared with the patient's images for anomalies. Phantom-based quality analysis include printing of imaging phantoms used to test image resolution in imaging systems or printing precisely drawn and measured test objects and shapes created using CAD software to ensure that the 3D print always conforms to the digital design.[14] Quality control should also include verification of the image acquisition parameters on CT and MRI, as this is an integral part of the 3D printing process.

Tips, Tricks, and Traps

In this section, we will discuss tips for creating and sustaining a successful 3D printing program for surgical planning and mention potential traps to look out for when planning a 3D printing laboratory.

One of the first steps in setting up a 3D printing service is to learn the basics of various software programs and the requirements to create an initial set of prints that can then be shown around to other colleagues to generate interest in like-minded clinical colleagues. This step can be accelerated by either visiting a facility that already does this or working through detailed websites and video tutorials created by various manufacturers and online communities on 3D printing using both proprietary and free, open source software (see examples of useful websites summarized in Table 3.3)

The other important element of successful 3D print laboratories is close communication between the members of the multidisciplinary team involved in the program. The team may be confined to a few members such as the orthopedic surgeon and the engineer in some cases or contain a large number of individuals when a model is complex and involve clinicians from other specialties, such as radiologists, material scientists, biomedical engineers, and artists. Communication of what the surgeon hopes to accomplish with the 3D printed model when starting the process is important as already mentioned.[1,3] In addition, a constant feedback loop should be maintained between the surgeon and engineering team throughout the process, including information about any delays, design issues (e.g., whether connectors need to be used to stabilize the model), cost, and time constraints. Furthermore, after a 3D print has been used for surgical planning, the team should be debriefed on how the model helped or, in some cases, did not help the surgical procedure. Any need for potential improvements at the different steps in the process for future prints should be noted at the time of this debrief. Engineers should be encouraged to observe the surgical procedures where their prints are used and attend multidisciplinary conferences where the models are used as an aid for discussion between various clinicians. This step is one of the advantages of developing an in-house printing service, even if the actual print is outsourced to a service bureau. There are several established and fairly economical print-on-demand services that allow physicians and engineers to upload files in various formats for 3D printing. The most commonly used service bureaus where physicians can upload print-ready files and get free quotes include Shapeways, i.materialise, Sculpteo, 3D Hubs, and MakeXYZ (Table 3.4). It is important to ensure that the data sent to these services are completely anonymized and any patient identifiable material is added to the model only after it is received from the printers. In case of in-house models, the medical record number and accession number of the study/studies used to print the model may be embedded into the model to ensure the correct model is used for a patient in the operating room.

A clear record of time spent by members working on a model and the time savings in the operating room due to use of the model in case of in-house models should be recorded meticulously in order to perform a cost-benefit analysis. Alternative methods of obtaining or displaying information should be explored before embarking on complex prints to ensure that the benefits of the print outweigh the cost.

TABLE 3.3
Educational Websites and Resources

Website	Type of Resource	What You Will Learn
http://www.materialise.com/en/medical/webinars	Live and recorded Webinars	Various facets of 3D printing from other Materialise users
embodi3D.com	Online community for biomedical 3D printing	Learn to 3D print with open source and proprietary software
Sculpteo.com	Written step-by-step tutorial and links to YouTube videos on Meshmixer	Modeling, correcting, and exporting 3D printed models to the Sculpteo print service
www.blender.org	Short videos describing specific features of Blender	Everything about Blender: from installation to modeling to rendering
https://www.slicer.org/wiki/Documentation/4.8/Training	Tutorials to various slicer modules: links to video and slides from presentation on segmentation for 3D printing	Segmentation for 3D printing using 3D slicer

TABLE 3.4
Service Bureaus for Outsourcing 3D Printing (Most Popular; Not Exhaustive)

Service	Materials	Printing Methods	Quotes
i.materialise	Metal, plastic, ceramic, resin, wood	PolyJet, FDM, SLA, SLS, Casting, ColorJet, CeramicJet	Instant quotes with worldwide shipping
Shapeways	Metal, plastic, ceramic, wax, sandstone	SLS, Binder, Jet Steel, wax casting	Instant quotes with worldwide shipping
3d Hubs	Metal, plastic, Paper, resin, stone, wax	FDM, metal sintering, PolyJet, SLA, SLS, Wax casting	Instant quotes with worldwide shipping
Sculpteo	Metal, plastic, ceramic, full color, resin, wax	SLA, SLS, casting, ColorJet	Instant quotes with worldwide shipping
MakeXYZ	Plastic, nylon, resin	FDM, SLA	Instant quotes with worldwide shipping
Axial³ᴰ	Plastic, resin, biocompatible, wax, full color, sandstone	SLA	Instant quotes with worldwide shipping

Reference for more services: https://all3dp.com/1/best-online-3d-printing-service-3d-print-services/. *FDM,* fused deposition modeling; *SLA,* stereolithography, *SLS,* selective laser sintering.

CONCLUSION

3D printing of anatomic models for surgical planning is now more accessible than ever, and there is increasing evidence these models can improve surgical outcomes and reduce uncertainty in the operating room.[1,7,17,18] Following a systematic approach, it is possible for surgeons and radiologists to create cost-effective and timely 3D printed models using an in-house or outsourcing approach. Quality control at various stages of production of the model and a feedback loop between the team creating the model and the surgeon are key elements to ensure an accurate print and in turn, a successful surgical procedure.

REFERENCES

1. Karlin L, Weinstock P, Hedequist D, Prabhu SP. The surgical treatment of spinal deformity in children with myelomeningocele: the role of personalized three-dimensional printed models. *J Pediatr Orthop B.* 2017;26(4):375–382.
2. Webb PA. A review of rapid prototyping (RP) techniques in the medical and biomedical sector. *J Med Eng Technol.* 2000;24(4):149–153.
3. Matsumoto JS, Morris JM, Foley TA, et al. Three-dimensional physical modeling: applications and experience at Mayo clinic. *Radiographics.* 2015;35(7):1989–2006.
4. Rogers-Vizena CR, Weinstock P, Livingston K, Prabhu SP. The current role of three-dimensional printing in plastic surgery. *Plast Reconstr Surg.* 2017;139(3):811e–812e.
5. Bucking TM, Hill ER, Robertson JL, Maneas E, Plumb AA, Nikitichev DI. From medical imaging data to 3D printed anatomical models. *PLoS One.* 2017;12(5):e0178540.
6. Tetsworth K, Block S, Glatt V. Putting 3D modelling and 3D printing into practice: virtual surgery and preoperative planning to reconstruct complex post-traumatic skeletal deformities and defects. *SICOT J.* 2017;3:16.
7. Papagelopoulos PJ, Savvidou OD, Koutsouradis P, et al. Three-dimensional technologies in orthopedics. *Orthopedics.* 2018;41(1):12–20.
8. Marro A, Bandukwala T, Mak W. Three-dimensional printing and medical imaging: a review of the methods and applications. *Curr Probl Diagn Radiol.* 2016;45(1):2–9.
9. Mitsouras D, Liacouras P, Imanzadeh A, et al. Medical 3D printing for the radiologist. *Radiographics.* 2015;35(7):1965–1988.
10. Heller M, Bauer HK, Goetze E, et al. Applications of patient-specific 3D printing in medicine. *Int J Comput Dent.* 2016;19(4):323–339.
11. Gargiulo P, Arnadottir I, Gislason M, Edmunds K, Olafsson I. New directions in 3D medical modeling: 3d-printing anatomy and functions in neurosurgical planning. *J Healthc Eng.* 2017;2017.
12. Shui W, Zhou M, Chen S, et al. The production of digital and printed resources from multiple modalities using visualization and three-dimensional printing techniques. *Int J Comput Assist Radiol Surg.* 2017;12(1):13–23.
13. Gillaspie EA, Matsumoto JS, Morris NE, et al. From 3-dimensional printing to 5-dimensional printing: enhancing Thoracic surgical planning and resection of complex tumors. *Ann Thorac Surg.* 2016;101(5):1958–1962.

14. Leng S, McGee K, Morris J, et al. Anatomic modeling using 3D printing: quality assurance and optimization. *3D Print Med.* 2017;3(1):6.

15. Guo K, Zou D, Chen X. 3D mesh Labeling via Deep Convolutional Neural Networks. *ACM Trans Graph.* 2015; 35(1):1−12.

16. George E, Liacouras P, Rybicki FJ, Mitsouras D. Measuring and establishing the accuracy and Reproducibility of 3D printed medical models. *Radiographics.* 2017;37(5): 1424−1450.

17. Boudissa M, Courvoisier A, Chabanas M, Tonetti J. Computer assisted surgery in preoperative planning of acetabular fracture surgery: state of the art. *Expert Rev Med devices.* 2018;15(1):81−89.

18. Guo F, Dai J, Zhang J, et al. Individualized 3D printing navigation template for pedicle screw fixation in upper cervical spine. *PLoS One.* 2017;12(2):e0171509.

CHAPTER 4

Economic and Regulatory Perspectives on Additive Manufacturing

GILBERT G. BERDINE, MD • MATTHEW DIPAOLA, MD • MICHAEL WEINBERG, JD

One can draw parallels between the impending manufacturing revolution that some forecasters contend additive manufacturing will augur in and the information revolution that the Internet has spawned. 3D printing has the potential to become a massive decentralizing force: moving manufacturing from industry to the individual, from the factory to the home. Just as the dawn of the Internet age made anyone with a laptop and an Internet connection a publisher, so too can 3D printing turn anyone with a 3D printer into a "manufacturer."

However, individuals that employ 3D printing and additive manufacturing do not operate in a vacuum. They operate within local, national, and sometimes worldwide economic and regulatory constraints that influence how, when, and where they can implement technology. As such it is important to consider how these constraints may influence the adoption, use, and reach of any technology in general.

From a legal and regulatory standpoint, 3D printing presents some unique challenges. While not completely new, 3D printing technology has only recently permeated the medical field, a field steeped in relatively static and far-reaching regulatory structures in most countries. At this point it is not clear whether its wider adoption will be absorbed quietly into existing regulatory frameworks or whether it will act as a disrupting force on those frameworks to upend much of what we know about how medical manufacturing is currently regulated.

The truth is that nobody knows for sure how 3D printing will ultimately change orthopedic practice from a broad contextual perspective. Instead, in this chapter we will attempt to help the reader understand how 3D printing technology fits into a broader economic and regulatory context. We will focus on the "macro" perspective where most of the rest of this book has focused on the "micro" perspective. We

hope the reader gains from the combination of theoretical and practical discussion that we will undertake.

Our first analysis will be somewhat more conceptual and theoretical in nature. We will briefly look at manufacturing from an economic standpoint and outline how 3D printing fits into an overall system of production. We will use a free market economic theory upon which to base our initial frame of reference and then branch into a more "real world" discussion of the landscape in which most of us currently operate.

3D PRINTING—SOME ECONOMIC CONSIDERATIONS

We have chosen to use a free market framework as a starting point upon which we will attempt to put the 3D printing movement into a broader systems-based context. We use the free market perspective not because that is what most of us currently operate under (most of us typically work in a system with a combination of both government and free market dynamics) but because we feel that it will give us the most basic model of how consumers and producers interact to meet their needs without some of the other more opaque influences at play. As such we will draw from the Austrian school of economics whose founding principles are the subjective basis of economic value and the theory of marginal utility (for a better understanding of free market principles please see Ref.[1]).

To begin, let us consider three models of production that exist along a continuous scale extending from a single source of production at one extreme to the opposite extreme of each consumer producing one's own goods.

Fig. 4.1 illustrates a centralized production scheme. There is one source of production and consumers must travel to this source in order to purchase the output. An example in the medical field would be a regional center that performs revision joint

3D Printing in Orthopaedic Surgery. https://doi.org/10.1016/B978-0-323-58118-9.00004-X

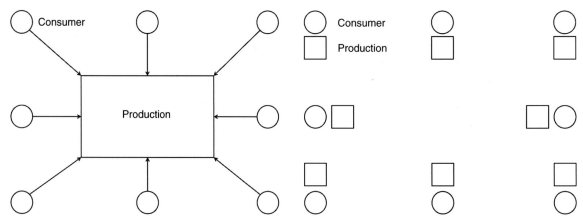

FIG. 4.1 Centralized Production Scheme

FIG. 4.2 Local Production or Decentralized Production Scheme

replacement. Although most community hospitals feature some form of orthopedic surgery, such as primary total joint replacement and basic fracture care, the regional center represents a central location for the production of a service to which consumers must travel in order to purchase that service. In this example, constraints such as surgeon expertise, implant inventory, and availability of complex ancillary services drive the concentration of revision joint replacement services to regional locations. In the manufacturing world, an example may be that one or only a few factories in the country produce a specific orthopedic implant due to the complexity and high cost of bringing together the resources necessary to build that specialized product.

There are pros and cons to a centralized production scheme. The pros are that it allows for a significant amount of specialization, control, and resource pooling to produce goods. The cons are that it may be subject to concentrated risks. For instance recently there has been a shortage of certain anesthetics in the world due to extreme hurricanes ripping through the Caribbean and taking Puerto Rican factories offline. One could argue that the production and distribution of these anesthetics was overly "centralized." A more decentralized system would have absorbed such a shock better by having a more distributed network of manufacturing in separate locations.

Fig. 4.2 illustrates a decentralized production scheme. Making toast is a simple example. Almost every household has a toaster. Production occurs at the location of the consumer and is regulated by the consumer. A surgical example would be sterile equipment. All modern hospitals and surgery centers have autoclave and other equipment that sterilize instruments. This allows the hospital (the end user) to regulate the delivery of sterile instruments in the operating room.

3D printing offers the possibility of fabricating equipment or supplies closer to the patient and expanding the role of the home in healthcare. In the abovementioned example, autoclaves could be produced at the point of use. While likely impractical in more industrially developed economies where transportation costs are low, one could imagine other environments where such local production of an autoclave would be advantageous. Consider a medical mission in a remote location or a space exploration mission to another planet. In both scenarios the transportation costs may limit the feasibility of bringing in a conventionally produced autoclave. If demand is high, at some cost the economic scales may tip in favor of producing that machine on site.

Fig. 4.3 is a hybrid scheme with centralized production and decentralized distribution. Most medications utilize this scheme. Medications are fabricated at a central location and distributed to local pharmacies where pharmacists regulate patient-specific dosages. Depending on your perspective, the autoclave example given in the previous section is a hybrid scheme. If you consider that the final product is a sterilized instrument, then you recognize that there are both centralized and decentralized production schemes at work in that process.

Another example of a hybrid system in orthopedics would be the production of anatomically fitting plates and screws for fracture fixation. An implant company typically produces a range of plate and screw sizes for any particular procedure. These are produced centrally in a factory and then brought to the hospital by a sales representative. Often the surgeon makes modifications to the implant prior to final implantation in order to

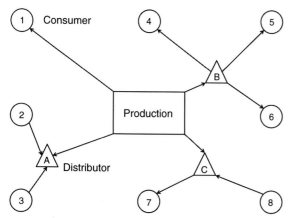

FIG. 4.3 Hybrid Production Scheme with centralized production, regional distribution and decentralized consumption

create a better anatomic fit. The surgeon modification would count as the decentralized portion of the production. Imagine that the surgeon creates a completely customized implant using a 3D printer at the hospital. This would be an example of a completely decentralized or "point-of-care" system of production.

The notion of fabricating parts to fit individual patients is not new. Prescription eyeglasses have been around a long time. The current system of measuring the patient locally, transmitting the prescription to a central optical laboratory or factory, distributing the eyeglasses from the central production facility back to the local retail outlet, and the customer buying the eyeglasses from the local retail outlet seems to work well.

Under current economic conditions it makes economic sense for such things as eyeglasses to be manufactured centrally. The process of shaping and polishing the material for the lenses requires sophisticated equipment, which is very expensive. The cost of this equipment must be distributed among many lenses. It would be impractical to make the lenses locally with a much smaller number of lenses to share the equipment costs. A toaster works in each household because the cost of the toaster is trivial. Thus we would be overreaching if we were to suggest that just because 3D printing *can* decentralize aspects of production that it automatically *will* decentralize most modes of production.

The degree to which 3D printing brings about a movement in manufacturing toward the point of the consumer will depend on many factors, not least of which will be the cost and convenience of the alternatives. And because value is subjective, that can be difficult to assess. For instance, it may be materially less

costly for a surgeon to produce a 3D printed surgical guide through a third-party company, but there may be value for the surgeon and the patient in creating and tailoring the guide locally that is not captured by comparison of costs alone.

Free market or Austrian economics is indifferent as to whether production is centralized or decentralized. It is concerned only that the choice of centralized production versus decentralized production is made by entrepreneurs risking their own capital, rather than dictated by government regulation. Mises, one of the founders of the Austrian economic school, discusses in *Human Action* the question of centralization (concentration) of production versus the decentralization of production as an entrepreneurial problem that must take into account many factors. The optimal degree of concentration of production "is not merely a mathematical problem which can be solved satisfactorily by all those familiar with the elementary rules of arithmetic. The main question is the determination of the money equivalents of the items which are to enter into the calculation. It is a mistake to assume, as many economists do, that these equivalents are given magnitudes, uniquely determined by the state of economic conditions. They are speculative anticipations of uncertain future conditions and as such depend on the entrepreneur's understanding of the future state of the market. The term *fixed* costs is also in this regard somewhat misleading."[2]

Free market economics is indifferent as to whether 3D printers making fracture prostheses are located in a single production center with decentralized distribution (Fig. 4.3) or whether 3D printers exist in each local hospital (Fig. 4.2) much like CT scanners. Free market economics is concerned only whether the entrepreneurial decision of choosing the production model is based on free market costs.

Consider this medical example from pulmonary medicine. For many years Medicare considered nebulized albuterol to be a supply for durable medical equipment rather than a prescription drug. Patients who used a nebulizer could receive albuterol solution at a discount of 80%−100% via Medicare subsidy. Prior to Medicare prescription coverage, it should not surprise anyone that many Medicare patients preferred nebulized albuterol to the use of a meter dose inhaler (MDI), which was not subsidized. After Medicare Part D went into effect, many patients switched to the MDI as the subsidies for the MDI and nebulized forms were similar and the MDI form was more convenient. Free market economics is opposed to choosing therapy based on subsidies rather than the free market costs of each option.

INNOVATION

Innovation is the production of ideas. As is the case with the production of goods, the production of ideas has costs. These costs include the time spent by the inventors and the equipment necessary to test those ideas. Figs. 4.1–4.3 are equally applicable to innovation as they were to the production of goods and services. Examples of centralized innovation would be Bell Labs or Google X. Advantages of centralized innovation include the application of multiple disciplines and points of view to the solution of problems.

Consider the problem of developing a new surgical hip prosthesis. Rather than finding an individual who is expert in both material science and orthopedic surgery, the centralized innovation center allows an expert in materials science to collaborate with an expert in orthopedic surgery. Disadvantages include higher costs. Larger buildings are more expensive than smaller buildings. Every project may not require the expertise of every researcher, so the time for some researchers may be idle. Higher costs mean that centralized innovation centers will limit their studies to big problems that offer the potential of big profits.

Medical innovation is often decentralized. New procedures often start with a single practitioner trying a new technique to solve the problem of a single patient. Decentralized innovation requires low cost fabrication for prototypes. 3D printing has the potential to decentralize innovation in medicine including orthopedic surgery. 3D printing makes it possible for individual practitioners to fabricate custom tools necessary for novel surgical techniques. The low cost of a 3D printer favors the decentralization of experimentation and innovation away from large research facilities. Pure free market economics is opposed to centralization made necessary by government regulation, patent monopoly, or expensive barriers to entry required by licensing agencies such as the Food and Drug Administration (FDA). As long as the entrepreneurial decision to try new innovative techniques is based on free market costs, pure free market principles are indifferent to the concentration of research and innovation.

Nevertheless, full realization of the innovation potential of 3D printing in orthopedic surgery will more likely depend on the nature of government regulation of medical 3D printing rather than the free market economic costs. There are many ways that regulation can hinder the decentralization of production or innovation in orthopedic surgery applications of 3D printing. Patent monopoly of 3D printers could make the costs too high for decentralized activity. Patent monopoly

of feedstock for 3D printers or copyright monopoly of blueprints could have the same effect.

Decentralization of innovation and production has important implications for charity care or indigent care as well. In economic terms, charity can be considered a market phenomenon based on voluntary contributions to solve the problems of needy customers. People make charitable contributions because they have more self-satisfaction or "happiness" by giving rather than keeping resources for their own material benefit. Low cost fabrication equipment favors decentralized charity versus centralized charity. A big issue for the viability of a charity is the tradeoff between quality and cost. All other things being equal, people prefer higher quality to lower quality. This is true even though quality is purely subjective. It is another objective truth that all other things being equal, including quality, people prefer the lower price item to the higher price item. Given a choice between a higher cost good of higher quality and a lower cost good of lower quality, however, it is entirely subjective whether an individual will choose high quality or low cost. Charities must try to maximize the good that they deliver given limited donations of time and money. Charities may very well choose low cost over high quality, especially if the alternative to low cost and low quality will be no care at all. Regulations that dictate minimal quality standards tend to centralize the production of goods as the higher quality standards require more inspection, more sophisticated equipment, and more production steps—all of which generate higher costs that need to be distributed over higher volume of sales.

3D printing, especially the lower cost 3D printing technologies, offers low cost options to the fabrication of parts and tools. An indigent patient might not be able to afford an expensive proprietary orthopedic prosthesis or implant. The local hospital might not be able or willing to donate the expensive proprietary part. A local orthopedic surgeon might be willing to donate his or her time to fabricate a lower cost and lower quality implant or prosthesis. The hospital might be willing to donate the lower cost of metal, ceramic, or plastic raw supplies. 3D printing offers the potential that the local healthcare system can deliver a low cost, low quality solution to the patient's problem which has the potential to be superior to no therapy at all. Quality regulations could preclude this decentralized, low cost option.

3D printing offers the potential to decentralize innovation and the production of goods in orthopedic surgery. Free market economic principles are indifferent to whether 3D printing is successful in decentralizing production and innovation as long as the decisions are based on free market economic costs. Free market principles are opposed to protecting centralized production and innovation by government legislation, government regulation, government licensing, patent monopoly, and copyright protection.

However, we do not live in a purely free market system. Particularly in medicine, we live in a system of tight government regulatory control in which all of the abovementioned regulatory mechanisms are at play. In our next section we will discuss what we know so far about the regulatory environment in which users of 3D printing technology will find themselves operating.

3D PRINTING: A REGULATORY PERSPECTIVE

General Principles of Regulation

In this section, we will consider general benefits and problems with regulation. Orthopedic implants will be used as an example to clarify these issues.

The stated purpose of regulation is safety and efficacy. Regulation explicitly decreases the available options for any need or problem. Ideally, regulation limits the available options to those that exceed some universally accepted minimum standard for efficacy and safety. The benefit for consumers is that they need not waste time evaluating options that they would automatically reject. In practice, however, the questions of how much safety and efficacy are enough to satisfy consumers are subjective in nature. This subjective nature can become problematic because compliance with regulations raises costs and limits competition. Furthermore, the environment of the regulation is important as we must always compare the safety and efficacy of a proposed solution to an alternative. The utility of regulation is much different for a new device that has no alternative versus a competing device that has a well-established alternative.

Consider hip prostheses as an example. The natural recovery from a hip fracture is usually poor. In the elderly, a hip fracture can significantly shorten life expectancy. The first hip prostheses had a very low bar to exceed in terms of safety and efficacy, as there were no good alternatives. 3D printed hip prostheses will have to compete against the well-established safety and efficacy record of existing implants. The long-term effects cannot be tested with short-term efficacy trials. Physicians will not adopt a new implant with unknown long-term side effects unless the new implant offers substantial improvements in efficacy, short-term safety, or both.

Modification of existing products introduces fewer uncertainties about performance than introducing totally new products. 3D printing applications that modify existing hip prostheses to better fit an individual may have fewer long-term uncertainties than the use of novel designs. Modification applications have to demonstrate less improvement in efficacy or convenience to be accepted. Scrutiny of modifications is different from the scrutiny of new products. A modification must be analyzed in terms of how the changes will alter the known properties of a device. The smaller the change introduced with the modification, the less expectation for unwanted results.

The benefits of minimum thresholds for efficacy and safety cannot be separated from the increased costs and decreased competition inherent in regulation. Regulations can be created with the intent of improving efficacy and safety, but regulations can also be created with the intent of raising barriers to competition and blessing current practices as safe or efficacious. Capture of the regulatory process by the regulated is always a concern for any regulatory process.

In the United States, options for orthopedic implants are filtered by both certification and licensure. The US FDA is the licensing agency that limits the available legal options. Licensing by the FDA does not guarantee use. Hospitals decide which implants will be available in their operating rooms. These decisions are made by orthopedic surgeons and the insurance companies who insure against liability. The health insurance companies who decide what patient benefits will be covered or paid for also play a role in the certification of options. The FDA has shown a willingness to tolerate off-label use of approved drugs for situations outside the boundary of approval when there are no good alternatives available. The off-label use of drugs model might be applied to some 3D printing modifications of already approved devices using already approved materials.

History of FDA Regulation of 3D Printing

This section outlines how the FDA is approaching questions related to 3D printing, including what types of considerations and concerns are driving the analysis. It will not—and cannot—provide comprehensive guidance for how regulators will evaluate any given 3D printed solution. This is in part because the regulatory processes are still evolving. Also, it is worth noting that nothing in this section is intended to be legal advice. If you have specific questions about specific solutions, prudence dictates seeking out a lawyer.

This is an evolving area of regulation. As discussed earlier, regulations inherently involve tradeoffs. Regulators at the FDA are tasked with protecting the public health by ensuring the effectiveness, quality, and security of drugs and medical devices. By their very nature new solutions bring both a potential for improvement and the risk of increased harm. Regulators must balance the value of moving forward with a new solution against the very real possibility that the new solution contains a hidden harm. The FDA Guidelines[3] must be considered in the light of these tradeoffs between benefits and costs.

Assumptions Underpinning Medical Regulation

Medical regulation traditionally assumes a degree of traceability and repeatability in regulated medical devices. 3D printing can challenge some of these assumptions. The FDA Guidelines[3] are an attempt to meet these challenges.

Traceability goes to the material chain, the design chain, and the manufacturing chain. It helps assure that the materials making up the object are safe and fit for purpose; the design of the object has been created by knowledgeable, responsible parties who understand the relevant factors that must be considered; and that the actual manufacturing process combines those safe materials and responsible designs into a device that will properly achieve its intended purpose. The FDA Guidelines explicitly acknowledge the abovementioned considerations with a flowchart that defines the scope of additive manufacturing (AM) or 3D printing process. This flowchart includes design, software workflow, material control, build, postprocessing, and final testing considerations as elements included within the AM or 3D printing process that will be regulated by the FDA.

Once those elements come together to create a single device, the entire process must be repeatable. The FDA Guideline states,

As with traditional manufacturing methods, design requirements drive the processes that can be used to reliably produce the device. It is therefore important to clearly identify key design parameters for your device, including, but not limited to, size range and available design or configuration options (e.g., range of angles between the trunnion and stem of the femoral component of a hip arthroplasty device).[3]

The FDA discussion of quality control uses an orthopedic implant as an example.

This repeatability serves the obvious purpose of creating devices that reliably achieve their intended purpose. It also serves the less obvious purpose of allowing for process-level and sample-based testing to verify safety. The Guidelines state,

The effects of the different steps in the AM processes can be seen in final device testing; however, determining the root cause of failures from manufacturing defects can be very difficult without a clear understanding of each step.[3]

The FDA Guideline makes it clear that all details related to the manufacturing process will be evaluated and must be properly documented. For example,

Each AM process may have different critical steps and identified risks. It is important to use all reasonably obtainable knowledge about your specific machine's capabilities to ensure the manufacturing process outputs meet defined requirements.[3] Additionally, the cumulative effects of prior processes on the final finished device or component should be incorporated into the development of each process step and documented.[3]

The detail of the Guideline includes consideration that a left-to-right print head motion may yield a significantly different result from a right-to-left print head motion.

While medical and surgical device manufacturers are accustomed to these FDA documentation requirements, 3D printing ventures may not necessarily comply with these requirements. Depending on the application, materials could come from nonverified sources, designs could be modified by nonexpert creators, and manufacturing can be done in smaller, less formal environments. Similarly, the 3D printers used to create the devices may not be optimized for the repeatability of traditional manufacturing methods. The FDA Guideline does not explicitly prohibit these possibilities, but the application for approval requires consideration how these issues would impact the overall result. Regardless of the source of 3D printing material, the documentation requires specification of minimum acceptable quality of material and consideration about how variation in quality would impact the final product.

Regulators may also find that 3D printing presents the opportunity for manufacturers that do not specialize in medical devices to meet some of the industry's needs. These general purpose manufacturers may not be interested in certifying compliance with medical-specific regulatory structures even though their existing standards would meet FDA requirements. This opportunity will require regulators to carefully evaluate which types of regulations are necessary in the context of specific solutions and when relying on existing industry practices is adequate. The FDA Guideline offers the possibility that general purpose 3D printing manufacturers could partner with medical and surgical device manufacturers where the device manufacturers could apply their expertise in process documentation to innovative ideas from smaller and more local 3D printing manufacturers. For example, a manufacturer of hip prostheses could partner with a university medical center to innovate a new interface between imaging technology and the manufacture of the individual prosthesis. The local innovator can supply the algorithm that achieves the desired result, and the device manufacturer can provide the documentation expertise to answer FDA questions about rounding errors, file conversion issues, and geometric interpolation.

Finally, medical device use relies on the nonregulatory (or quasi-regulatory) structure of insurance reimbursement codes. As solutions are created and approved, consensus will need to be reached regarding the proper codes to apply to given solutions. Resolving this challenge will require cooperation between Medicare, private insurance companies, and the device entrepreneurs.

The FDA Review Process

The FDA has been exploring regulatory questions related to 3D printing since 2014. One of the recurring challenges of the exploration has been attempting to distinguish between uses of 3D printing that focus on communicating with and educating patients (categories that would involve a lesser degree of regulatory scrutiny) and those that focus on diagnosis, measurement, and treatment (categories that would involve a higher degree of regulatory scrutiny).

For example, a 3D printing application might convert a patient's radiographic image into a model of the proposed prosthesis and patient-specific anatomy. This model could be used to illustrate to the patient the proposed individualized procedure. Such an application might aid or improve the informed consent process. Educational applications have far fewer safety issues and would have lower barriers to entry for small ventures lacking expertise in process documentation.

In October of 2014 the FDA held an initial workshop on 3D printing entitled "Additive Manufacturing of Medical Devices: An Interactive Discussion on the Technical Considerations of 3-D Printing."[4] The workshop was an initial exploration of the topic by the FDA and attempted to examine issues such as

- material chemistry
- physical properties
- recyclability
- part reproducibility
- process validation
- printing process characterization

- software used in the process
- postprocessing steps (hot isostatic pressing, curing)
- additional machining
- cleaning/excess material removal
- effect of complexity on sterilization and biocompatibility
- final device mechanics
- design envelope
- verification

These initial topics encompass many issues that would recur in discussion surrounding 3D printing regulation going forward. As one might expect, the topics focus on making sure that the physical device is safe, even if it is manufactured via a relatively novel technique. They also suggest the FDA's relative lack of foundational information about the process and its applications.

In August of 2017 the FDA presented an updated view on its role with regard to 3D printing.[5] In a presentation to the Radiological Society of North America, the FDA announced that software used to generate models for diagnostic purposes would be regulated as Class II medical devices.[6] This focus on the software would be prioritized over regulating specific printers or individual models. If the software was certified, at least in theory, it could be used on a number of specific printers.

While clear in theory, these distinctions can become muddied in practice. Although the focus is on software, in practice that software often must be validated in the context of specific 3D printing technologies and materials. As a result, software validation can often become a proxy for validation for the larger ecosystem.

There is also ambiguity regarding the distinction between models created for diagnostic purposes and those created for nondiagnostic purposes. As only the former requires regulatory compliance, there is an incentive for vendors to advertise educational software packages with at least a tacit understanding that some models created by those packages may also be used for diagnostic purposes.

FDA Guidance in December 2017

The FDA's review culminated in the publication of "Technical Considerations for Additive Manufactured Medical Devices" in December of 2017, over a year after the initial draft was circulated.[7] This guidance focuses on the same types of concerns raised during the 2014 workshop. It reiterated the importance of validation, documentation, and awareness of how various steps in the 3D printing process can introduce variation into final products.

In light of the variability in 3D printing technologies and the fact that many 3D printed objects will be customized to the patient, the document highlights the importance of identifying key design parameters that can be tested before the printed object is used. Once manufacturing has been controlled, the FDA also advises on best practices for testing and labeling the finished device.

The guidance is intended as a complement to, not a replacement for, existing regulation that might cover a specific advice. This approach is consistent with an understanding that, while 3D printing is a novel method of creating devices, it does not suspend the types of regulations or concerns that would govern other similar types of devices.

> *It is anticipated that AM devices will generally follow the same regulatory requirements and submission expectations as the classification and/or regulation to which a non-AM device of the same type is subject. In rare cases, AM may raise different questions of safety and/or effectiveness. In addition, this guidance only addresses manufacturing considerations related to the AM process.[3]*

In other words, regulation of 3D printed devices will not be less stringent than regulation of devices manufactured by traditional methods.

Conclusions

The 2017 FDA Guideline presents a number of considerations that any manufacturer or user of 3D printing must take into account when bringing a solution to market. While these considerations are familiar to those involved in the manufacture of medical and surgical devices generally, the guidance provides 3D printing–specific details that serve to highlight the way that 3D printing differs from traditional manufacturing. The FDA Guideline indicates that the scrutiny of 3D printed devices will be at least as great as traditional medical and surgical devices. It also suggests ways that the FDA may be willing to accommodate differences between 3D printing and traditional manufacturing going forward. 3D printing ventures will either have to develop the process documentation expertise necessary to meet FDA standards or they will have to partner with traditional medical device manufacturers. The FDA Guideline appears to favor partnerships between innovators with more established actors in the medical and surgical device field. The FDA Guidelines may evolve, but the existing environment favors a hybrid production scheme with centralized process documentation and 3D printing innovators solving individual patient problems with local manufacturing.

The guidance provides an important first step toward bringing 3D printing–based solutions into the medical mainstream. In the coming months and years, it is likely to be tested and revised as specific solution providers attempt to apply it to specific solutions.

It will also remain to be seen if 3D printing–based solutions emerge from nontraditional actors. It is possible that 3D printing makes it easier for players outside the traditional medical device field to develop and provide important solutions. If this pattern does begin to manifest itself, it also remains to be seen if the FDA can accommodate these new players. It is always easier for a regulatory agency to interface with producers that are accustomed to the agency's existing processes and expectations. The opportunities for new players to enter the market for 3D printing solutions to orthopedic surgery problems will be greatest where the FDA has indicated the most flexibility: patient education.

Incremental expansion of new players would most likely be in the arena of modification of existing devices. The documentation requirements in this area are less daunting as the manufacturer must only convince the FDA they have not broken something that has already passed FDA scrutiny for safety and reliability. New players are not prohibited from entering the arena of implant manufacture, but the high barrier to entry presented by the process documentation requirements will likely lead new players to partner with traditional device manufacturers who already have the process documentation expertise. Finally, the FDA has, in the past, been more flexible to accommodating innovation where no viable solution already exists. A regulatory model analogous to off-label drug use might evolve to handle situations where there are no good alternatives.

REFERENCES

1. What is Austrian Economics? [Internet]. Available from: https://mises.org/about-mises/what-austrian-economics.
2. Mises L. *Human Action. The Scholar's Ed.* Ludwig von Mises Institute; 1998.
3. https://www.fda.gov/downloads/MedicalDevices/DeviceRegulationandGuidance/GuidanceDocuments/UCM499809.pdf.
4. https://www.gpo.gov/fdsys/pkg/FR-2014-05-19/html/2014-11513.htm.
5. https://www.fda.gov/downloads/MedicalDevices/NewsEvents/WorkshopsConferences/UCM575719.pdf.
6. http://raps.org/Regulatory-Focus/News/2017/09/01/28381/3D-Printed-Anatomical-Models-FDA-Explains-Regulatory-Framework/.
7. https://www.fda.gov/ucm/groups/fdagov-public/@fdagov-meddev-gen/documents/document/ucm499809.pdf.

CHAPTER 5

Additive Manufacturing of Arthroplasty Implants

WILLIAM M. MIHALKO, MD, PHD

Additive manufacturing (AM), also commonly known as 3D printing, has been used in medical applications for over 10 years, often in surgical subspecialties such as cranio-maxillo-facial surgery, cardiothoracic surgery, and orthopedic surgery. Other technologies using 3D bioprinting techniques has been successfully used for fabrication of tissue engineering scaffolds and vascular surgery grafts, which may change the way we treat many pathological issues in the near future. Other applications for AM have included models for surgical planning for complicated procedures and patient-specific instruments and certain aspects of arthroplasty implants. AM technology has the capability to foster a more personalized approach to produce implants and may be the best method for developing prototypes and implants for complex anatomical geometries. While AM of entire components of arthroplasty implants currently has several roadblocks, it certainly may add a key component to a personalized approach to knee replacement surgery in the not so distant future. Currently, the total knee arthroplasty implant manufacturers' approach to designing implants uses average bony morphology and designs sizes to fit patients into certain categories. These techniques to design implants, along with current surgical techniques, seem to allow an 85% patient satisfaction rate. But many surgeons believe that the design limitation is a shortcoming in the functional and personal aspects of our current treatment approach and that is the main reason for lower patient satisfaction scores compared to total hip replacement.[5] Certainly AM may allow for personalized algorithms to be used to manufacture implants during surgery that will allow surgeons to use techniques and implants that make a patient feel that their knee replacement is more like their knee was

before their arthritis progressed. Although the use of AM to produce a personalized arthroplasty implant is somewhat limited by materials and in some cases by a lengthy postprocessing window, the use of AM is estimated to grow at an annual rate of nearly 16% by 2020.[1,2,10]

THE BASICS

According to the American Society for Testing Material (ASTM), AM is "*a powder bed fusion process used to produce objects from powdered materials using one or more lasers to selectively fuse or melt the particles at the surface, layer by layer, in an enclosed chamber.*"[12–20] Four techniques of powder bed fusion are commonly used: selective laser sintering (nonmetal SLS), selective laser melting (SLM), direct metal laser sintering (DMLS), and electron beam melting (EBM).[1,2]

SLM fuses metal powder with a laser, and a re-coater sweeps a fine layer onto the part for fusion or melting onto the previous 2D layer. This technique works well with composites made of one material, such as pure titanium or steel, rather than many mixed components such as most plastics. When the part is completed, it goes for the required heat treatment and postproduction processing.

With DMLS a laser is used to microweld powdered metals and alloys from computer-aided design data. Made from materials such as Inconel, aluminum, stainless steel, and titanium, DMLS parts are strong, durable, and heat-resistant. They also are typically denser than investment-casted metal parts.

The EBM technique is similar to DMLS but uses an electron beam instead of a laser beam. An advantage of this technique is the production of less thermal stress

3D Printing in Orthopaedic Surgery. https://doi.org/10.1016/B978-0-323-58118-9.00005-1

in parts and less warping of smaller geometries. Surfaces may not be as smooth as those produced with DMLS, but these can be treated during postprocessing.[1,2,10]

ADDITIVE MANUFACTURING IN MEDICAL APPLICATIONS

AM in the medical applications market is segmented into stereolithography, EBM, and droplet deposition manufacturing. Of these, EBM, which is composed of photopolymerization and laser beam melting, has dominated the market. 3D Systems Corporation, Voxeljet Technology GmbH, EnvisionTEC GMbH, EOS GmbH, Electro-Optical Systems, Stratasys Ltd., Nanoscribe GmbH, and Materialise NV are the most prominent players in the AM marketplace today.

The different types of metals currently used in AM are steel, stainless steel, pure titanium, titanium alloys, aluminum alloys, nickel-based alloys, cobalt chrome alloys, and copper-based alloys. Most AM laser-sintered metal products have a lower elastic modulus, yield strength, and tensile strength than plain casted steel, and there are a number of common issues with metal 3D printing (3DP), including warping (corners of print lift and detach from the platform), elephant foot deformity of edges (lowest layers flare out), layer misalignment, missing layers, cracks in tall objects, pillowing (top surfaces not closed properly or come out bumpy), and stringing (unwanted strands of metal span across the print) (Fig. 5.1).

Postprocessing protocols are aimed at relieving areas of stress and strengthening the metal in parts that are created using AM due to the fused and layered nature of the processing itself. Depending on the design and shape of the part, stress relief may be necessary to avoid deformation of areas during removal of supportive surrounding material. Parts are kept at high temperatures typically for over an hour and then are air-cooled to prevent stress areas from being weak points in the part. Through stress relief, the alloy or metal returns to the annealed state. Hot isostatic pressing, solution heat treatment, and precipitation hardening treatment are types of postprocessing that are used on an AM product to strengthen the metal to a near wrought property state (a state after forging to improve crystallinity and material properties of the alloy). In many cases these postprocessing protocols can increase material density from 95% to nearly 100%.[1,2,10]

Additive Manufacturing of Custom and Patient-Specific Arthroplasty Implants

Cost is still an issue when determining if AM is feasible because 3D imaging studies and preprocessing are needed to create custom arthroplasty blocks. These custom or personalized cutting jigs involve technician time to process either a magnetic resonance imaging or computed tomography (CT) scan to construct a wire mesh model that in turn must be used to create the topography to match the distal femur and proximal tibia which is then included in the cost of

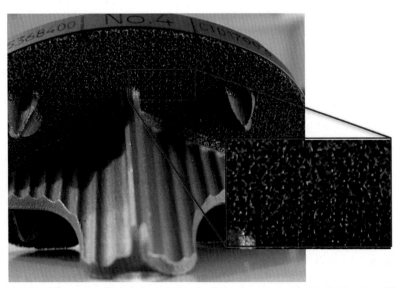

FIG. 5.1 A total knee baseplate that was created using AM processes. In the fine intricacies of the ingrowth surfaces inaccuracies are not as important as long as porosity is maintained. *AM*, additive manufacturing.

manufacturing a patient-specific block. In addition, there are very few studies reporting outcomes.[3,4,7,9,11] Studies that have shown improved alignment with a custom cutting block have not been able to show differences in functional outcomes or postoperative lower extremity alignment, while other studies have found no difference in mechanical alignment.

So why might companies choose to pursue AM for certain products? Custom, patient-specific instruments, and implants may produce better outcomes in patients with abnormal anatomy, complex fractures, or neoplasms for whom traditional manufacturing methods are unable to produce an implant.[6,8,10] Also, in the future if scaffolds with cellular products can be fashioned using bioprinting methods, then exact surface morphometry may be produced for a biologic implant and resurfacing of the joint.

In the 1990s, Techmedia used CT scans to produce custom femoral total hip arthroplasty implants, but with high costs and no improvement in outcomes. Other short-stem implants have been used in a custom manner, but costs remained an issue.[21] Currently patient-specific implants that are produced from CT scans by manufacturers are primarily used for patients with conditions that result in abnormal anatomy, such as fibrous dysplasia, acromegaly, dwarfism, posttraumatic deformity, and musculoskeletal oncologic conditions. Problems with creating these custom implants have included manufacturing issues, poor bone quality that may hamper proper sizing, imaging software accuracies and modeling variables, and the necessity for robotic techniques for implantation.

Although the ASTM International and the International Standards Organization (ISO) have established standards for 3DP systems, the Federal Drug Administration (FDA) has found its standards and guidance document creation for approval processes, as well as quality assurance measures, outpaced by the rapid development of the technology. The ASTM and ISO created an AM standards structure (Fig. 5.2) to combat overlap in committee endeavors.[12-20]

This new structure is expected to (1) help guide the work of global experts and standards development organizations involved in AM standardization,

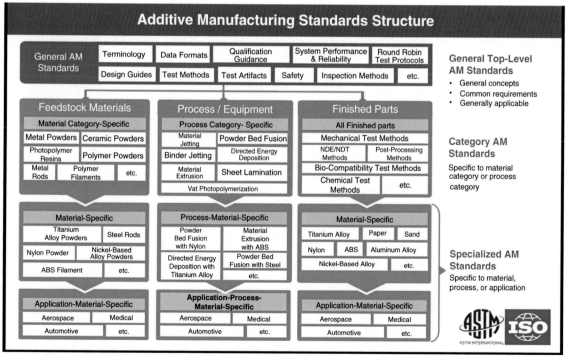

FIG. 5.2 ASTM and ISO plans for AM standards activity. These plans aim to make certain overlap does not occur across the many different committees and industrial applications. *AM,* additive manufacturing; *ASTM,* American Society for Testing Material; *ISO,* International Standards Organization.

(2) identify standards-related gaps and needs in the AM industry, (3) prevent overlap and duplicative efforts in AM standards development, (4) insure cohesion among AM standards, (5) prioritize AM standards areas, and (6) improve usability and acceptance among the AM community, including manufacturers, entrepreneurs, consumers, and others. Based on this structure, standards can be developed at three levels: general standards (e.g., concepts, common requirements, guides, and safety), standards for broad categories of materials (e.g., metal powders) or processes (e.g., powder bed fusion), and specialized standards for a specific material (e.g., aluminum alloy powders), process (e.g., material extrusion with acrylonitrile butadiene styrene [ABS]), or application (e.g., aerospace, medical, automotive).

Currently, there are dozens of ASTM/ISO standards directed at AM, most of which deal with defining terminology in the field, proper assessment/characterization of the powder forms used as the base material, and characterization of the mechanical properties of the post-processed devices. While several other fields, such as the automotive and aerospace industries, have been using AM to produce parts, the standards organizations have tried to assure that duplication of standards does not occur to provide consistency among applicable fields of manufacturing.

Currently, implants created by AM must meet the same standards/guidance measures set forth by the FDA for standard implants. The postprocessing required after AM implants are produced (e.g., bearing surfaces need significant polishing), along with quality assurance measures, may prohibit approval of on-site processing methods at a hospital or surgery center for many years. Once these techniques become standardized and material properties and implant quality have been tested and improved, manufacturers may be able to change over to a system that can produce implants on-site on a personalized basis. Because bearing surfaces from an AM technique may not be established for quite some time due to the extensive postprocessing that is needed to polish and then sterilize the implant, there are currently other aspects of arthroplasty implants such as ingrowth surfaces that make the most sense right now to be produced by AM techniques (Fig. 5.2). Most of these implants that utilize AM techniques do not involve bearing surfaces, so issues with lower strength of AM implants compared to casted or forged implants does not seem to be an issue.

In today's cost-conscious healthcare environment, it is attractive to think that 3D printing can deliver customized solutions in a time-efficient, reliable,

and cost-effective manner. In combination with other technologies in the future, such as instant anatomic registration and robotics, it may be conceivable to register total joint arthroplasty implant geometry on-site, build a 3D model and print on-site, use real-time surgical planning to insert the device, and use a full-service computer application to allow a fully personalized approach.

There are, however, considerable start-up costs for 3D printing technology, ongoing maintenance and operation issues, as well as regulatory issues, and the ultimate applications may require technology advancements that may not be realized for quite some time. We must not allow technology to outpace regulatory and standards/guidance documents and potentially compromise quality and patient safety moving forward.

In the standards organizations, there has been significant activity in the aircraft and manufacturing sectors. These endeavors are being used as a platform for the medical industry so that there is little overlap of standards and new activities are only being started where necessary.

WHERE ARE WE HEADING? THE FUTURE OF AM IN TOTAL JOINT IMPLANTS

If newer materials can be used, some of these postprocessing issues could be averted in the near future. One material that may have promise is poly ether ketone (PEEK), an organic thermoplastic polymer in the polyaryletherketone family that has been used in engineering and medical applications over the last decade. If this material can be used as a bearing surface in total knee arthroplasty, this may be processed on-site in a personalized implant design. Currently, one company is utilizing PEEK as a bearing surface, and this may show promise for use in the arthroplasty field. If on-site or corporate-based postprocessing can be used to make a bearing surface that can live up to the current implant standards set forth by ISO/ASTM and the FDA, then a leap in AM may be realized.

The next technological leap in 3D printing for arthroplasty may actually come from bioprinting. The use of collagen matrices is now possible using current bioprinting technology as well as the combination of different cell types cultured from the patient. If imaging technologies can be used to construct patient-specific articular cartilage geometry with articular cartilage cells cultured from the patient, then true biologic 3D printed resurfacing may be realized in the next few decades.

REFERENCES

1. Anderson PA, Mihalko WM, Golish SR, Jakus A, Hsu W. 3D Printing applications in orthopedic surgery. *Instr Course Lect.* 2018. In press.
2. Anderson PA, Hsu WK, Golish SR, Jakus A, Mihalko WM. 3D Printing applications in orthopaedic science and oncology. *Instr Course Lect.* 2018. In press.
3. Camarda L, D'Arienzo A, Morello S, Peri G, Valentino B, D'Arienzo M. Patient-specific instrumentation for total knee arthroplasty: a literature review. *Musculoskelet Surg.* 2015;99(1):11−18.
4. Chotanaphuti T, Wangwittayakul V, Khuangsirikul S, Foojareonyos T. The accuracy of component alignment in custom cutting blocks compared with conventional total knee arthroplasty instrumentation: prospective control trial. *Knee.* 2014;21(1):185−188.
5. Gibon E, Goodman MJ, Goodman SB. Patient satisfaction after total knee arthroplasty: a realistic or imaginary goal? *Orthop Clin N Am.* 2017;48(4):421−431.
6. Luo W, Huang L, Liu H, et al. Customized knee prosthesis in treatment of giant cell tumors of the proximal tibia: application of 3-dimensional printing technology in surgical design. *Med Sci Monit.* 2017;23:1692−1700.
7. Qui B, Liu F, Tang B, et al. Clinical study of 3D imaging and 3D printing technique for patient-specific instrumentation in total knee arthroplasty. *J Knee Surg.* 2017;30(8):822−828.
8. Smith KE, Dupont KM, Safranski DL, et al. Use of 3D printed bone plate in novel technique to surgically correct hallux valgus deformities. *Tech Orthop.* 2016;31:181−189.
9. Spencer-Gardner L, Pierrepont J, Topham M, Baré J, McMahon S, Shimmin AJ. Patient-specific instrumentation improves the accuracy of acetabular component placement in total hip arthroplasty. *Bone Joint J.* 2016;98-B(10):1342−1346.
10. Tetsworth K, Block S, Glatt V. Putting 3D modeling and 3D printing into practice: virtual surgery and preoperative planning to reconstruct complex post-traumatic skeletal deformities and defects. *SICOT J.* 2017;3:16.
11. Wong TM, Jin J, Lau TW, et al. The use of three-dimensional printing technology in orthopaedic surgery: a review. *J Orthop Surg (Hong Kong).* 2017;25(1):1−7.

Web references

12. F2924. *Standard Specification for Additive Manufacturing Titanium-6 Aluminum-4 Vanadium with Powder Bed Fusion;* 2018. https://www.astm.org/Standards/F2924.htm.
13. F2971. *Standard Practice for Reporting Data for Test Specimens Prepared by Additive Manufacturing;* 2018. https://www.astm.org/Standards/F2971.htm.
14. F3122. *Standard Guide for Evaluating Mechanical Properties of Metal Materials Made via Additive Manufacturing Processes;* 2018. https://www.astm.org/Standards/F3122.htm.
15. F3049. *Standard Guide for Characterizing Properties of Metal Powders Used for Additive Manufacturing Processes;* 2018. https://www.astm.org/Standards/F3049.htm.
16. ISO/ASTM52900-15 *Standard Terminology for Additive Manufacturing − General Principles − Terminology;* 2018. https://www.astm.org/Standards/ISOASTM52900.htm.
17. ISO/ASTM52910-17 *Standard Guidelines for Design for Additive Manufacturing;* 2018. https://www.astm.org/Standards/ISOASTM52910.htm.
18. ASTM F3055-14a *Standard Specification for Additive Manufacturing Nickel Alloy (UNS N07718) with Powder Bed Fusion;* 2018. https://www.astm.org/Standards/F3055.htm.
19. ASTM F3056-14e1 *Standard Specification for Additive Manufacturing Nickel Alloy (UNS N06625) with Powder Bed Fusion;* 2018. https://www.astm.org/Standards/F3056.htm.
20. ASTM F3049-14 *Standard Guide for Characterizing Properties of Metal Powders Used for Additive Manufacturing Processes;* 2018. https://www.astm.org/Standards/F3049.htm.
21. OrthopedicsOne. *Techmedica Custom Stem;* 2018. http://www.orthopaedicsone.com/display/ODR/Techmedica+Custom+Stem.

FURTHER READING

1. Lee SH, Song EK, Seon JK, Seol YJ, Prakash J, Lee WG. A comparative study between patient-specific instrumentation and conventional technique in TKA. *Orthopedics.* 2016;39(suppl 3):S83−S87.
2. Morrison RJ, Kashlan KN, Flanagan CL, et al. Regulatory considerations in the design and manufacturing of implantable 3D-printed medical devices. *Clin Transl Sci.* 2015;8(5):594−600.
3. Nam D, Park A, Stambough JB, Johnson SR, Nunley RM, Barrack RL. The Mark Coventry Award: Custom cutting guides do not improve total knee arthroplasty clinical outcomes at 2 years followup. *Clin Orthop Relat Res.* 2016;474(1):40−46.
4. Woolson ST, Harris AH, Wagner DW, Giori NJ. Component alignment during total knee arthroplasty with use of standard or custom instrumentation: a randomized clinical trial using computed tomography for postoperative alignment measurement. *J Bone Joint Surg Am.* 2014;96(5):366−372.

3D Printing for Education and Surgical Planning in Orthopedic Surgery

PAUL A. ANDERSON, MD

INTRODUCTION

Three-dimensional printing, also known as additive manufacturing, is a disruptive technology that has gained widespread use in orthopedic surgery. The most common applications thus far have been as an adjunct to medical education and surgical planning. The ability to rapidly progress from CT DICOM images to 3D printing using low-cost printers and materials has opened the use of 3D printing to a range of applications. The availability of a variety of materials allows optimization for mechanical properties to match specific needs.

This chapter will focus on the use of 3D printing in medical education as it applies to orthopedic surgery. 3D printed models can be used for students, residents, and even experienced surgeons. It may aid patients to gain a better understanding of their disease and planned treatment and assist them in making treatment decisions. Specific applications of 3D printing will be reviewed, including use as a substitute for cadavers in teaching anatomy, 3D models to practice surgical techniques, and the use of sterilizable guides to improve performance at the time of surgery.

Systematic Reviews

Several investigations have examined the use, identified advantages, and disadvantages of 3D printing in surgery. Martelli performed a qualitative analysis across 20 domains examining the advantages and disadvantages of 3D printing in surgery.[1] The most common types of printers were fuse deposition modeling and selective laser sintering (SLS). The reported advantages of 3D printing include preoperative planning, anticipation of anatomic variance, high degree of accuracy for guides and templates, decreased operating time, aides to intraoperative navigation, use for patient education, training of experienced medical personnel, low cost, and availability of a variety of suitable materials. The disadvantages were increased time and expense, disruption of work flow, high cost of initial equipment, in some cases poor accuracy, unproven indications, lower efficiencies than other methods (such as injection molding), and poor performance of mechanical properties.

Hoang et al. also performed a systematic review and found a significant publication increase on 3D printing starting in 2013.[2] The majority of publications was in craniofacial and cardiovascular surgery. They identified two primary purposes for 3D printing. First is for anatomic models that were useful in preoperative planning, simulation training, surgical guides, and to aid in identifying areas of resection. Second was for education based on patient-specific anatomy and as a substitute for dissection.

Tack performed a systematic review and identified 227 papers on the use of 3D printing in surgery.[3] Although all surgical specialities had utilized 3D printing, the most common was orthopedic surgery, which included 45% of the papers. In orthopedics, the knee, hip, shoulder, and hand were the most commonly utilized subspecialties. Most papers utilized 3D printing to develop surgical guides. Other indications were models for surgical planning, custom implants, models to be used for implant shaping, and teaching. One important advantage of 3D printing was reduction of surgical operating time. Tack reported that 3D printing resulted in a 45-min reduction in OR time in spine surgery, 12 min for ankle, and 6 min for knee surgery.[3] Other surgical disciplines such as maxillofacial and cranial showed even greater reductions in surgical time.

EDUCATION

Surveys of patients, medical trainees, and surgeons have shown the potential usefulness of 3D models in understanding disease processes. Jones surveyed 51

3D Printing in Orthopaedic Surgery. https://doi.org/10.1016/B978-0-323-58118-9.00006-3

medical students and surgeons finding that 96% wanted models to aid in explanation of disease to patients.[4] Although cost was a concern, 83% still found significant value in the models when priced less than $500. Naftulin surveyed patients and neurosurgeons after visualizing 19 personalized 3D printed brain and cranial specimens.[5] Among the surgeons, 64% felt the personalized brain specimens would be helpful, while 53% of patients found them to be helpful or extremely helpful. The general opinion of the authors of these investigations was that 3D printing was a disruptive technology that will be of increasing use in educating patients, in surgical planning, and in improving surgeon education.

Patient Education

There has been an increased emphasis on shared decision-making and improved informed consent. Patients have difficulty understanding verbal descriptions of their pathology or even two-dimensional images that might be displayed on a computer. The use of 3D printed models that are patient-specific has the potential to greatly improve the patients' understanding and therefore potentially their decision-making ability. Patient education models have largely been used in liver and renal disease and in craniofacial surgery. Bernhard assessed the effectiveness of 3D printed models of seven patients with renal carcinoma.[6] After exposure to the 3D models, patients demonstrated improved understanding of basic kidney pathology, anatomy, and understanding of their planned surgical resection. Silberstein 3D printed models of carcinomatous kidneys and found patients had an improved understanding of the proposed resection.[7] Yang also found patients and families (7 children and their 14 parents) gained improved understanding of hepatic tumors and planned surgical resections.[8] In contrast, Biglino examined the impact of 3D printing on 103 parents of children with congenital heart disease.[9] Although the parents and the cardiologists found models useful and helped engage the family in the discussion of their heart disease, it did not improve the understanding of the child's condition.

Madrazo reported two cases utilizing SLS 3D printing.[10] In one case, a 62-year-old male with cervical foraminal stenosis significantly improved his understanding of his disease and eventually consented to surgery only after visualizing his pathology on the 3D model. In a second case, a 3D printed model of a solid lumbar fusion resulted in the patient understanding that he had healed, which resulted in improvement of his chronic back pain.

Anatomy Education

Recently there has been a de-emphasis of cadaveric dissection in medical school education. Instead there is reliance on cross-sectional anatomy from CT and MRI. 3D printing of anatomic specimens may be a compromise as these are relatively low cost and avoid the risks of handling biologic tissues, but still provide the feel and look of a cadaveric dissection. In addition, these models could be printed with patient-specific pathology.

McMenamin determined the accuracy of 3D printed models for anatomic specimens.[11] Objects that were larger than 10 mm in size had an average of 1.5% inaccuracy. Smaller dimensional objects had greater inaccuracies of up to 15%. The technique, however, was quite reproducible when multiple specimens using the same model were printed. He also compared the cost of 3D printed models to plasterized cadaveric specimens and found them to be significantly lower in cost. AbouHashem utilized 3D surface scans from bones of the Macquarie University Skeletal Collection and then duplicated them using a 3D printer. The students felt they had excellent visual and haptic feel of real tissue and the dimensional accuracy was excellent. The authors noted that utilizing CT DICOM images would be a time-saving step, possibly increasing resolution of the printing and could also reproduce the internal architecture of the bones.[12]

Preece performed a randomized trial in third-year veterinary medical students to measure the understanding of MRI of the equine hind foot.[13] Students were randomized to physical models, textbooks, and 3D computer models. The MRI assessment scores were significantly higher in the 3D printed physical models compared with textbook and computer models. Lim performed a similar trial in medical students to learn cardiac anatomy.[14] He found that students had improved learning on the 3D printed models over cadaveric dissection and even combined cadaveric dissection and 3D models.

Teaching Pathoanatomy

In addition to using 3D printed models as a substitute for cadaveric dissection, another application has been to demonstrate pathoanatomy. Classification of severity and disease morphology is a cornerstone of treatment of most orthopedic conditions. Unfortunately, many classification systems have poor intra- and interobserver reliability and may be difficult for students to master. Acetabular fracture classifications are particularly difficult as they occur in multiple planes that are not orthogonal to the standard planes. In addition, they are 3D injuries not easily visualized by 2D imaging. Hurson used 3D printing of 20 acetabular fractures.[15] The 3D models were then compared with standard radiographs and CT by experienced traumatologists and registrars. There was moderate agreement about classification based on radiographs and CT; however, this improved to substantial agreement with the use of 3D modeling. Brouwers performed a similar study of 20 surgeons with varying levels of experience.[16] The use of 3D printed models resulted in significant improvement in fracture classification reliability for all groups except interns.

Surgical Simulation

Surgical training using simulation has been recognized as an adjunct to the more traditional "learn by repetitive practice" on live patients. Surgical simulation has a number of advantages. Training can be done repetitively under controlled circumstances. Learning and retention are significantly improved when training occurs over multiple events over a period of time rather than a short course, such as a weekend cadaveric course. Trainees during simulation can have immediate feedback by faculty. In addition, patient-specific pathology can be added to the training process using modern techniques such as 3D printing. The model should have a similar feel to bone which would include mechanical properties such as hardness, acoustic and vibrational properties during drilling, smell, visual appearance, and an overall suitability. Traditional 3D printing is excellent at printing surfaces but does not include internal structures. To overcome this, Hochman infiltrated 3D printed temporal bone with various acrylic compounds and found that these significantly improved the fidelity of the specimens as determined by otolaryngology surgeons.[17] In addition, the mechanical properties of a sheep femur were nearly identical between the 3D printed bone and the real anatomic specimens.

The University of Wisconsin's Department of Orthopedics has investigated 3D printed material for suitability in orthopedic surgery training. Twenty-eight different 3D printed materials were assessed for their suitability for various surgical applications including drill tapping, sawing, biting, and shaving with osteotomes. We found that materials required higher melting points so that drilling did not melt the material. Readily available and cheap acrylonitrile butadiene styrene (ABS) and ABS copolymers have suitable mechanical properties for most orthopedic machining operations.

One application is for spine surgery simulation. The method involves segmentation from a CT of the lumbar or cervical spine and 3D printing of the vertebrae independently (Fig. 6.1A and B). The vertebrae are then reconstructed with foam glued to simulate the intervertebral disc and the anterior longitudinal ligament simulated using duct tape (Fig. 6.1C and D). In the lumbar spine, rubber bands placed along the transverse process helped to stabilize the specimen (Fig. 6.2A, cervical spine example). A simulated dural tube of lambskin latex-free condom can be inserted. The student can then perform a cervical laminoplasty and reconstruction with laminoplasty plates (Fig. 6.2B–D). For the lumbar spine, a simple laminectomy can be practiced. In addition, a controlled dural incision is made and repair done using fine 6.0 suture. A hydraulic test can assess quality of the dural repair.

Rose evaluated multiple materials for 3D printed models for temporal bones surgical simulation using a 5-point Likert scale.[18] He found that multicolored compared with monocolored materials offered significant improvements in face validity. The simulated specimens rated 4.5 to 5 over 10 domains including bony detail, soft tissue anatomy, likeness to drilling, ease of use, safety, and overall value. O'Reilly compared 3D printed bone, vessels, and simulated muscle to older casting methods.[19] The vascular anatomy could be cannulated and fluid pumped through them and used to simulate intervascular access and endovascular surgery. Waran used a 3D printed cranial model to teach neuronavigation.[20] The models were able to be registered, validated, and navigation performed in a laboratory simulation center. All models were spatially accurate and the navigation system was unable to differentiate between the model and the corresponding patient anatomy. Da Cruz evaluated face and content validity of 3D printed temporal bone.[21] Mean rating for depth, recession, and anatomic structures was greater than 4 out of 5 on a 5-point scale. Tissue feel was 4.0, while drill tone was 3.7 and color contrast 3.2. The trainees felt that the task-based usefulness was excellent. Overall, the trainees strongly agreed that this was a useful model for teaching anatomy, planning surgical, improving hand-eye coordination, and as an overall training tool. Waran tested 3D printed cranial models for their efficacy in utilization in the entire process of surgical navigation in eight residents.[22] In this case, the models included pathoanatomic diseases of a patient. The model was useful to measure the duration required for successful registration on two different navigation platforms and the number of attempts to achieve successful biopsy of a simulated tumor. Unlike in live patient surgery, where less experienced surgeons are allowed to only do part of the procedure, the simulation model allowed trainees to perform the entire

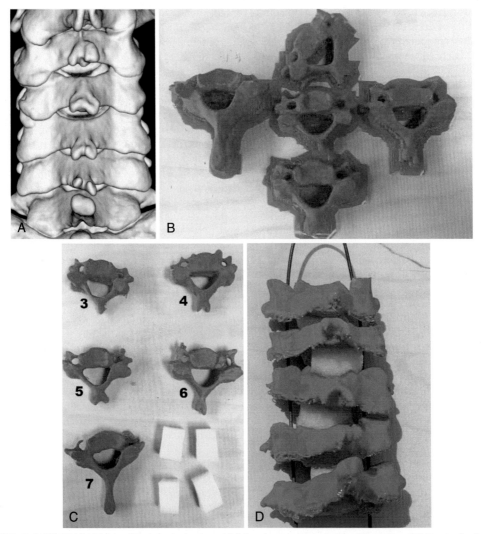

FIG. 6.1 **(A)** 3D Model from CT of cervical spine which has been segmented for 3D printing. **(B)** Cervical spine (C3–C7) 3D printed full size. The individual vertebrae are printed individually but are loosely connected and need to be separated. **(C)** C3–C7 3D printed vertebrae separated and simulated discs created from foam. **(D)** Epoxy glue is used to glue the foam as simulated disc to allow the cervical segment to be created. Further stabilized is done with a wire in the transverse neuroforamen.

procedure starting with registration and proceeding to completion of the biopsy.

The use of 3D printed models for simulation training in orthopedic surgery has been rarely reported. Based on the experience of craniofacial surgeons, these models show promise for overcoming the normal time constraints of residency and, more importantly, allow a more structured learning process that is consistent with modern theories of education; that is, proctored learning done repetitively in a controlled environment is much more conducive to skill building than the standard preceptorship-type training on patients.[23]

3D MODELS FOR SURGICAL PLANNING

A common use of 3D printing is to aid in surgical planning. In orthopedic surgery, 3D printing has been used across all subspecialties for this purpose. 3D printing of anatomic models allows the development of surgical

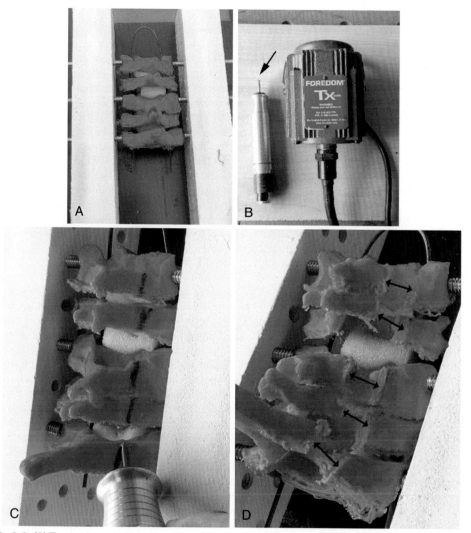

FIG. 6.2 **(A)** To simulate a laminoplasty, the 3D printed cervical spine is placed in a special holder. **(B)**. A Foredom TXH440 wood carver approximate cost $360 is used to simulate surgical burr. A 1/8 in round cutting burr is selected. **(C)**. The junction of the lateral mass and lamina is marked with lines and the burr is used to create a complete osteotomy on the right side. **(D)** An incomplete osteotomy on the opposite side (not seen) was performed and lamina is opened by spinous process rotation to the left. The *arrows* indicate opening. Laminoplasty plates can be added to complete the simulation.

approaches and testing the feasibility of procedures. 3D models can be used as templates to prebend fixation plates and theoretically allow for less invasive surgery. In more complex cases, the effect on planned surgery such as osteotomy can be assessed ex vivo. Furthermore, the 3D modeling process can be used to design customized drilling and cutting templates. Examples of the use in various subspecialties will be described in the following section.

Spine

Misplacement of pedicle screws has been reported to occur in up to 15% of cases, placing neurovascular structures at risk. Screw placement is more difficult in patients who have preexisting disease such as scoliosis or prior surgery. Several approaches using 3D printed models have been utilized to aid surgeons in screw placement. Yang used 3D printed models in 50 patients to practice screw placement before surgery and compared accuracy to a cohort using standard methods.[24] Preoperative planning with 3D models resulted in shorter operative time and less blood loss; however, there was no difference in pedicle screw accuracy or clinical outcome. However, when curves were greater than 50 degrees there was an improvement in accuracy. Wu performed rapid prototyping in 62 patients with congenital scoliosis undergoing hemivertebrae resection.[25] These models were sterilizable and were available at the time of surgery to aid pedicle screw fixation. Accuracy improved from 86% to 95% with the 3D models. In addition, there was shorter operative time and improved scoliosis correction.

Several authors have designed 3D printed drill guides to aid in the insertion of pedicle screws.[26,27] Using software such as Mimics, a 3D model is rendered from CT DICOM images and then customized drill guides for each vertebra is designed and subsequently 3D printed. This can be sterilized and available at the time of surgery. Sugawara utilized this by inserting 58 pedicle screws in thoracic spines which resulted in 100% accuracy: the actual to planned starting points all were within 0.8 mm of deviation.[27]

Trauma
Understanding the three-dimensional anatomy of complex fractures or bony defects using radiographs or even CT is challenging. At surgery, a more extensive exposure that further devitalizes bone and soft tissues is required resulting in increased complication rates and slower healing. 3D models can aid in understanding and facilitate minimally invasive surgery. Jeong (Archives of Orthopedic Trauma) created mirror images of clavicle fractures which allowed him to prebend the internal fixation. This facilitated the MIS fixation. Zeng utilized 3D models to plan fixation and prebend plates in complex acetabular pelvic ring injuries.[28,29] This aided reduction at the time of surgery and placement of the fixation. They found that 7 of the 10 reductions were within 1 mm, while 3 out of 10 were between 2 and 3 mm. 3D printed models have shown effectiveness in preoperative planning and improves doctor-patient communication in elbow, trimalleolar, and pilon fractures.[30−33]

Orthopedic Oncology
3D printing aids orthopedic oncology by allowing visual display of the tumor where bony resection margins can be identified. Further reconstruction methods can be planned and custom implants, if needed, be designed and subsequently made available for surgery. In addition, the use of spinal navigation can be

optimized. Tam reported a case of a chondrosarcoma of the scapula where unexpectedly the 3D models showed tumor involvement of the chest wall and proximal humerus.[34] The surgeons felt that "the 3D model aided their visualization of the lesion, helping plan the approach and reassure them in regard to the level of serratus anterior resection." Internal pelvectomy for management of tumors is a formidable operation and results in significant disability to the patient. Oftentimes this is not reconstructed and the limb is left flail. Liang reported on custom 3D printed prostheses in 35 patients who had partial hemipelvectomy for tumors.[35] The prostheses could include acetabular cups for reconstruction of the hip as well as fixation to allow sacral iliac and iliac fixation. Wide resection occurred in 32 patients and 35 were ambulatory after surgery.

Sports Medicine
Michalik utilized 3D printing based on CT arthrography to assess cartilage defects in the knee.[36] He found that the 3D model differed by less than 5% than when actually measured and was more accurate than MRI and CT arthrography. Arciero utilized 3D printed models of patients with Hill-Sachs lesions to create specific defects in human cadavers. These were used in biomechanical studies to determine the effects of location and the size of the defect on glenohumeral stability.[37] Sheth utilized a 3D printed model of the glenohumeral joint in a young patient with recurrent anterior shoulder instability.[38] The 3D printed model allowed the surgeon to determine the degree of abduction and external rotation in which the Hill-Sachs lesions engaged. Based on their 3D printed models, in addition to a Bankart repair, a remplissage procedure would be required and planned suture anchors placement. The procedure went uneventfully and the patient had an excellent clinical outcome.

Joint Preservation
Preservation of the hip is new technology that requires identification of dynamic pathoanatomy such as femoral acetabular impingement. 3D printed models from patients' CTs allow identification of impingement of cam lesions and allow surgeons to plan surgical resection. Periacetabular osteotomies for treatment of developmental dysplasia require careful planning and execution. Using 3D printed models, Fukushima performed the planned osteotomy.[39] When range of motion was checked, anterior impingement occurred which allowed the surgeon to change the plan prior to surgery to improve the outcome.[39]

Proximal tibial osteotomy is used for patients with medial knee joint arthritis and varus deformity. The realignment of the limb or and joint surface requires proper location and orientation of the osteotomy and correct sizing of the opening wedge. 3D printed models are ideally suited to allow testing of feasibility and assessment of the operative plan. In addition, fixation can be planned. Kwun performed high tibial osteotomy in 10 porcine knees using open source software.[40] The osteotomies were planned and the osteotomy gap opened until the desired tibial slope was reached. The planned opening wedge was 3D printed and the osteotomy performed in the porcine tibias using the wedge as a template for the insertion of a wedge and planned fixation. The results showed that the authors were able to execute their plan nearly perfectly.

Total Joint Arthroplasty

In complex cases of hip replacement, patients have a poorly formed or eroded acetabulum and will require additional iliac bony reconstruction. There are numerous surgical options available to surgeons and 3D printed models allow the surgeons to practice with the exact implants to be used during surgery to reconstruct these bony defects. Hughes used 3D printed models of acetabular bony defects following failed total hip arthroplasty to test the feasibility of various standard available reconstructive techniques as well as design of custom implants. He then practiced these in the 3D printed bones and was able to execute the plans.[41] Similarly Xu obtained CT scans in 15 patients with developmental dysplasia.[42] The surgical plan was devised using custom software, the models were 3D printed, and the surgeon practiced the planned surgery on these models identifying the location of the new acetabulum as well as the size and orientation. This was subsequently performed in the patient. Radiographically, the planned and practiced procedure had a high concordance with what actually occurred at the time of surgery.

Pediatric Orthopedic Surgery

Pediatric orthopedic surgery oftentimes requires design of patient-specific techniques to treat deformities, coalitions, and other congenital anomalies. 3D printing of these models has been shown for long bone deformities, tarsal coalitions, hip dysplasia, pelvic abnormalities, and congenital fusion and spinal abnormalities. The general approach has been to obtain a CT scan, 3D print the bones, and practice a planned surgery including the choice of implant and prebending the implants. One example was by Park who analyzed the ability of commercially available intermedullary nails to be used in a patient with extreme anterior bowing of the femur.[43] None of the nails were suitable in a

simulated fracture reduction because of their mismatch between the radius and curvature of the implant and the femur. The authors demonstrated the need for customized implants for this case.

Foot and Ankle Surgery

Tarsal coalition can be difficult to visualize and plan surgery accordingly. 3D printing of the tarsal coalition gives the surgeon the opportunity to actually see where the coalition exists and plan a less invasive surgical procedure. Similarly, forefoot osteotomies are needed and 3D printing can be useful to achieve correct alignment. Hirao designed pre-op drill guides that placed K-wires above and below the osteotomy that, when properly pronated, achieved the desired correction.[44]

CONCLUSION

3D printing is transformative technology and results in improved training of students and young surgeons, the development of new treatment methods, and the ability to test the feasibility of surgical procedures. In addition, patient-specific 3D models provide better patient understanding of disease. The low cost of 3D printers and low-cost materials make this technology available to almost every surgeon. Segmentation of bone from CT can be easily learned and is available using open source software. A variety of materials can be 3D printed, which allows the surgeon to choose the desired material properties required.

REFERENCES

1. Martelli N, Serrano C, van den Brink H, et al. Advantages and disadvantages of 3-dimensional printing in surgery: a systematic review. *Surgery*. 2016;159(6):1485−1500.
2. Hoang D, Perrault D, Stevanovic M, Ghiassi A. Surgical applications of three-dimensional printing: a review of the current literature & how to get started. *Ann Transl Med*. 2016;4(23):456.
3. Tack P, Victor J, Gemmel P, Annemans L. 3D-printing techniques in a medical setting: a systematic literature review. *Biomed Eng Online*. 2016;15(1):115.
4. Jones DB, Sung R, Weinberg C, Korelitz T, Andrews R. Three-dimensional modeling may improve surgical education and clinical practice. *Surg Innov*. 2016;23(2): 189−195.
5. Naftulin JS, Kimchi EY, Cash SS. Streamlined, inexpensive 3D printing of the brain and skull. *PLoS One*. 2015;10(8): e0136198.
6. Bernhard JC, Isotani S, Matsugasumi T, et al. Personalized 3D printed model of kidney and tumor anatomy: a useful tool for patient education. *World J Urol*. 2016;34(3): 337−345.

7. Silberstein JL, Maddox MM, Dorsey P, Feibus A, Thomas R, Lee BR. Physical models of renal malignancies using standard cross-sectional imaging and 3-dimensional printers: a pilot study. *Urology.* 2014;84(2):268–272.

8. Yang T, Tan T, Yang J, et al. The impact of using three-dimensional printed liver models for patient education. *J Int Med Res.* 2018: 300060518755267.

9. Biglino G, Capelli C, Wray J, et al. 3D-manufactured patient-specific models of congenital heart defects for communication in clinical practice: feasibility and acceptability. *BMJ Open.* 2015;5(4):e007165.

10. Madrazo I, Zamorano C, Magallon E, et al. Stereolithography in spine pathology: a 2-case report. *Surg Neurol.* 2009; 72(3):272–275; discussion 275.

11. McMenamin PG, Quayle MR, McHenry CR, Adams JW. The production of anatomical teaching resources using three-dimensional (3D) printing technology. *Anat Sci Educ.* 2014;7(6):479–486.

12. AbouHashem Y, Dayal M, Savanah S, Strkalj G. The application of 3D printing in anatomy education. *Med Educ Online.* 2015;20:29847.

13. Preece D, Williams SB, Lam R, Weller R. "Let's get physical": advantages of a physical model over 3D computer models and textbooks in learning imaging anatomy. *Anat Sci Educ.* 2013;6(4):216–224.

14. Lim KH, Loo ZY, Goldie SJ, Adams JW, McMenamin PG. Use of 3D printed models in medical education: a randomized control trial comparing 3D prints versus cadaveric materials for learning external cardiac anatomy. *Anat Sci Educ.* 2016;9(3):213–221.

15. Hurson C, Tansey A, O'Donnchadha B, Nicholson P, Rice J, McElwain J. Rapid prototyping in the assessment, classification and preoperative planning of acetabular fractures. *Injury.* 2007;38(10):1158–1162.

16. Brouwers I, Pull ter Gunne AF, de Joung MAC, et al. The value of 3D printed models in understanding acetabular fractures. *3D Print Addit Manuf.* 2018;5(1).

17. Hochman JB, Rhodes C, Wong D, Kraut J, Pisa J, Unger B. Comparison of cadaveric and isomorphic three-dimensional printed models in temporal bone education. *Laryngoscope.* 2015;125(10):2353–2357.

18. Rose AS, Webster CE, Harrysson OL, Formeister EJ, Rawal RB, Iseli CE. Pre-operative simulation of pediatric mastoid surgery with 3D-printed temporal bone models. *Int J Pediatr Otorhinolaryngol.* 2015;79(5):740–744.

19. O'Reilly MK, Reese S, Herlihy T, et al. Fabrication and assessment of 3D printed anatomical models of the lower limb for anatomical teaching and femoral vessel access training in medicine. *Anat Sci Educ.* 2016;9(1):71–79.

20. Waran V, Pancharatnam D, Thambinayagam HC, et al. The utilization of cranial models created using rapid prototyping techniques in the development of models for navigation training. *J Neurol Surg A Cent Eur Neurosurg.* 2014; 75(1):12–15.

21. Da Cruz MJ, Francis HW. Face and content validation of a novel three-dimensional printed temporal bone for surgical skills development. *J Laryngol Otol.* 2015;129(suppl 3): S23–S29.

22. Waran V, Narayanan V, Karuppiah R, et al. Injecting realism in surgical training-initial simulation experience with custom 3D models. *J Surg Educ.* 2014;71(2): 193–197.

23. Palter VN, Orzech N, Reznick RK, Grantcharov TP. Validation of a structured training and assessment curriculum for technical skill acquisition in minimally invasive surgery: a randomized controlled trial. *Ann Surg.* 2013;257(2): 224–230.

24. Yang M, Li C, Li Y, et al. Application of 3D rapid prototyping technology in posterior corrective surgery for Lenke 1 adolescent idiopathic scoliosis patients. *Med Baltim.* 2015;94(8):e582.

25. Chana-Rodriguez F, Mananes RP, Rojo-Manaute J, Gil P, Martinez-Gomiz JM, Vaquero-Martin J. 3D surgical printing and pre contoured plates for acetabular fractures. *Injury.* 2016;47(11):2507–2511.

26. Kaneyama S, Sugawara T, Sumi M. Safe and accurate mid-cervical pedicle screw insertion procedure with the patient-specific screw guide template system. *Spine (Phila Pa 1976).* 2015;40(6):E341–E348.

27. Sugawara T, Higashiyama N, Kaneyama S, Sumi M. Accurate and simple screw insertion procedure with patient-specific screw guide templates for posterior C1-C2 fixation. *Spine (Phila Pa 1976).* 2017;42(6): E340–e346.

28. Zeng C, Xiao J, Wu Z, Huang W. Evaluation of three-dimensional printing for internal fixation of unstable pelvic fracture from minimal invasive para-rectus abdominis approach: a preliminary report. *Int J Clin Exp Med.* 2015; 8(8):13039–13044.

29. Zeng C, Xing W, Wu Z, Huang H, Huang W. A combination of three-dimensional printing and computer-assisted virtual surgical procedure for preoperative planning of acetabular fracture reduction. *Injury.* 2016; 47(10):2223–2227.

30. Shuang F, Hu W, Shao Y, Li H, Zou H. Treatment of intercondylar humeral fractures with 3d-printed osteosynthesis plates. *Med Baltim.* 2016;95(3):e2461.

31. Yang L, Grottkau B, He Z, Ye C. Three dimensional printing technology and materials for treatment of elbow fractures. *Int Orthop.* 2017;41(11):2381–2387.

32. Zheng W, Chen C, Zhang C, Tao Z, Cai L. The feasibility of 3D printing technology on the treatment of pilon fracture and its effect on doctor-patient communication. *Biomed Res Int.* 2018;2018:8054698.

33. Yang L, Shang XW, Fan JN, et al. Application of 3D printing in the surgical planning of trimalleolar fracture and doctor-patient communication. *Biomed Res Int.* 2016; 2016:2482086.

34. Tam MD, Laycock SD, Bell D, Chojnowski A. 3-D printout of a DICOM file to aid surgical planning in a 6 year old patient with a large scapular osteochondroma complicating congenital diaphyseal aclasia. *J Radiol Case Rep.* 2012; 6(1):31–37.

35. Liang H, Ji T, Zhang Y, Wang Y, Guo W. Reconstruction with 3D-printed pelvic endoprostheses after resection of a pelvic tumour. *Bone Joint J.* 2017;99-b(2):267–275.

36. Michalik R, Schrading S, Dirrichs T, et al. New approach for predictive measurement of knee cartilage defects with three-dimensional printing based on CT-arthrography: a feasibility study. *J Orthop.* 2017;14(1):95—103.
37. Arciero RA, Parrino A, Bernhardson AS, et al. The effect of a combined glenoid and Hill-Sachs defect on glenohumeral stability: a biomechanical cadaveric study using 3Dimensional modeling of 142 patients. *Am J Sports Med.* 2015; 43(6):1422—1429.
38. Sheth U, Theodoropoulos J, Abouali J. Use of 3-dimensional printing for preoperative planning in the treatment of recurrent anterior shoulder instability. *Arthrosc Tech.* 2015;4(4):e311—e316.
39. Fukushima K, Takahira N, Uchiyama K, Moriya M, Takaso M. Pre-operative simulation of periacetabular osteotomy via a three-dimensional model constructed from salt. *Sicot J.* 2017;3:14.
40. Kwun JD, Kim HJ, Park J, Park IH, Kyung HS. Open wedge high tibial osteotomy using three-dimensional printed models: experimental analysis using porcine bone. *Knee.* 2017;24(1):16—22.
41. Hughes AJ, DeBuitleir C, Soden P, et al. 3D printing aids acetabular reconstruction in complex revision hip arthroplasty. *Adv Orthop.* 2017;2017:8925050.
42. Xu J, Li D, Ma RF, Barden B, Ding Y. Application of rapid prototyping pelvic model for patients with DDH to facilitate arthroplasty planning: a pilot study. *J Arthroplasty.* 2015;30(11):1963—1970.
43. Park JH, Lee Y, Shon OJ, Shon HC, Kim JW. Surgical tips of intramedullary nailing in severely bowed femurs in atypical femur fractures: simulation with 3D printed model. *Injury.* 2016;47(6):1318—1324.
44. Hirao M, Ikemoto S, Tsuboi H, et al. Computer assisted planning and custom-made surgical guide for malunited pronation deformity after first metatarsophalangeal joint arthrodesis in rheumatoid arthritis: a case report. *Comput Aided Surg.* 2014;19(1—3):13—19.

CHAPTER 7

3D Printing for Commercial Orthopedic Applications: Advances and Challenges

JERRY D'ALESSIO, PHD • ANDY CHRISTENSEN, BS

HISTORY OF 3D PRINTING IN MEDICINE AND ORTHOPEDIC APPLICATIONS

3D printing has been known by many different terms since it first arose in the 1980s. The very beginning of this field involved Chuck Hull inventing the first 3D printing process in 1983 which he coined "stereolithography." (SLA)[1] The technique utilized photocuring a liquid resin in a layered fashion with a platform that moved in the up and down (z) direction and a laser which cured the resin in sequential layers (x and y), stacking layers on top of layers.[2] The standard file format still used today for 3D printing is called STL and this was also developed by Hull's group in the 1980s. The SLA technique was commercialized in 1986 by 3D Systems in Valencia, California. Interestingly, in the first shipment of beta SLA machines was a unit delivered to Baxter Healthcare (Round Lake, IL), making clear that the broader healthcare market saw the possible impact of these technologies very early on.

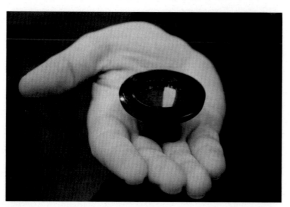

FIG. 7.1. Chuck Hull invented the stereolithography process in 1983. This was the first stereolithography part ever produced, he called it an "eye cup". (3D Systems, Rock Hill, South Carolina, USA.)

The larger field was originally coined rapid prototyping, which stuck as the most used term from the 1980s through the 1990s with Advanced Digital Manufacturing and Additive Manufacturing also being used. The consensus term today for the group of manufacturing processes which produce three-dimensional parts by means of laying down layers of material is Additive Manufacturing.[3] The term 3D printing is also used extensively today and is a synonym for Additive Manufacturing for most applications. Applications for heavy manufacturing in aerospace and for implants still typically use the term Additive Manufacturing but for the purposes of this text the term 3D printing or 3DP will be used.

Automotive, aerospace, and consumer products were the industries which fueled early development of 3D printing. To understand why these industries were drawn to the possibilities that 3DP promised, you have to understand the way that products are developed in mostly large companies such as Ford, Boeing, and General Motors.

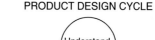

PRODUCT DESIGN CYCLE

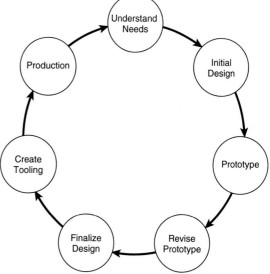

Understand Needs → Initial Design → Prototype → Revise Prototype → Finalize Design → Create Tooling → Production → Understand Needs

3D Printing in Orthopaedic Surgery. https://doi.org/10.1016/B978-0-323-58118-9.00007-5

This will be familiar to most, but the area to focus on here would be in the prototype phase. With tight timelines looming, there is always a crunch to move through the prototype phase to ensure that production can begin on time. That means there is a squeeze for design to be completed fully, but often ahead of being the best possible solution because of the timing. If designs can be iterated over and over again with reduced cost and with little time, the designs will benefit. This is exactly where 3D printing fits, it allows for many more iterations of designs to be performed before finalization and heading to production. That is the reason the processes were originally called rapid prototyping and still today one of the largest uses of the technology. The original focus was not using these techniques for manufacturing, whereas today this is much more of the pie chart and where a lot of the future potential of these techniques lies.

Industrial applications versus medical applications of 3D printing are still somewhat different today. While industrial applications benefitted from iterative prototyping in a new, responsive way to fuel shorter product design cycles, medical applications benefitted from the ability of these technologies to make a "lot size" of one, or in other words "personalized." By allowing personalized designs for individual patients, the ability to make one-off designs was the initial driving force for the clinical and surgical applications of 3D printing. As the adoption of 3D printing has increased, designs not otherwise manufacturable have been produced in larger batches.

The most commonly used techniques in use today include SLA (3D Systems, Valencia, CA, USA, 1987), Fused Deposition Modeling (Stratasys, Eden Prairie, MN, USA, 1989), Selective Laser Sintering (DTM Corporation, Austin, TX, USA, 1989, now part of 3D Systems), 3D printing (Z Corporation, Woburn, MA, USA, 1995, now part of 3D Systems), Multi-Jet Modeling (Objet Technologies, Rehovot, Israel, 2000, now part of Stratasys), Digital Light Synthesis (Carbon, Redwood City, CA, USA, 2015), and Multi-Jet Fusion (Hewlett Packard, 2016). Several additive metal processes capable of producing biocompatible metallic components were developed and commercialized, namely Electron Beam Melting (EBM) (Arcam, Mölndal, Sweden, 2003, now part of GE Additive) and Direct Metal Laser Sintering (DMLS), produced by several companies including EOS (Krailling, Germany 1989) and Concept Laser (Frankfurt, Germany 2000, now part of GE Additive).[4]

Today the ISO/ASTM standard for Additive Manufacturing[3] calls out seven different, high-level processes as follows:
1. Vat Photopolymerization (SLA, DLP, CDLP)
2. Powder Bed Fusion (SLS, SLM/DMLS, EBM, MJF)
3. Material Extrusion (FDM, FFF)
4. Material Jetting
5. Binder Jetting
6. Direct Energy Deposition
7. Sheet Lamination

Several of these types of processes have very few commercialized options, and most of this chapter will focus on Vat Photopolymerization, Powder Bed Fusion, Material Extrusion, and Material Jetting.

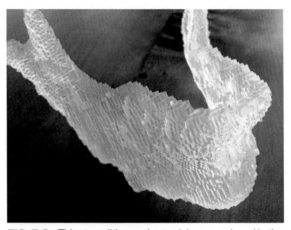

FIG. 7.2. This stereolithography model was produced in the early 1990's of a mandible and shows what look to be "cubic" elements which represent the high intensity voxels of the CT scan without interpolation (averaging, smoothing). (Andy Christensen, Littleton, Colorado, USA.)

Surgical applications were an immediate fit for 3D printing. Even before its advent, researchers in Europe and the United States were forming 3D objects for surgical planning by subtractively milling shapes from foam, plastic, and other materials.[5,6] In 1988 researchers, led by Dr. Nicholas Mankovich at UCLA Medical Center, produced the world's first 3D printed structure of human anatomy.[7] In this case, they modeled bone structure of the cranium imaged from a computed tomography (CT) scan, producing the model with the newly commercialized SLA process. The collaboration between Dr. Mankovich at UCLA and 3D Systems for producing these early SLA models involved direct work with Chuck Hull and one of his senior engineers, Scott Turner. CT scans are inherently two and a half dimensional, namely that the slices of the CT themselves are 2D representations taken at known cross sections with a known distance between each cross section. Thus they are 2D slices that can be oriented in space, thus the extra half D. The process of taking the two and a half dimensional CT scan slices and creating a file that would be possible to build using the SLA process proved difficult, but this small team figured it out, creating individual STL files for each slice of the CT scan produced. The purpose of this first model was to enable patient-matched cranial implant creation for a patient with a large cranial defect.[8] This application has stood the test of time and today most of the large (>6 cm diameter) cranial defects which are treated around the world by neurosurgeons are reconstructed with patient-specific cranial implants.[9] Some of these implants are directly 3D printed[10] but most are digitally designed and created using other manufacturing technologies enabled by 3D printed templates, molds, or models.

Over the course of the last 30 years, the orthopedic surgical uses for 3D printing have fallen into five main categories as follows:

1. Presurgical Anatomic Modeling (late 1980s to now)
2. Patient-Matched Implants (early 1990s to now)
3. Total Joint Arthroplasty Templating (mid-2000s to now)
4. Corrective Osteotomy and Fixation Templating (late 2000s to now)
5. 3D printing for Off-the-Shelf Implants—Metal or Polymeric (late 2000s to now)

Presurgical Anatomic Modeling

Medical-image-based anatomic modeling was an early use case for harnessing the power of 3D printing in the surgical space.[7,11] Typically made of hard tissue anatomy (i.e., bones) from CT scans, these models are usually produced in rigid plastic materials. In the orthopedic surgery space, the typical anatomic modeling case might involve visualization of a difficult fracture/subsequent deformity, a large bone-invading lesion and surrounding vital structures, or congenital defect requiring reconstructive surgery.[12–15] The data from a standard CT should be sufficient to model the bony anatomy but other times contrast agents will be used to highlight vasculature. The combination of a magnetic resonance imaging (MRI) study with a CT image data set can be used to better visualize soft tissue structures such as a tumor or articular cartilage. The models have reportedly provided benefits to

surgeons including (1) reduced surgical time, (2) increased surgeon confidence, (3) better operative results.[7,12] Typical uses for anatomic models include (1) presurgical visualization, (2) hands-on simulation of surgery/osteotomies, (3) plate bending, (4) device choice before surgery, and (5) intraoperative reference.

1. Presurgical Visualization

   The most prevalent use of anatomic models by themselves to date has been for presurgical visualization of an individual patient's anatomy. Typically, these are for complex reconstructive surgery cases where more spatial awareness will benefit the surgeon in preparing for the surgery. When a model is held in the hand, the scale of the structures becomes immediately apparent, something that is not possible with other 3D imaging technologies such as static 3D reconstructions common from CT scans. This better understanding of the relationships of the bony anatomy and surrounding vital structures along with a better sense of scale help to provide more assurance to the surgeon before the surgery. Many times the model will be used to explain the procedure to the patient and the surrounding medical staff, a bonus benefit to using a life-sized model of the individual patient for planning and teaching.

2. Hands-On Simulation of Surgery/Osteotomies

   With a 1:1 model in hand the surgeons can now simulate in a tactile way some of the major aspects of the bony portions of the surgery. This could be for excision of a tumor or realignment of fractured segments or correction of a congenital deformity.

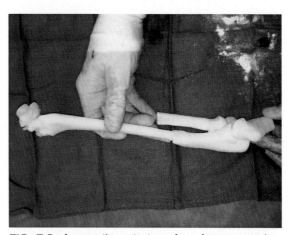

FIG. 7.3. A corrective osteotomy for a forearm case has been planned physically using a 3D printed stereolithography model. (James P Higgins, MD, Curtis National Hand Center, Baltimore, Maryland, USA.)

Sometimes mirror-imaged models will be produced alongside of the as-scanned anatomy to allow for comparison to the patient's contralateral anatomy. This additional rehearsal for surgery is reported to provide greater three-dimensional understanding of the patient's case, which should lead to a more efficient surgery.

3. Fixation Plate Choice and Prebending

   If the osteotomies are simulated in a physical way and the different segments of the model can be realigned to their desired positions, it makes sense that fixation devices can be predetermined. Choosing the right plate for the case is the first step, but the more helpful step is to actually prebend the plate to the patient's anatomy. This can save precious time in surgery, which benefits the patient. Prebending fixation plating can also provide for a more predictable shape of the plate to passively rest against the patient's anatomy, again providing for a more streamlined surgery and increased surgeon confidence.

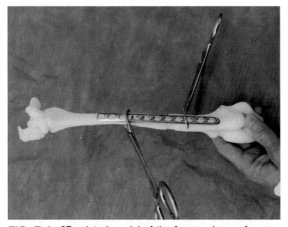

FIG. 7.4. 3D printed model of the forearm in use for pre-bending a reconstruction plate. The osteotomies were physically simulated and the plate bent by hand to the resultant anatomy. (James P Higgins, MD, Curtis National Hand Center, Baltimore, Maryland, USA.)

4. Total Joint/Distraction Device Choice Before Surgery

   For total joint arthroplasty applications where the surgeon has a 1:1 physical model of the anatomy in hand, it becomes possible to choose the device or size before surgery. In distraction osteogenesis within orthopedics and the craniomaxillofacial arenas, the use of models to preplan vectors, positioning and fixation has been critical to attaining an optimized outcome.

5. Intraoperative Reference

   If the model is produced in a material which is biocompatible and able to be sterilized, it can be used within the operating room for reference. In surgery there are other factors such as the soft tissue and surgical exposure which complicate the visualization of the bony anatomy. If the model can sit on the table during surgery and be used as reference, there are likely benefits for reference to exact locations of different parts of the anatomy. For cases involving graft material, the surgeon may also choose to fit autogenous or alloplastic grafts to the anatomic model on the back table before inserting into the final position, reducing back and forth "fitting" sessions for graft shape/size.

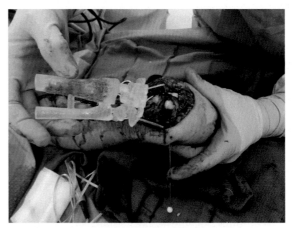

FIG. 7.5. Wrist model in use for reference during surgery produced using a biocompatible and sterilizable stereolithography model. (James P Higgins, MD, Curtis National Hand Center, Baltimore, Maryland, USA.)

Patient-Matched Implants

Patients with needs falling outside of the bell curve for traditional sizes of implants are oftentimes left with few options. Patient-matched implants help provide the optimal size and shape best suited to the individual patient's reconstruction.[16–19] For many of these applications, surgery time is shortened dramatically with the benefit of the optimal reconstruction with fewer components (think revision total joint components and reducing numbers of augments). Direct production of implants with 3D printing in biocompatible materials has only progressed in the last 5 years. Previously the 3D printed model of the anatomy was the key to designing the implant which would be created using more typical techniques of investment casting, machining, or milling. Application areas abound for patient-matched implants today and the future is bright as 3D printing technologies become easier to use, cheaper, and with a wider choice of materials.

Patient-Matched Primary Total Joint Components

By volume this is likely the largest application for patient-matched implants happening in orthopedics today.[20] 3D printing, to the authors' knowledge, is still not used for production of the implant component itself but is used for the patient-specific instrumentation and the sacrificial pattern for the femoral component which is investment cast cobalt-chrome alloy. Investment casting starts with a wax pattern of the component which is invested in plaster and subsequently burned out, leaving a shell with the pattern inside. Molten metal is "cast" into the pattern and then the plaster is broken away revealing the metal component. It is possible that the femoral component could be directly 3D printed in the future. The tibial components in titanium alloy and UHMWPE (ultra-high molecular weight polyethylene) are machined from the digitally designed files to perfectly fit the patient and align with the patient-specific instrumentation used for bony preparation. This is a common commercial use today and utilized by companies such as Conformis (Billerica, MA) in patient-matched implant systems for knee and hip.

Patient-Matched Revision Total Joint Components

Each revision surgery of a total joint leaves less and less bone stock to work with. 3D printed patient-matched revision components are a very nice fit for the technology. For revision acetabular cases, the expanding circumference of the bony cavity poses a challenge for maintaining stability of the entire construct along with optimal orientation of the cup.[21] When designing a patient-matched component for this application, the priority can be placed where it should be—on the proper, ideal position of the cup. Once the cup is in its proper position, the fixation of the cup to the surrounding bone can be carried out as it needs to for the specific patient's condition. A single, patient-matched augment can be designed to fill this space and allow for ideal location of screw fixation to the surrounding bone where it is best suited. A large benefit is that the augment can then be attached to the cup and produced with 3D printing as a singular component, reducing the number of different components needed. Instead of being a puzzle with an unknown solution, the surgeon has a precisely fitting implant which will guide positioning of the structure against the patient's anatomy. Reducing the part count of components for revision cases should have an impact on simplifying surgery but also, more importantly, on removing another place where failure or wear could happen at interfaces between components.

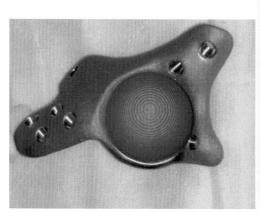
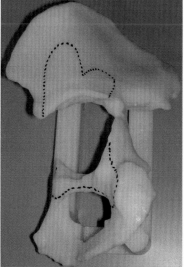

FIG 7.6. The anatomical model shows a patient with severe bone loss following revision total hip replacement. A patient-matched acetabular cup will allow spanning gaps and providing the optimal position for the cup. (P. James Burn, MD and Paul Morrison, Ossis Ltd, Christchurch, New Zealand.)

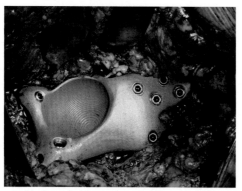

FIG. 7.7. One benefit of patient-matched implants is in the reduction of surgical time for what are typically very complex reconstruction cases. Here a personalized revision acetabular cup is placed during surgery using screws, depths and trajectories pre-established in the surgical planning phase. (P. James Burn, MD and Paul Morrison, Ossis Ltd, Christchurch, New Zealand.)

Patient-Matched Oncologic Reconstruction Components

Perhaps the best example of the benefits that patient-matched implants can have is in oncologic reconstruction cases.[22-24] These cases can involve abnormal anatomy and typically large defects created after removal of malignant tissue. In addition, stability of surrounding structures, including joints, becomes extremely challenging. Owing to the fact that imaging is a requirement to adequately identify the tumor and that reconstruction is dependent on identifying the appropriate margins, the 3D model is nearly always possible from an imaging standpoint. This allows for more personalized planning. Much like the application for combination of joint components and augments mentioned previously, oncologic cases can benefit from dramatically reducing part count and increasing stability for large segmental defects, a critical factor for future success. Many times these cases involve defects which otherwise have no other ideal reconstruction, and thus have immense patient benefit potential.

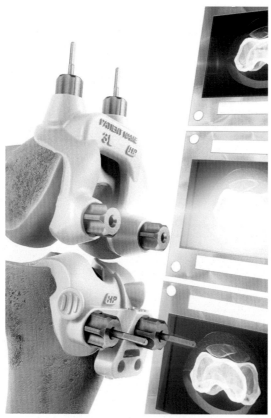

FIG. 7.8. Preoperative planning combined with patient-specific surgical guides for total knee arthroplasty allow for clinical transfer of the digital plan to the patient during surgery. (DePuy Synthes, a Johnson & Johnson Company, Warsaw, Indiana, USA.)

Patient-Matched Fixation Plates

Once surgical planning is predicted in a computer simulation, it is possible to also predict the placement and indeed the shape of the fixation plate for corrective osteotomies.[25,26] Powerful tools exist to allow transfer of the plan to the patient, a technique some call "Clinical Transfer." If the position of the plate and screws is known to a high degree of accuracy, the surgeon can use a template to predrill the screw holes and then use a patient-matched plate to align the screw holes, basically aligning the digital placement of the segments with the physical world.

Total Joint Arthroplasty Planning and Templating

Starting back in the early 2000s Dr. Steve Howell was trying to attain anatomic alignment of the knee using milled cutting guides, forming the company OtisMed (later sold to Stryker in 2009). The concept was to place off-the-shelf total knee components in a patient-specific manner using two enabling technologies: (1) digital presurgical planning and (2) patient-matched, physical template for use during surgery.[27] The patient-specific templating approach for total knee alignment did not really take off until the technique was more broadly applied for mechanical alignment of the knee using 3D printing, a more flexible manufacturing technique. Many device manufacturers offer these solutions today for total joint reconstruction of the knee,[5,28,29] shoulder,[30] and hip.[31] A rough overview of the workflow is as follows.

PRODUCT DESIGN CYCLE

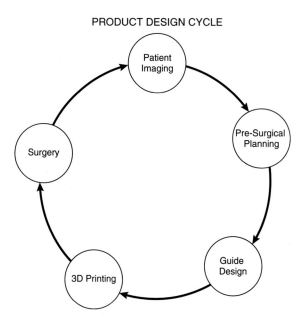

Step 1: Patient Imaging

The presurgical planning is done digitally using either the patient's CT or an MRI. Because the guide will sit on both bone and cartilage for positioning and registration, the complete anatomic picture is needed. CT scans do great at imaging bone but do not image cartilage structures well. In contrast, MRI scans do very well at soft tissue and cartilage delineation but are typically poor at imaging bone. Different manufacturers take different approaches, some use CT scans and estimate cartilage and some use MRI scans and estimate the bony structure. The word "estimate" is not exactly what happens, but through sophisticated algorithms looking at the patient anatomy and other databases of anatomy, these scans become more complete.

Step 2: Computer-Based Presurgical Planning

Once the medical imaging is done, typically a service provider or the orthopedic device company will segment the anatomy and prepare for surgical planning in a digital fashion. For the knee, the largest application area in orthopedic surgery today, the beginning of the planning starts with isolating the structures and then determining anatomic landmarks that will be used for mechanical alignment. The target knee alignment is determined by the surgeon and the total joint components are sized for the patient. The implants are placed into the three-dimensional space in optimal position and then compared to the underlying bone structures. Once final alignment has been achieved, the digital representations of the implants are used to create the underlying bony osteotomies on the femur and tibia. These osteotomy planes will then guide the design of the patient-matched cutting guides used to translate these osteotomies from the computer to the patient in surgery.

Step 3: Template/Guide Design

Once the total joint planning has been accomplished, the guide design work can begin. The goal for the guide is to help the surgeon position the off-the-shelf implant devices in a way that has been predetermined for the specific patient. Because the guides will be produced using 3D printing, the typical constraints for design are reduced and there is more design freedom. The guides will either orient the osteotomies, the positioning pins, or both. For many of these guides, they will incorporate metal sleeves for drilling through the 3D printed plastic components. Metal sleeves are used to limit plastic debris and guide the osteotomy more accurately.

The guide can be designed within a number of hours, and the surgeon can be involved in both the design and/or the approval of the design prior to production.

Step 4: 3D Printing of Template/Guide

Most guides for total knee arthroplasty (TKA) are produced using the laser sintering 3D printing technique in a nylon material. The reasons for this are many, but primary reasons include high strength of the final parts, biocompatibility of the material, and ease of sterilization. A few companies use SLA as the production technique, and this also can work well given the slight drawbacks of reduced strength (as compared with laser sintering) and a more complex biocompatibility path. Advantages of SLA parts include their more substantial weight, surface smoothness, and slightly increased level of detail possible. It is expected that in the future the use of the newest 3D printing techniques, Digital Light Synthesis and Multi-Jet Fusion, will be used for applications needing biocompatible parts.

Step 5: Surgery

Guidance for TKA typically includes a surgical guide that will fit onto bone/cartilage and guide either aligning holes or osteotomies for both femur and tibia or femur alone. Typically, the guide is not meant to replace all of the cutting blocks but augment the blocks by guiding first cut(s) and/or positioning holes. Some of these guides are provided nonsterile to the hospital and require cleaning and sterilization and some are provided sterile.

Because of the preplanning that occurs, the surgeon knows with high assurance which size implant will be needed for the case. Instead of sending in 20 sizes to the surgery, the surgeon gets a reduced kit of perhaps three, the planned size, and one size up and down. As time progressed, the orthopedic industry realized that presurgical planning of total joint components could not only hold benefits for the patient (better joint orientation) but also the surgeon (reduced surgical time), the hospital (reduced instrument cleaning/sterilization requirements, simplified operating room setup), and even the device manufacturer (reduced capital outlay for implants and instruments). For total joints, an important desired benefit would be increased prosthetic longevity due to better sizing or orientation. Most of the work done to date centers around TKA, but applications also exist in total hip arthroplasty and for placement of pedicle screws.[32,33,34] In all of these instances the implants are off the shelf, and the personalization of fit is performed using a combination of digital presurgical planning and 3D printed surgical guides. Studies have been done to illustrate these benefits,[29] but for some applications the jury is still out on whether the guidance technologies are providing meaningful benefit to the patient's outcome.

Today the largest application for template-guided total joint surgery is for total knee replacement and it is estimated that 10% of all total knee cases performed in the United States today utilize presurgical planning and 3D printed templates. The concept of Bundled payments under the Medicare Comprehensive Care for Joint Replacement directive has incentivized everyone involved in providing care to look at the total cost for the entire episode of care for common procedures such as total hips and knees to achieve continued growth in this area, the benefits will clearly need to outweigh the extra costs involved in procuring the medical imaging studies and the planning and templates themselves.

Robotics is having an impact as a competitive force against physical templating for procedures such as total knees and total hips. One can think of robotics as being a *digital* guide versus what 3D printing provides, which is a *physical* guide.[35] There are other differences in what is possible between robotics-guided procedures and template-guided procedures. It is still very early days for robotic assistance, and it will be interesting to see how these two technologies coexist in the future surgeon's armamentarium.

Corrective Osteotomy/Fixation Planning and Templating

This category includes implant components which are off the shelf and guides which are personalized versus a completely personalized implant system. For most applications, a corrective osteotomy of some type is planned digitally. The resultant guides/templates for surgery may also include a prebent or personalized fixation plate that becomes an integral part of the surgical guidance. There are many ways to get to a personalized fixation plate, but a very simple way is to digitally plan a desired corrective osteotomy result, 3D print a model of that desired result, and manually prebend a reconstruction plate. The plate would then be sterilized and used in surgery. Other, more elaborate techniques include direct 3D printing of a plate in metal or printing of a template for further bending of a plate by machine or human. For orthopedics, the technique has been successfully applied to acetabular osteotomies,[36–40] tibial

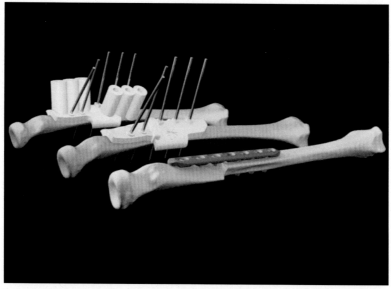

FIG. 7.9. The combination of digital surgical planning for osteotomies and patient-matched cutting guides provides a path to accurately transfer the digital plan to the operating room. The guides shown here were produced with the laser sintering technology and transferred screw holes and osteotomy planes to the patient for a distal radius case. (Materialise, Leuven, Belgium.)

osteotomies,[41] distal radius osteotomies,[42–44] hip dysplasia corrective osteotomies, and many other long bone or extremity procedures where accuracy of the cut or final placement are of critical importance to surgical success. Many good applications also exist in craniomaxillofacial surgery for use of these techniques for planning corrective osteotomies of the cranium, midface, and mandible.[45–47]

3D Printing for Off-The-Shelf Implants (Metal or Polymeric)

The largest impact, by volume, of metal 3D printing in the orthopedic industry is for production of off-the-shelf total joint and spinal fusion implants. Acetabular cups, tibial baseplates, spinal cages, and augments of many types have been the largest users of this technology to date. In the United States, the first Food and Drug Administration (FDA) clearance for a 3D printed metal implant of any kind was for an acetabular cup product produced by Exactech[48] in 2010. In the last 7 years since that first approval, it is estimated that the FDA has cleared dozens of implant products produced by 3D printing in metals.[49] EBM and DMLS are the two main methods in use today for producing these implants in titanium, titanium alloy, and cobalt-chrome alloy.

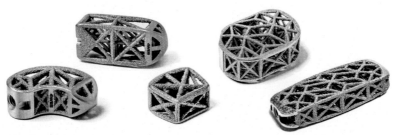

FIG. 7.10. The FDA cleared the first 3D printed titanium spinal cages in 2012 and since then this market has expanded dramatically. Here showing the 4WEB truss technology as applied across multiple types of spinal cages, produced by 3D printing using a powder bed fusion technique. (4Web Medical, Frisco, Texas, USA.)

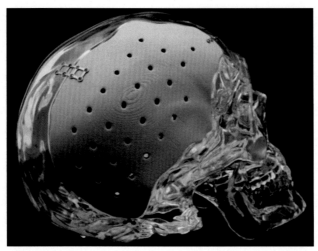

FIG. 7.11. Laser sintering of polyetherketoneketone (PEKK) has been used for various implant applications, including the patient-matched cranial plate shown here. (Oxford Performance Materials, South Windsor, Connecticut, USA.)

Additionally, there are several 3D printed polymeric implants which are cleared by the FDA. Polyetherketoneketone (PEKK) components made by laser sintering have been cleared by the FDA as far back as 2013 for craniomaxillofacial applications[10] and for spine cages in 2015.[50]

One might ask why 3D printing is being used for implants versus the more traditional methods of milling, forging, and investment casting. The primary answer lies in the fact that 3D printing can produce extremely complex parts as easily as simple parts and in some cases even more cost and time effectively as compared with the standard techniques. The ability to print a single implant part, such as an acetabular cup, with both the solid component and the porous bone ingrowth surface component at one time, in the same material has been the propelling force for these applications. The cost of small components, like spinal cages, can be dramatically less than other manufacturing methods, whereas the cost for larger parts like large-diameter acetabular cups may actually be more expensive than the traditional methods. As 3D printer machine speed continues to improve, the cost of the components will continue to drop. There is no doubt that 3D printing can continue to make an impact in the production of off-the-shelf orthopedic implant components.

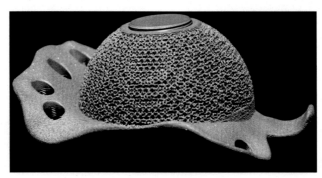

FIG. 7.12. Patient-matched revision hip cup, 3D printed in titanium alloy using the Electron Beam Melting process allows porous bone ingrowth structure to be produced at the same time as the solid substrate. (P. James Burn, MD and Paul Morrison, Ossis Ltd, Christchurch, New Zealand.)

REASONS FOR TODAY'S HIGH INTEREST IN 3D PRINTING IN MEDICINE
Mainstream Knowledge of 3DP

The world came to know 3D printing more in the 2012—14 period, with 3D printers promoted to make everything from human organs to wedding cake toppers.[51] This time period had a lot to do with exposing people from all areas with this 30 year old technology for the first time. Even though 3D printing has been used (in volume) for guidance-based surgical products such as knee templates from the late 2000s, it was not until 2013—15 that 3D printing was used in advertising and promotion of these products. As if it suddenly became "cool," these products were now being branded as 3D printed and this carried some weight, at least in marketing.

3D Printed Products Impacting the Consumer Market

In 2018 consumers can look around and find many professionally designed and produced 3D printing products impacting their lives. These include hearing aid shells, which are more than 90% 3D printed today,[52] and dental aligners, made using a process which involves 3D printing.[53] These are areas where the technology is used to make millions of distinctly different forms every year. Dentistry is evolving completely digital pathways to produce items ranging from dental implants to sleep apnea devices to dentures and teeth. No longer does a patient need to have physical impressions taken with rubber materials in the mouth. Much of this market has already transitioned to intraoral scanning for acquiring the anatomy and then directly digital methods of outputting the data into long-term devices used in the mouth.

In the last year new materials and new players in the 3D printing ecosystem have enabled some breakthrough products in more mainstream markets. Products such as Adidas Futurecraft 4D tennis shoes,[54] Snugs custom-fit earphones,[55] and HOYA Yuniku personalized eyewear[56] are all available in 2018 and are all powered by 3D printing. One main driver why many of these applications, especially the personalized product applications, are able to be delivered to the consumer market is that the technology for personalizing them has gotten more accessible. This is not just about cost of equipment but about lightweight technology and increasing speed and automating workflows for items like custom-fit earphones.

In-Hospital 3D Printing (Point-of-Care Manufacturing) Opening up Discussion/Applications

Over the last 5 years there has been an increasing number of hospitals installing 3D printing laboratories. Most of these new centers have come under the auspices and supervision of the radiology department with an initial aim of producing anatomic models. The key clinical specialties which are driving this effort are oral surgery, otolaryngology, craniofacial surgery, orthopedic surgery, and cardiac surgery. The concept is that faster and closer geographic access to anatomic models will open up new use cases and allow better collaboration between surgeons and radiologists. Institutions such as the Mayo Clinic and Boston Children's Hospital are building on early success and branching out into 3D printing of different materials for different applications, including surgical guides, templates, and models.[57]

The Radiological Society of North America (RSNA), in response to their members and the entry of 3D printing into the hospital, has formed their first Special Interest Group on 3D printing.[58] Formed in 2016, this group has interest in tackling some of the larger problems which come alongside provision of 3D anatomic models, including reimbursement, regulatory, and quality issues.

Materials Expansion

The choices today for 3D printing materials span a wide gamut, including: (1) rigid to flexible (and all in-between with "digital materials"), (2) translucent to opaque, (3) single to full color, (4) single to multiple materials, (5) visualization only to fully functional for surgical rehearsal, implant prebending, etc., (6) biocompatible plastics for guides, templates, and models, and (7) biocompatible metals. Digital materials refer to the ability of some multi-jet printing processes to take two or more materials and blend them "on the fly" to create an entirely new third material, called a digital material. Each set of two materials could potentially have different properties based on blending percentages.

There are many good applications whereby a very flexible (think silicone) material would be the perfect fit for body-contacting applications, but this is a weak point today for 3D printing materials. In general, there are relatively few biocompatible materials which can withstand cleaning and sterilization and stand up to rigor in the operating theater. The dental industry is one to watch in this area as they forge ahead to replace many of the dental laboratory materials in a 3D printable form.

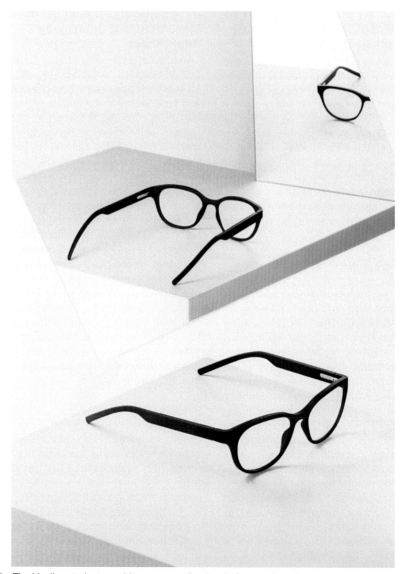

FIG 7.13. The Yuniku product combines personalized style for eyeglass frames along with scanning of the wearer's face prior to 3D printing using the laser sintering technique in nylon. (HOYA Vision Care, Tokyo, Japan & Materialise, Leuven, Belgium.)

FDA Regulation of Medical Devices

The FDA has been an agency of the US federal government focused on protecting consumers since the mid-1800s.[59] Although the agency was not always formally known by their current name and their responsibilities have undergone changes since its inception, its mission to protect the public health has not wavered. Although the FDA has jurisdiction and responsibility over various consumer products, the major focus of this discussion will be on the regulation of medical devices.

A historical representation of the major FDA milestones modified from Sweet et al.[60] is displayed in Fig. 7.15. The changes represent the agencies' response to consumer demands from those time periods. In 1906 the Federal Food and Drug Act was passed which prohibited interstate commerce of misbranded or adulterated foods and drugs. In addition, it required that the

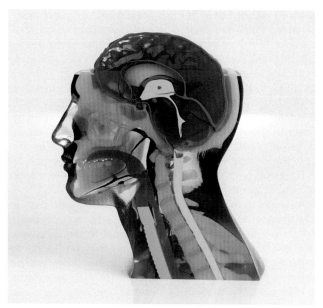

FIG. 7.14. High resolution full color cranial model printed on the Stratasys J750 3D printer using the polyjet material jetting process. (Stratasys, Ltd., Eden Prairie, Minnesota, USA.)

strength and purity of the drug be represented. Misbranded or adulterated products are those that are being marketed, sold, or used for a purpose other than that which is was cleared for by the agency. Although this initial act was an important step to assure consumers, it did not require any information to be submitted to the FDA for review prior to distribution of the drug. In 1912, the Sherley Amendment was passed prohibiting manufacturers from labeling medications with false therapeutic claims intended to defraud the consumer.[60] The next major change came in 1938 with the passing of the Federal Food, Drug, and Cosmetic Act (FDCA). This required drug manufacturers to submit applications for

approval prior to commercializing a pharmaceutical. Although this required manufacturers to prove the drug was safe, no requirements for their efficacy were established.

Approximately 30 years later, the Kefauver Harris Drug Amendment required this efficacy to be established as well as safety. This act was a direct response to the European tragedy where babies were born with birth defects after their mothers were given the sleeping pill thalidomide. This amendment applied to all drugs (prescription and over the counter). It required a drug's efficacy to be proved through a well-conducted and controlled clinical study. Furthermore, rules were

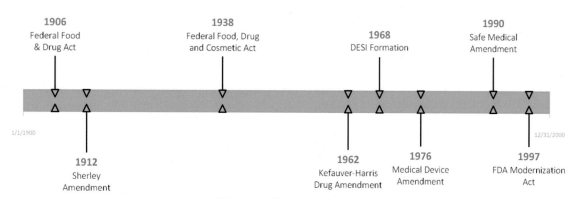

FIG. 7.15 Historic FDA events.

established for informed consents so patients could be adequately aware of potential side effects and their rights under the research.

Although the FDA regulated drugs and medical devices in such ways as prohibiting the distribution of misbranded or adulterated products, it was not until the passage of the Medical Device Amendment in 1976 that manufacturers were required to submit and register with the FDA on their medical device prior to commercial distribution. Also, they now had to follow quality control standards prior to marketing the device. As with the Kefauver Harris Drug Amendment, this regulation was in response to a public health concern where thousands of women were injured by the Daikon Shield intrauterine device. Manufacturers were now also required to gain approval or clearance from the FDA prior to the commercialization of their products. Essentially, the medical device companies now were under the same rigor as the drug companies. The last two major amendments made were in 1990 and 1997. The Safe Medical Device Act of 1990 required manufacturers to implement postmarketing surveillance procedures along with adverse event reporting. Finally, the Food and Drug Administration Modernization Act of 1997 provided some of the largest changes since the 1930s. Regulation of advertising for unapproved (off-label) uses for drugs and devices was added, which resulted in a growing number of warning letters to manufacturers for off-label promotion. It also provided for accelerated reviews of drugs and medical devices using less stringent thresholds for products used to treat very rare diseases (i.e., orphan drugs) or serious medical conditions for which there are no currently available treatment options (e.g., treatment-resistant malignancies). Also, it incorporated fees on manufacturers of drugs to provide additional funding to the FDA for the new product review process along with time windows for review.

The Center for Devices and Radiological Health (CDRH) is the branch of the FDA that primarily regulates the medical device industry. A medical device is defined in the Food, Drug and Cosmetic Act Section 201(h)[61] as:

an instrument, apparatus, implement, machine, contrivance, implant, in vitro reagent, or other similar or related article, including a component part, or accessory which is:

1. recognized in the official National Formulary, or the United States Pharmacopoeia, or any supplement to them,
2. intended for use in the diagnosis of disease or other conditions, or in the cure, mitigation,

treatment, or prevention of disease, in man or other animals, or intended to affect the structure or any function of the body of man or other animals, and which does not achieve its primary intended purposes through chemical action within or on the body of man or other animals and which does not achieve its primary intended purposes through chemical action within or on the body of man or other animals and which is not dependent upon being metabolized for the achievement of its primary intended purposes. The term "device" does not include software functions excluded pursuant to section 520(o).

Several FDA approval or clearance pathways exist for medical device manufacturers. Although certain pathways do not require clinical evaluations of the products prior to commercialization, the FDA has become more rigorous in their review and more demanding on the information proving the risks and benefits of new medical devices.[60] Although the passage of the Medical Device Amendment in 1976 required approval or clearance prior to commercialization, the FDA noted that not all devices require the same level of regulation. As such, the FDA established a class system to acknowledge low risk to higher risk devices. Table 7.1 outlines the class system and definitions. Furthermore, any device sold prior to 1976 was initially grandfathered in, and no submission was required, at least initially. Some of these devices became known as predicate devices and were used to provide a comparison for new devices during the approval process.

There are two general pathways for FDA clearance of a medical device, the 510(k) pathway and the Pre-Market Approval (PMA) pathway. Generally, Class II devices follow the 510(k) route and are referred to as FDA-cleared. Devices which follow the Class III PMA and Humanitarian Device Exempt route (HDE, to be discussed later) are referred to as "FDA-Approved." All medical devices regardless of classification require many of the same regulations to be followed. These include the company to be registered with the FDA and list their products, to follow Good Manufacturing Practice (GMP)/Quality System Regulation (QSR), and adherence to not adulterating or misbranding devices. Most of the Class II and some Class III devices will undergo a traditional 510(k) submission, which requires the manufacturer to prove substantial equivalence to a predicate device. Substantial equivalence means the device performance and intended use are similar to a previously cleared device.

The PMA route requires more stringent controls and a larger burden of proof that the device is both safe and

TABLE 7.1
FDA Medical Device Classification System

Class	Definition
I	• Lowest risk device • Generally exempt from 510(k) processes (no clearance required before commercialization) • Examples include surgical gloves, dental floss, Band-Aids • Requirements: General Controls (Labeling, Manufacturer Registration, Device Listing, Adherence to QSRs, Reporting)
II	• Slightly higher risk devices than Class I devices and therefore require more stringent regulatory controls to provide assurance of their safety, but less/no focus on proven effectiveness • Devices must show substantial equivalence to a legally marketed and FDA-cleared predicate device • Usually no clinical trials needed, Premarket Notification 510(k) is the process for clearance • Examples include powered wheelchairs and orthopedic implants • Requirements: General Controls (Labeling, Manufacturer Registration, Device Listing, Adherence to QSRs, Reporting), 510(k) Clearance
III	• Highest risk devices requiring the most stringent regulatory controls to provide assurance of their effectiveness and safety • Premarket Approval (PMA) process is the path for regulatory approval • Most require data through IDE clinical trials to prove safety along with effectiveness • Examples include implantable pacemakers, orthopedic implants with novel biomaterials/bearing surfaces • Requirements: General Controls (Labeling, Manufacturer Registration, Device Listing, Adherence to QSRs, Reporting), PMA Approval, Post-Market Surveillance (typically) • Only Class III products with an approved PMA can claim "FDA-Approved"

effective. As a result of the need to demonstrate effectiveness, clinical data are often required. These data can come from countries in which the device is cleared or approved for use, but normally they come from studies in the United States. In order to study the device, it must be commercialized in some fashion. Therefore, manufacturers are required to submit for Investigation Device Exemption (IDE) study approval so the device can be commercialized to be included in the controlled clinical study. Although an IDE allows for the components to be shipped and used, it is restricted to the clinical trial only. Currently only about 2% of medical devices follow the Class III PMA pathway.

Humanitarian Use Devices

The HDE provision is intended to provide a regulatory pathway for treating rare diseases where there are limited numbers of people affected.[62,63] The Humanitarian Use Device is a medical device intended to benefit patients in the treatment or diagnosis of a disease or condition that affects or is manifested in not more than 8000 individuals in the United States per year (Section 3052 of the 21st Century Cures Act (Pub. L. No. 114–255). An HDE

is exempt from the effectiveness requirements of Sections 514 and 515 of the FDCA and is subject to certain profit and use restrictions. The manufacturer only has to show that the probable benefits outweigh the risks.

Practice of Medicine

As discussed earlier, the FDA regulates medical device and drug manufacturers; however, they do not directly regulate a practicing physician or hospital.[63] Physicians are expected to consider and ensure the safety and efficacy of the device, as proven by the manufacturer, is not compromised. Furthermore, the physician must have a working knowledge of the device instructions and labeling for its cleared indications. If a physician deems that the use of a medical device is necessary for an unapproved condition, they may act in their best judgment in their practice of medicine. Although the FDA does not control the off-label use of a device by a physician, it does have the authority to take action if the off-label use has the potential to harm patients. Furthermore, the FDA prohibits the promotion of off-label use of manufacturers. A physician may publish reports of this use but cannot formally study a device for an area that has not had clearance.

Custom Devices Versus Patient-Matched Devices

Note that while patient-matched or patient-specific devices (PMDs) are sometimes colloquially referred to as "customized" devices, they are not custom devices meeting the FDCA custom device exemption requirements unless they comply with all of the criteria of section 520(b).[64] For a device to be considered a custom device it must not be generally available, must be designed to treat a unique pathology or condition on the order of a physician, and must not be available elsewhere. In other words, if the surgeon request describes a device that is not available at manufacturer A, but is available at manufacturer B, then the device is not custom and cannot be produced. Furthermore, the FDA mandates only five of a device type can be produced each year if the requirements for custom are met. A process or procedure for designing a PMD can be cleared through the FDA utilizing the 510(k) or PMA pathways. Manufacturers are required to study the safety of the device. Often an envelope of maximum and minimum conditions is established in the clearance. If for some reason a patient's needs fall outside the clearance, the device cannot be produced under the current clearance.

Expanded Access/Compassionate Use

Expanded access, sometimes called "compassionate use," is the use outside of a clinical trial of an investigational medical product (i.e., one that has not been approved by FDA).[65] The FDA is committed to increasing awareness of and knowledge about its expanded access programs and the procedures for obtaining access to human investigational drugs (including biologics) and medical devices.

Wherever possible, use of an investigational medical product as part of a clinical trial is preferable because trials can generate data that may lead to the approval of products and, consequently, to wider availability. However, when patient enrollment in a clinical trial is not possible, e.g., a patient is not eligible for any ongoing clinical trials, or there are no ongoing clinical trials, patients may be able to receive the product, when appropriate, through expanded access. The expanded use or compassionate use process requires manufacturers to submit to the FDA prior to allowing the device to be commercialized. This process involves several steps. First, the patient and licensed physician must be willing to participate. Next, the surgeon must describe the need for the device with an explanation of why no commercially available device is suitable. An independent physician, one not affiliated with the surgeon's practice or hospital system, must concur with the original assessment. The FDA will review the application and assess if the benefits outweigh the risks and provide acceptance for the device to be used. The remaining items for the use of the device are that the institutional review board at the physician's hospital approve the use of the device and that the physician provides the monitoring plan. Unlike cleared or approved devices, the health and status of the patient must be reported to the FDA at specific time points based on the plan submitted and agreed upon by the FDA.

FDA Guidance on 3D Printing

In the area of 3D printing the US FDA has taken a keen interest in this technology, clearing some 100+ 3D printing-related devices over the last 10 years.[49] In 2014, the FDA held a public forum[66] attended by more than 500 industry attendees on the topic and in May 2016 published a draft guidance document entitled, "Technical Considerations for Additive Manufactured Medical Devices" which outlined their collective thinking on the topic. The draft guidance was made final on December 5, 2017 and is now the "law" for medical device manufacturers to consult when working on a 3D printed medical device from a regulatory and quality assurance standpoint.[67] The fact that 3D printing is gaining so much interest today has been positively impacted by the FDA acknowledgment of the technology and its importance in the future of manufacturing for many medical devices, some personalized and some off the shelf. Although these medical devices must follow the same pathway mentioned earlier (510(k) or PMA) for clearance, the guidance document provides further clarification on the information that the FDA is wanting to see in the application specific to 3D printed medical devices.

Technological Advancements Ahead

Breaking down personalized surgery technologies into large subunits would leave you with Software (image processing, surgical planning, design tools), 3D printing hardware, and 3D printing materials. Software advancements will come through more powerful algorithms used to automate tasks which today are still too time consuming. A typical clinical case today for a patient-matched implant design or templating for total joint arthroplasty may take 10−15 hours of an engineer's time. The reasons for this are many, but key to making these technologies more accessible will be reduction of the time a human needs to "touch" the patient's data. Artificial intelligence and deep learning computer techniques will allow the automation of these processes to not only reduce human time but also add repeatability and precision, something that can obviously vary between human operators today. Reducing time and automating tasks will also have the impact of making the software portions of these systems more lightweight and able to be pushed closer to the surgeons using the technologies.

3D printing technologies and materials continue to evolve and today in 2018 we are seeing a lot of development efforts in both faster processes and more functional materials. Techniques such as digital light synthesis and jet fusion have come about in the past few years due to the desire to take the industry beyond making 10, 100, or 1000 parts, and push it forward to make tens of thousands of parts and beyond. For personalized medicine these numbers may not be the key, but that the processes are fast, each part can be unique, and the materials are appropriate for real-world applications. Faster processes equal less amortization of the equipment cost per part, which equals better economy in general. Functional materials will enable thinner parts to have the same strength as thicker, bulkier parts and retaining all of the key benefits, such as biocompatibility, important in medicine.

Future Directions and Conclusions

3D printing has made inroads into many aspects of orthopedic surgery over the past 10 years. Most visibly the applications for total joint templating and for personalized implants have impacted tens of thousands of clinical cases over that time period. Less visible but just as powerful is use of metal 3D printing to directly produce implants in titanium, such as spinal cages, acetabular cups, and augments. The direct output of complex reconstructive devices in biocompatible materials is definitely a major step forward and one that we will continue to see progress over the coming years.

Regarding personalized surgery techniques and methods for guiding surgery, it is still early and more work will be done to apply these techniques to a larger number of procedures in a time and cost-effective manner. In the future, it may be possible to create a more personalized surgical plan which combines off-the-shelf and patient-matched components to allow for the most efficient workflow to meet the desired objective. This varies from today's workflows by adding in patient-matched implants where they fit, but only where they add value to the process. Hospital-based 3D printing, or "point-of-care manufacturing," is on the rise and will make an impact in the next 5 years. Patient-matched templates that were too expensive, too time consuming, or too complex may soon be produced at your local hospital when you need it and for a reasonable price. Hospital-based manufacturing of certain types of devices will happen, for instance, anatomic models and personalized templates, and the spread of knowledge within the hospital will empower new groups of surgeons. Reimbursement is a key issue. With some effort and better documented studies, the authors believe broader reimbursement for personalized surgery technology will start to trickle in during the next 5 years.

The US FDA has made the pathways for 3D printed medical devices clearer than ever before, ushering in a new wave of technologies which are rooted in 3D printing. Building on success in using these techniques for patient-matched implants and surgical guides, we will see further progress being made as cost and time is reduced for use of these technologies. Further democratization of the technology through the on-site production of models, guides, and even perhaps implants will be an interesting progression to watch.

REFERENCES

1. Hull C. *Apparatus for Production of Three-dimensional Objects by Stereolithography US Patent No. 4575330 A*. 1986.
2. Jacobs PF. *Rapid Prototyping & Manufacturing: Fundamentals of StereoLithography*. Society of Manufacturing Engineers; 1992.
3. ISO. *ISO/ASTM 52900:2015. Additive Manufacturing—General Principles—Terminology*; 2015. https://www.iso.org/standard/69669.html.
4. Redwood B, Schoofer F, Garret B. *The 3D Printing Handbook: Technologies, Design and Application*. 1st ed. 3D Hubs; November 2017.
5. Chareancholvanich K, Narkbunnam R, Pornrattanamanee wong C. A prospective randomised controlled study of patient-specific cutting guides compared with conventional instrumentation in total knee replacement. *Bone Joint J*. 2013;95(3):354–359.
6. Lambrecht JT. *3-D Modeling Technology in Oral and Maxillofacial Surgery*. Chicago, IL: Quintessence Publishing Co; 1995.
7. Mankovich NJ, Cheeseman AM, Stoker NG. The display of three-dimensional anatomy with stereolithographic models. *J Digit Imaging*. 1990;3(3):200–203.
8. Stoker NG, Mankovich NJ, Valentino D. Stereolithographic models for surgical planning: preliminary report. *J Oral Maxillofac Surg*. 1992;50(5):466–471.
9. Eppley BL, Sadove AM. Computer generated patient models for reconstruction of cranial and facial deformities. *J Craniofac Surg*. 1998;6:548.
10. FDA. Oxford Performance Materials 510(k) K121818 Osteo Fab™ Patient-specific Cranial Device. https://www.accessdata.fda.gov/cdrh_docs/pdf12/K121818.pdf.

11. Erickson DM, Chance D, Schmitt S, Mathts J. An opinion survey of reported benefits from the use of stereolithographic models. *J Oral Maxillofac Surg.* 1999;57:1040.

12. Brown GA, Firoozbakhsh K, DeCoster TA, Rayna Jr JR, Monein M. Rapid prototyping: the future of trauma surgery? *JBJS.* 2003;85(suppl 4):49–55.

13. Mulford JS, Babazadeh S, Mackay N. Three-dimensional printing in orthopaedic surgery: review of current and future applications. *ANZ J Surg.* 2016;86(9):648–653.

14. Hurson C, Tansey A, O'Donnchadha B, Nicholson P, Rice J, McElwain J. Rapid prototyping in the assessment, classification and preoperative planning of acetabular fractures. *Injury.* 2007;38(10):1158–1162.

15. Bizzotto N, Tami I, Tami A, Spiegel A, Romani D, Corain M, et al. 3D printed models of distal radius fractures. *Injury.* 2016;47(4):976–978.

16. Luo W, Huang L, Liu H, et al. Customized knee prosthesis in treatment of giant cell tumors of the proximal tibia: application of 3-dimensional printing technology in surgical design. *MedSci Monit.* 2017;23:1691–1700.

17. Kim D, Lim JY, Shim KW, et al. Sacral reconstruction with a 3d-printed implant after hemisacrectomy in a patient with sacral osteosarcoma: 1-year follow-up result. *Yonsei Med J.* 2017;58(2):453–457.

18. Wei R, Guo W, Ji T, Zhang Y, Liang H. One-step reconstruction with a3D-printed, custom-made prosthesis after total en bloc sacrectomy: a technical note. *Eur Spine J.* 2017;26(7):1902–1909.

19. Wong KC, Kumta SM, Geel NV, Demol J. One-step reconstruction with a3D-printed, biomechanically evaluated custom implant after complex pelvic tumor resection. *Comput Aided Surg.* 2015;20(1):14–23.

20. Beckmann J, Steinert A, Zilkens C, et al. [Partial replacement of the knee joint with patient-specific instruments and implants (ConforMIS iUni, iDuo)]. *Orthopade.* 2016;45(4):322–330.

21. Taunton MJ, Fehring TK, Edwards P, Bernasek T, Holt GE, Christie MJ. Pelvic discontinuity treated with custom triflange component: a reliable option. *Clin Orthop Relat Res.* 2012;470(2):428–434.

22. Dai KR, Yan MN, Zhu ZA, Sun YH. Computer-aided custom-made hemipelvic prosthesis used in extensive pelvic lesions. *J Arthroplasty.* 2007;22(7):981–986.

23. Ma L, Zhou Y, Zhu Y, et al. 3D-printed guiding templates for improved osteosarcoma resection. *Sci Rep.* 2016;6:23335.

24. Hamid KS, Parekh SG, Adams SB. Salvage of severe foot and ankle trauma with a 3D printed scaffold. *Foot Ankle Int.* 2016;37(4):433–439.

25. Chana-Rodríguez F, Mañanes RP, Rojo-Manaute J, Gil P, Martínez-Gómiz JM, Vaquero-Martín J. 3D surgical printing and pre contoured plates for acetabular fractures. *Injury.* 2016;47(11):2507–2511.

26. Shuang F, Hu W, Shao Y, Li H, Zou H. Treatment of intercondylar humeral fractures with 3d-printed osteosynthesis plates. *Med Baltim.* 2016;95(3):e2461.

27. Howell SM, Kuznik K, Hull ML, Siston RA. Results of an initial experience with custom-fit positioning total knee arthroplasty in a series of 48 patients. *Orthopedics.* 2008;31(9):857–863.

28. Slamin J, Parsley B. "Evolution of customization design for total knee arthroplasty". *Curr Rev Musculoskelet Med.* 2012;5(4):290–295.

29. McLawhorn AS, Carroll KM, Blevins JL, DeNegre ST, Mayman DJ, Jerabek SA. Template-directed instrumentation reduces cost and improves efficiency for total knee arthroplasty: an economic decision analysis and pilot study. *J Arthroplasty.* 2015;30(10):1699–1704.

30. Gauci MO, Boileau P, Baba M, Chaoui J, Walch G. Patient-specific glenoid guides provide accuracy and reproducibility in total shoulder arthroplasty. *Bone Joint J.* 2016;98-B(8):1080–1085.

31. Qiu B, Liu F, Tang B, et al. Clinical study of 3D imaging and 3D printing technique for patient-specific instrumentation in total knee arthroplasty. *J Knee Surg.* 2017;30(8):822–828.

32. Sakai T. Patient-Specific Surgical Guide for Total Hip Arthroplasty. In: Sugano N, ed. *Computer Assisted Orthopaedic Surgery for Hip and Knee.* Singapore: Springe; 2018.

33. Liu K, Zhang Q, Li X, et al. Preliminary application of a multi-level 3D printing drill guide template for pedicle screw placement in severe and rigid scoliosis. *Eur Spine J.* 2017;26(6):1684–1689.

34. Wang YT, Yang XJ, Yan B, Zeng TH, Qiu YY, Chen SJ. Clinical application of three-dimensional printing in the personalized treatment of complex spinal disorders. *Chin J Traumatol.* 2016;19(1):31–34.

35. Jaffry Z, Masjedi M, Clarke S, Harris S, Karia M, Andrews B. Cobb J.Unicompartmental knee arthroplasties: robot vs. patient specific instrumentation. *Knee.* 2014;21(2):428–434.

36. Chen X, Chen X, Zhang G, et al. Accurate fixation of plates and screws for the treatment of acetabular fractures using 3D-printed guiding templates: an experimental study. *Injury.* 2017;48(6):1147–1154.

37. Du H, Tian XX, Li TS, et al. Use of patient-specific templates in hip resurfacing arthroplasty: experience from sixteen cases. *Int Orthop.* 2013;37(5):777–782.

38. Otsuki B, Takemoto M, Kawanabe K, et al. Developing a novel custom cutting guide for curved peri-acetabular osteotomy. *Int Orthop.* 2013;37(6):1033–1038.

39. Cartiaux O, Paul L, Francq BG, Banse X, Docquier PL. Improved accuracy with 3D planning and patient-specific instruments during simulated pelvic bone tumor surgery. *Ann Biomed Eng.* 2014;42(1):205–213.

40. Cernat E, Docquier PL, Paul L, Banse X, Codorean IB. Patient specific instruments for complex tumor resection-reconstruction surgery within the pelvis: a series of 4 cases. *Chir (Bucur).* 2016;111(5):439–444.

41. Chung KJ, Huang B, Choi CH, Park YW, Kim HN. Utility of 3D printing for complex distal tibial fractures and malleolar avulsion fractures: technical tip. *Foot Ankle Int.* 2015;36(12):1504–1510.

42. de Muinck Keizer RJO, Lechner KM, Mulders MAM, Schep NWL, Eygendaal D, Goslings, JC. Three-dimensional virtual planning of corrective osteotomies of distal radius malunions: a systematic review and meta-analysis. *Strateg Trauma Limb Reconstr*. 2017;12(2): 77–89.

43. Honigmann P, Thieringer F, Steiger R, Haefeli M, Schumacher R, Henning JA. Simple 3-dimensional printed aid for a corrective palmar opening wedge osteotomy of the distal radius. *J Hand Surg Am*. 2016;41(3): 464–469.

44. Schweizer A, Fürnstahl P, Nagy L. Three-dimensional correction of distal radius intra-articular malunions using patient-specific drill guides. *J Hand Surg Am*. 2013; 38(12):2339–2347.

45. Mardini S, Alsubaie S, Cayci C, Chim H, Wetjen N. Three-dimensional preoperative virtual planning and 717 template use for surgical correction of craniosynostosis. *J Plast Reconstr Aesthet Surg*. 2014;67(3):336–343.

46. Hirsch DL, Garfein ES, Christensen AM, Weimer KA, Saddeh PB, Levine JP. Use of computer-aided design and computer aided manufacturing to produce orthognathically ideal surgical outcomes: a paradigm shift in head and neck reconstruction. *J Oral Maxillofac Surg*. 2009;67: 2115–2122.

47. Gateno J, Xia J, Teichgraeber J, et al. Clinical feasibility of computer-aided surgical simulation in the treatment of complex cranio-maxillofacial deformities. *J Oral Maxillofac Surg*. 2007;65:728–734.

48. FDA. Exactech 510(k) K102975 Exactech Novation Crown Cup with InteGrip Acetabular Shell. https://www. accessdata.fda.gov/cdrh_docs/pdf10/K102975.pdf.

49. Di Prima M, Coburn J, Hwang D, Kelly J, Khairuzzaman A, Ricles L. Additively manufactured medical products— the FDA perspective. *3D Printing Med*. 2016;2(1). https://doi.org/10.1186/s41205-016-0005-9.

50. FDA. Oxford Performance Materials 510(k) K152005 Clearance for SpineFab Vertebral Body Replacement. https:// www.accessdata.fda.gov/cdrh_docs/pdf14/K142005.pdf.

51. The Economist Journal, Cover Story (2011), Print me a Stradivarius. The Economist February 10, 2011. http://www.economist.com/node/18114327

52. Sharma R. *The 3D Printing Revolution You Have Not Heard About*. Forbes; July 8, 2013. https://www.forbes.com/sites/ rakeshsharma/2013/07/08/the-3d-printing-revolution-you-have-not-heard-about/#5249f4c01a6b.

53. Vlaskalic V, Boyd RL. Clinical evolution of the Invisalign appliance. *J Calif Dent Assoc*. 2002;30(10):769–776.

54. Vincent, J. Adidas Reveals the First 3D-printed Shoe It'll Mass-produce. The Verge. https://www.theverge.com/ 2017/4/7/15216724/adidas-3d-printed-sneaker-futurecraft. Accessed January 5, 2018.

55. Westbrook A. *I've Seen the Future of Hearables—and It Involves a Lot of Lube*. The Memo; January 6, 2017. https:// www.thememo.com/2017/01/06/snugs-earphones-review-3d-printing-lube-hearables/.

56. Hoya Vision Care Europe. *Hoya Launches Yuniku, a Global First in Vision-centric*. 3D Tailored Eyewear; September 23, 2016. https://www.prnewswire.com/news-releases/hoya-launches-yuniku-a-global-first-in-vision-centric-3d-tailored-eyewear-594546501.html.

57. Matsumoto JS, Morris JM, Foley TA, et al. Three-dimensional physical modeling: applications and experience at Mayo clinic. *Radiographics*. 2015;35(7):1989–2006.

58. RSNA. *RSNA Introduces 3-D Printing Special Interest Group*; December 15, 2016. http://www.rsna.org/News.aspx? id=20955.

59. FDA. *History of the Food and Drug Administration*; 2017. https://www.fda.gov/AboutFDA/WhatWeDo/History/.

60. Sweet BV, Schwemm AK, Parons DM. Review of the processes for FDA oversight of drugs, medical devices, and combination products. *J Manag Care Pharm*. 2011;17(1): 40–50.

61. FDA. https://www.fda.gov/MedicalDevices/DeviceRegulation andGuidance/Overview/ClassifyYourDevice/ucm051512. htm.

62. FDA. Humanitarian Device Exemption. https://www.fda. gov/medicaldevices/deviceregulationandguidance/howto marketyourdevice/premarketsubmissions/humanitari andeviceexemption/default.htm.

63. Maisel WH. Medical device regulation: an introduction for the practicing physician. *Ann Intern Med*. 2004;140(4): 296–302.

64. FDA. Custom Device Exemption Guidance for Industry and FDA Staff. Document issued on September 24, 2014. https://www.fda.gov/downloads/ medicaldevices/deviceregulationandguidance/ guidancedocuments/ucm415799.pdf

65. FDA. Expanded Access (Compassionate Use). https:// www.fda.gov/NewsEvents/PublicHealthFocus/Expanded AccessCompassionateUse/default.htm#Investigational_ Medical_Devices..

66. FDA. *Public Workshop—Additive Manufacturing of Medical Devices: An 729 Interactive Discussion on the Technical Considerations of 3D Printing*; October 8–9, 2014. http://wayback. archive-it.org/7993/20170111083117/http://www.fda.gov/ MedicalDevices/NewsEvents/WorkshopsConferences/ ucm397324.htm.

67. FDA. Technical Considerations for Additive Manufactured Medical Devices, Guidance for Industry and FDA Staff. https://www.fda.gov/downloads/MedicalDevices/ DeviceRegulationandGuidance/GuidanceDocuments/ UCM499809.pdf.

CHAPTER 8

3D Printing in Orthopedics: Upper Extremity Trauma and Deformity

SEAN GAO, DO • JOSEPH DALLIS STEPHENS, DO • CALEB PIATT, DO • TAYLOR HOCKMAN, DO • ANDREW HILLS, DO • JAY THOMPSON, DO • MORGAN SMITH, DO • DAVID MARTINEAU, MD • H. BRENT BAMBERGER, DO

INTRODUCTION

Three-dimensional (3D) printing technology is increasingly becoming a popular topic in medicine due to its versatility in creating custom components.[1] Some significant advantages 3D printing offers include increased access to supplies from any location, revolutionizing personalized medicine, and integration with tissue engineering and regenerative medicine.[2] For orthopedics, 3D printing enables a next level of personalized patient care by creating custom orthopedic instruments and hardware.[3] In this chapter we will examine the current literature on 3D-printed orthopedic tools for upper extremity trauma and deformities. The chapter is further divided into subchapters on (1) 3D-printed guides and plates for primary fracture fixation, (2) 3D-printed osteotomy guides for malunion correction, (3) 3D-printed models, and (4) 3D-printed tools, and prosthesis.

3D-PRINTED GUIDES AND PLATES FOR PRIMARY FRACTURE FIXATION

Scaphoid Fracture

Displaced scaphoid fractures are treated surgically with screw fixation because they have a high rate of avascular necrosis if treated nonoperatively. Surgical technique can include percutaneous screw fixation for minimally displaced fractures or open reduction and internal fixation (ORIF) with screws for displaced fractures. A challenge to ORIF is achieving anatomic reduction of the

fragments, whereas a challenge to percutaneous fixation is orienting the screw along the central axis of the scaphoid to provide the highest construct stiffness.[4] Patient-specific 3D-printed guides for scaphoid fractures can aid in solving both these issues.

A case-control study with 22 patients out of Switzerland compared outcomes of scaphoid fixation for nonunion with and without patient-specific guides for fracture reduction.[5] These reduction guides were produced by using selective laser sintering, a manufacturing technique using a laser to heat polyamides. During surgery these guides are fixed to the scaphoid to reduce the two fragments (Fig. 8.1). The authors found that the patient-specific guide group achieved a more accurate fracture reduction with average residual displacement of 7 degrees versus 26 degrees in the control. However, nonunion rates were not significantly different with one of nine nonunion in the patient-specific guide group and 2 of 13 in the traditional group. In this small study, patient-specific guides for scaphoid fracture reduction were superior to traditional methods in achieving anatomic reduction, although they did not significantly affect nonunion rates.

A separate technique article out of Shanghai in 2017 examined using a 3D-printed surgical guide for a "one-shot" percutaneous scaphoid screw fixation.[6] During surgery a custom 3D-printed guiding template that resembles a glove is placed over the patient's wrist. The guiding template has a special guide wire—aiming tube designed to position the K-wire through the center

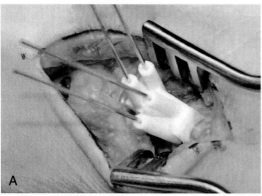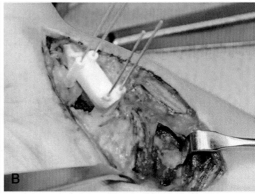

FIG. 8.1 3D Printed Guide for Scaphoid Fracture Reduction and Fixation. **(A)** Setting K-wires with the prereduction guide. **(B)** Reduction is achieved with application of the reduction guide. (Schweizer A, Mauler F, Vlachopoulos L, Nagy L, Fürnstahl P. Computer-assisted 3-dimensional reconstructions of scaphoid fractures and nonunions with and without the use of patient-specific guides: early clinical outcomes and postoperative assessments of reconstruction accuracy. *J Hand Surg Am*. 2016;41(1):59—69. https://doi.org/10.1016/j.jhsa.2015.10.009.)

axis of the scaphoid. A partially threaded cannulated screw can then be advanced along the k-wire to stabilize the fracture. Although this is a technique article and does not provide clinical outcome data, the theoretical advantage for this procedure is a quicker and more reliable method for percutaneous screw fixation of scaphoid fractures. A separate radiological study comparing the anatomic alignment using this one-shot technique and traditional technique is required to demonstrate efficacy of each technique.

Distal Radius Fracture Fixation With 3D-Printed Plates

Distal radius fractures are commonly treated with volar locking plates for their ability to provide strong fracture fixation and their limited rate of tendon complications. There are several volar distal radius plate designs including fixed angled, proximal fit, distal fit, and fragment specific, all with the goal of obtaining rigid fracture fragment fixation.[7]

A 2017 biomechanical study out of Korea compared the strength of 3D-printed volar plates using titanium alloy powder and conventional volar plates (Fig. 8.2).[8] They found that the 3D-printed plates had higher stiffness and a higher yield strength of 1043N than 876N in traditional plates. The authors theorized that higher yield strength in the 3D plates could be due to the titanium alloy powder or due to the 3D plate's ability to better match the bony anatomy and allow for better screw purchase in the distal fragment. An additional potential benefit of creating 3D-printed plates with titanium powder is the ability to adjust each plate's stiffness by adjusting the thickness of the plate. Taken as whole, it is questionable whether the difference in ultimate yield strength in 3D plates versus conventional plates is clinically significant. For reference the max load on the distal radius at max grip strength is roughly 1926N. Although the 3D-printed plate is biomechanically superior, a surgeon would have to weigh the cost of the 3D-printed implant against the marginal benefit.

Distal Humerus Fracture Fixation With a 3D-Printed Plate

Intraarticular distal humerus fractures can have a very complex fracture pattern, especially when there is comminution. Surgical treatment of these fractures is open reduction, internal fixation (ORIF) with plates and screws. O'Driscoll outlines several principles for successful plate and screw fixation including maximizing distal fragment fixation with as many screws as possible.[9] The earliest plates used were simple reconstruction plates that were bent by the surgeon in surgery to match the contour of the bone. These plates evolved into precontoured locking compression plates (LCPs) that offer more rigid fracture fixation. However, fractures that have a short distal fragment may not have good distal fragment screw fixation which can lead to construct failure.[10] 3D-printed plates for distal humerus fractures offer an option to create plates to maximize distal humerus distal fragment fixation.

A small randomized control trial with 13 patients out of Nanchang China in 2016 compared operative time, functional outcome, and Mayo elbow

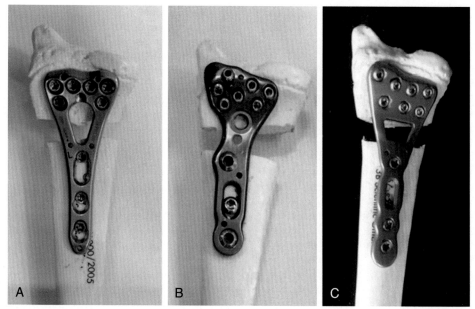

FIG. 8.2 Plate preparation. **(A)** Synthesis; the variable angle LCP-2 column distal radius plate. **(B)** Acumed Acu-Loc plate (Hillsboro, OR). **(C)** 3-Dimensional printed volar locking plate. (Kim S-J, Jo Y-H, Choi W-S, et al. Biomechanical properties of 3-dimensional printed volar locking distal radius plate: comparison with conventional volar locking plate. *J Hand Surg Am.* 2017;42(9):747.e1–747.e6. https://doi.org/10.1016/j.jhsa. 2017.05.009.)

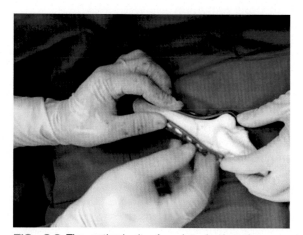

FIG. 8.3 The optimal site for plate implantation was determined using the 3D-printed model. (Shuang F, Hu W, Shao Y, Li H, Zou H. Treatment of intercondylar humeral fractures with 3D-printed osteosynthesis plates. *Medicine (Baltimore).* 2016;95(3):e2461. https://doi.org/10.1097/MD. 0000000000002461.)

performance score (MEPS) between 3D-printed plates and conventional plates for distal intercondylar fractures (Fig. 8.3).[11] They found that operative time was on average 21.7 min shorter for the 3D-printed group

with no significant difference in elbow active range of motion or MEPS. Additionally, bony union was seen at the last follow-up in all patients. A major advantage the authors mention about the 3D plates was the ease in performing the surgery. Some limitations of 3D-printed plates include the CT scan of the fracture to design the plate not being able to differentiate severely comminuted fragments and the time it takes to print a 3D plate. Although this study has a small sample size, it demonstrates that functional outcomes between 3D-printed plates and conventional plates for distal intercondylar fractures are similar and that it may be possible to save operating room time with the 3D-printed plates.

3D OSTEOTOMY GUIDES FOR UPPER EXTREMITY MALUNION CORRECTION
Upper extremity bony deformities and malunions after trauma can be surgically corrected with precise osteotomies to restore normal anatomical alignment. These surgeries can be complex. 3D-printed osteotomy guides offer a way to create customized cuts for each patient's unique malunion pattern. The literature offers examples of using 3D-printed guides to perform

correctional osteotomies for fracture malunion after supracondylar, elbow, both bone, Monteggia, and distal radius fractures.

Supracondylar Malunion, Cubitus Varus, and Cubitus Valgus

Supracondylar fractures are a common pediatric orthopedic fracture. The most common deformity complication in supracondylar fractures is cubitus varus and is believed to be due to uncorrected or recurrent medial tilting of the distal fracture fragment.[12] There are many osteotomies to correct cubitus varus, with lateral closing wedge osteotomy being the most common.[13]

A small case series from Osaka Japan in 2013 with several cases of cubitus varus, cubitus valgus, and forearm shaft malunion examined the use of plate fixation for 3D-printed correction osteotomy for these malunited upper extremity fractures.[14] The main advantage of these 3D-printed guides over a traditional osteotomy done by eye is the ability to better execute an osteotomy with a full understanding of the 3D anatomy of the deformity. When surgeons correct a cubitus varus malunion using traditional methods for example, there may be a tendency to preferentially focus on the coronal plane to only correct varus or valgus deformity. 3D-printed guides allow the surgeon to not only correct the coronal varus deformity but also the sagittal hyperextension and axial internal rotation in a reliable manner. Additionally, these 3D guides allow direct visualization of the fracture during surgery.

The authors in this Osaka study measured clinical outcome and accuracy of correction for their cubitus valgus, cubitus varus, and forearm shaft malunion. At 22-month follow-up they showed improvement in forearm rotation range of motion, grip strength, and pain secondary to deformity. They also found the osteotomies to be accurate within 3 mm and 2 degrees as calculated by comparing the difference between the preoperative simulation and postoperative CT scan. Despite their small sample size and grouping the outcomes from different fracture types together, this study demonstrates that the 3D osteotomy guides can provide accurate cuts that result in improved anatomical and clinical outcomes.

A second 2013 small case series with 33 patients from Osaka Japan examined the use of 3D-printed surgical cutting guides to perform correctional osteotomies in cubital varus deformity after supracondylar malunion (Fig. 8.4).[15] Using this technique, they were able to correct an average 18.2 degrees varus deformity to 5.8 degrees of valgus alignment, hyperextension deformity of more than 20 degrees to neutral,

and internal rotation from 13.6 to 0.5 degrees. At 12-month follow-up, they found excellent radiographic results in 90% of their patients and defined the humerus-elbow-wrist angle as within 5 degrees of the normal side. Complications included one case of plate breakage and one patient with early loss of correction with recurrent cubitus varus. Overall, this study provides evidence that 3D-printed correctional osteotomy guides for cubitus varus can reliably and accurately restore normal anatomy.

Distal Humerus Correctional Osteotomy

A possible issue with using 3D osteotomy guides for distal humerus correctional osteotomy is the accuracy of guide placement onto the bone to create the predicted outcome. This was investigated by Omori et al. in 2014 by 3D-printed osteotomy for artificially created distal humerus and distal radius fractures in cadavers.[16] They found that guide placement was within 1 mm of the intended position and correctional osteotomy within 2 degrees of the predicted correction. Although this study looked at osteotomies in cadavers without bony deformities, it provides more provisional evidence that 3D osteotomy guides can produce accurate and reproducible cuts within a relatively small margin of error.

Both-Bone Malunion

Both-bone forearm fractures are common in the pediatric population and often treated through closed reduction and casting. However, malunion and deformity can occur resulting in pain, decreased range of motion, and distal radial ulnar joint (DRUJ) instability.

A case series published in 2015 out of Shriners hospital examined seven patients with forearm malunion treated with osteotomy with 3D-printed correctional guides. Their results showed an average increase in forearm supination and pronation by 25 degrees and total rotation greater than 120 degrees[17] A separate case series out of Osaka Japan with 20 patients with symptomatic malunited forearm fractures treated with osteotomies by 3D-printed osteotomy guides found an average doubling of forearm arc range of motion from 76 to 152 degrees and mildly improved grip strength from 82% to 94% compared to normal side.[18] Both these case series show how 3D-printed osteotomy guides can produce positive clinical results with increased range of motion and function.

Monteggia Malunion

A case report by Oka et al. examined two patients with malunion and chronic radial head dislocation after a both-bone fracture treated nonoperatively initially

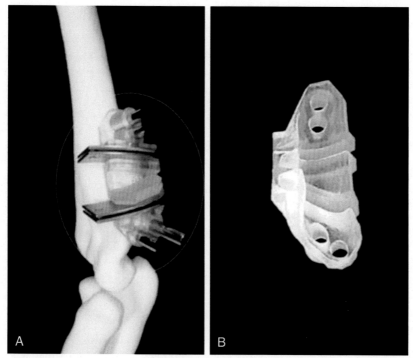

FIG. 8.4 3D osteotomy guide for UE Malunion. Photographs of the custom-made osteotomy template. **(A)** The template, with two metal osteotomy sites and four metal sleeves, on a full-scale plastic bone model. **(B)** The bone-contact side of the template. (Takeyasu Y, Oka K, Miyake J, Kataoka T, Moritomo H, Murase T. Preoperative, computer simulation-based, three-dimensional corrective osteotomy for cubitus varus deformity with use of a custom-designed surgical device. *J Bone Joint Surg Am*. 2013;95(22):e173. https://doi.org/10.2106/JBJS.L.01622.)

with closed reduction and casting.[19] Again, 3D osteotomy guides were created to perform correctional osteotomies. Follow-up at 42 and 54 months for each patient showed restoration of forearm rotation and resolution of elbow pain.

Distal Radius Malunion

Surgeons are implementing 3D custom guides for distal radius malunion correction on a more widespread basis. A 2017 systematic review article and metaanalysis out of the Netherlands looked at studies examining 3D planning for corrective osteotomies of distal radius malunions.[20] The majority of studies (10/15) used custom-made osteotomy template with guiding holes and an osteotomy slit. The majority of osteotomies were based on the contralateral normal side. Functional outcomes after surgery showed significantly improved mean flexion-extension, pronation-supination, and grip strength. Postoperative radiographic correction of alignment showed improvement of palmar tilt, and radial inclination improved to within 5 degrees of their normal in all but three cases. Complications occurred in 11 patients (16%) including loose screw, partial laceration of extensor pollicis longus (EPL) tendon, distal radioulnar subluxation persistence, or hardware removed due to pain or discomfort.

The accuracy of 3D-printed osteotomy guides for distal radius malunions was examined by a small retrospective case series out of Belgium in 2013.[21] The authors recorded radiographic measurements before and after surgery including volar tilt, radial inclination, ulnar variance, and articular surface step off and compared them to the computer model−predicted measurements. Of these values, volar tilt was most difficult to correct with an average of −6+/6 degrees of undercorrection. Radial inclination was corrected to within -1+/-5 degrees ulnar variance 0 ± 1 mm, and articular step off 1.1 ± 0.6 mm. Overall, this small case series demonstrates fairly precise correction of distal radius malunions with radial inclination and articular step off while volar tilt was less reliably restored. Additionally, one difficulty the authors noted with the 3D-printed guides was the need for a wider bone exposure and visual field obscured by soft tissue, making optimal placement more difficult than when testing on a dry cadaver bone. A cadaver study investigating the accuracy of 3D corrective osteotomies guides found that they were able to get plate fixation within 1 degree of flexion and 1 mm of displacement.[16] Additional randomized control trials are underway specifically examining outcomes for corrective osteotomy for malunited distal radius fractures with and without preoperative computer-assisted planning and patient-specific surgical guides.[22]

3D-PRINTED MODEL

3D printing of fractures has also been used to generate physical models used for preoperative planning. These physical fracture models can be used to prebend plates, whereas the computer models can aid greatly in visualizing the fracture pattern and for preoperative planning.

Clavicle Fracture Models and Prebending Plates

Treatment of displaced midshaft clavicle fractures has recently become a popular topic for debate. Classical literature by Neer found good clinical results with nonoperative treatment, whereas newer data from the Canadian Orthopedic Trauma Society have found support for surgery in some patients, citing improved functional outcomes within 1 year.[23] The more recent Canadian Orthopedic Trauma Society study on operative versus nonoperative treatment of clavicle fractures recommends surgical treatment for displaced midshaft clavicle fractures because they have a lower malunion and nonunion rate at 1 year than nonoperative treatment.[24] A common surgical technique for clavicle fractures is ORIF with plates and screws.

A 2014 article out of Chunbgbuk South Korea discusses a technique for using 3D-printed models of fractures to allow for prebending plates for clavicle fractures.[25] These 3D-printed clavicle plates allow for enhanced plate contouring each patient's unique clavicle "S" shape which can have substantial variation based on gender and race. Additionally, this technique allows for easier fracture reduction, minimizing soft tissue dissection. Finally the cost of these plates was only $20 and took 3 h to print. Although this chapter does not provide clinical outcome data, it does offer a novel,

quick, and relatively inexpensive way to treat clavicle fractures.

Proximal Humerus Fracture Model

You et al. studied the effect of using 3D-printed proximal humerus fracture models in preoperative planning on operative time, time to union, blood loss, and intraoperative fluoroscopy use for 66 isolated proximal humerus fracture cases.[26] The authors found that the preoperative 3D model group had on average a 14-min decrease in OR time, 46-mL lower blood loss, and three less fluoroscopic images. There was no significant difference for time to union between the two groups. This study shows that preoperative planning with 3D models can enhance OR performance, although traditional methods produced the same patient outcome with time to union.

Elbow Fracture Model

Yang et al. examined the use of 3D-printed models in preoperative planning for 40 patients with complex elbow fractures.[27] In the 3D group, the surgical plan was preoperatively developed based on the creation of a 3D-printed fracture model that was used to apply plates and check for screw placement and orientation. The 3D model group had a surgical approach, plate position, screw implantation direction, and length that were all highly consistent with the preoperative plan. The average operation time decreased about 21 minutes in the 3D model group when compared to the control group while the average intraoperative blood loss was 22 mL. The average MEPS postoperatively was 88 and 82. Although the 3D-printed model preoperative planning had modest decreases in OR time and blood loss, the final patient outcomes were similar between the two groups.

Radial Head Fracture Model

Radial head fractures can be classified by the Mason classification with Broberg modification. This classification is useful as it can help guide treatment of patients with Mason I treated nonoperatively, mason II ORIF, and mason III with radial head arthroplasty.[28] The interobserver classification for the Mason classification with Hotchkiss modification was examined by Sheps et al.[29] who found moderate reliability with a mean percent agreement of 72.3%.

Guttion et al. published a prospective study examining the use of 3D-printed models to classify radial head fractures with the Mason classification with Broberg Morrey modification.[30] In their study, senior attendants, fellows, and residents were asked to classify different radial head fractures first with plain radiographs followed sequentially by 3D CT, 3D models, and intraoperative visualization. They found that the interobserver reliability for 3D-printed models and intraoperative visualization was similar at a kappa of 0.37 and 0.38, respectively. However, there was no difference between having a 3D CT or a printed 3D model for identifying a fracture line. Overall, this study demonstrates that 3D-printed models allow for reliable diagnosis of radial head fractures by the Mason classification with Broberg Morrey modification.

3D-PRINTED INSTRUMENTS, AND PROSTHESES

Instruments

3D printing has not only allowed surgeons to better characterize fracture patterns and conceptualize proper anatomic reduction and fixation but also been used successfully to create instruments for more efficient intraoperative usage. Fuller et al. used 3D printing to create reduction clamps for hand fractures.[31] Individualized clamps were able to be created relatively quickly based on physician preference, experience, and design (Fig. 8.5). As 3D printing has become more affordable and more easily attainable, using software to create personalized instruments for reduction has improved patient care and nurtured advances in orthopedic surgery of the upper extremity.

3D-Printed Prosthesis

A 2016 review article in the Journal of Hand Surgery by Burn et al. examines the use of 3D printing for prosthetic hands in children.[32] The main advantage of 3D printing is its ability to create custom and varied orthotic designs (Fig. 8.6). Additionally, body-powered prosthesis or myoelectric prosthesis can be very costly and require frequent repairs. The authors suggest that the best candidates for 3D-printed hand prosthesis are those with unilateral congenital or traumatic limb reductions at the distal carpal or transmetacarpal level. The candidate should also have an active wrist flexion and extension arc of 30 degrees to power composite grasp.

Contraindications specific to 3D prosthesis are lack of wrist motion, a small residual carpal segment, and the presence of partial or complete fingers which existing designs cannot accommodate. Measurement for 3D templating is achieved by simple measurements of the recipient's bilateral limbs. After a hand design is selected, the design file can be downloaded, and the appropriate measurements are adjusted. The 3D printer can then print the pieces for the prosthesis, which are then assembled together. Some challenges to these 3D-printed prostheses are obtaining a good first layer fit or failure at load-bearing areas. Overall the authors concluded that these 3D-printed hand prostheses offer a low-cost lightweight, and easily replaced prosthesis for pediatric patients.

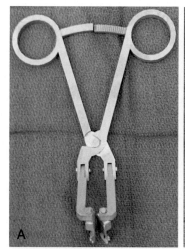 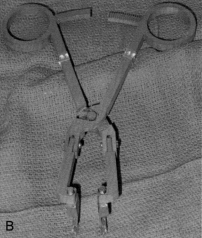

FIG. 8.5 3D printed surgical instruments: **(A)** Plastic prototype. **(B)** Final stainless-steel instrument. (Fuller SM, Butz DR, Vevang CB, Makhlouf MV. Application of 3-dimensional printing in hand surgery for production of a novel bone reduction clamp. *J Hand Surg Am.* 2014;39(9):1840–1845. https://doi.org/10.1016/j.jhsa.2014.06.009.)

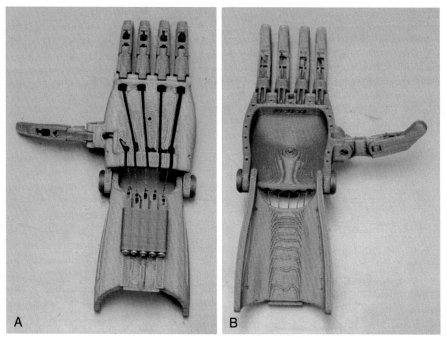

FIG. 8.6 3D Printed Hand Prosthesis: Raptor reloaded hand by e-NABLE: A) Dorsal view; B) palmar view.

CONCLUSION

There are a variety of applications for 3D printing in upper extremity orthopedic trauma and deformity including but not limited to 3D guides for primary fracture fixation, 3D osteotomy guides for malunion correction, 3D-printed models for preoperative planning, and 3D-printed surgical tools, and prosthesis. They offer new avenues for innovation in creating patient-specific treatments.

Preliminary studies looking at 3D printing technology for primary fracture fixation of scaphoid, distal humerus, and distal radius fractures have shown promise. However, these studies often involve small sample sizes and fail to signify superior functional outcome to traditional fracture treatment methods. The malunion studies with 3D-printed correctional osteotomy guides also show accurate postoperative anatomic alignment as demonstrated by radiographs. Again, there are few case control studies comparing 3D-printed osteotomy guides to osteotomies done by hand.

Several advantages of 3D printing technology for upper extremity orthopedic trauma and deformity include making technically challenging preoperative plans more concrete, improving visualization in the OR, reducing OR time, having superior biomechanical constructs, and making technology for instruments, plates, and prosthesis available to anyone across the world with a 3D printer. It offers an exciting new frontier for bottom-up orthopedic surgical equipment development and will certainly challenge the existing treatment paradigm of upper extremity trauma treatment in the years to come.

REFERENCES

1. Michalski MH, Ross JS. The shape of things to come: 3D printing in medicine. *JAMA.* 2014;312(21):2213−2214. https://doi.org/10.1001/jama.2014.9542.
2. Maruthappu M, Keogh B. How might 3D printing affect clinical practice? *BMJ.* 2014;349:g7709.
3. Wong TM, Jin J, Lau TW, et al. The use of three-dimensional printing technology in orthopaedic surgery. *J Orthop Surg (Hong Kong).* 2017;25(1):2309499016684077. https://doi.org/10.1177/2309499016684077.
4. McCallister WV, Knight J, Kaliappan R, Trumble TE. Central placement of the screw in simulated fractures of the scaphoid waist: a biomechanical study. *J Bone Joint Surg Am.* 2003;85-A(1):72−77.

5. Schweizer A, Mauler F, Vlachopoulos L, Nagy L, Fürnstahl P. Computer-assisted 3-dimensional reconstructions of scaphoid fractures and nonunions with and without the use of patient-specific guides: early clinical outcomes and postoperative assessments of reconstruction accuracy. *J Hand Surg Am.* 2016;41(1):59−69. https://doi.org/10.1016/j.jhsa.2015.10.009.

6. Yin H-W, Xu J, Xu W-D. 3-Dimensional printing-assisted percutaneous fixation for acute scaphoid fracture: 1-shot procedure. *J Hand Surg Am.* 2017;42(4):301.e1−301.e5. https://doi.org/10.1016/j.jhsa.2017.01.017.

7. Alluri RK, Hill JR, Ghiassi A. Distal radius fractures: approaches, indications, and techniques. *J Hand Surg Am.* 2016;41(8):845−854. https://doi.org/10.1016/j.jhsa.2016.05.015.

8. Kim S-J, Jo Y-H, Choi W-S, et al. Biomechanical properties of 3-dimensional printed volar locking distal radius plate: comparison with conventional volar locking plate. *J Hand Surg Am.* 2017;42(9):747.e1−747.e6. https://doi.org/10.1016/j.jhsa.2017.05.009.

9. O'Driscoll SW. Optimizing stability in distal humeral fracture fixation. *J Shoulder Elbow Surg.* 2005;14(1 suppl S):186S−194S. https://doi.org/10.1016/j.jse.2004.09.033.

10. Jayakumar P, Ring D. A pitfall in fixation of distal humeral fractures with pre-contoured locking compression plate. *Arch Bone Joint Surg.* 2015;3(2):130−133.

11. Shuang F, Hu W, Shao Y, Li H, Zou H. Treatment of intercondylar humeral fractures with 3D-printed osteosynthesis plates. *Medicine (Baltimore).* 2016;95(3):e2461. https://doi.org/10.1097/MD.0000000000002461.

12. Labelle H, Bunnell WP, Duhaime M, Poitras B. Cubitus varus deformity following supracondylar fractures of the humerus in children. *J Pediatr Orthop.* 1982;2(5):539−546.

13. Srivastava AK, Srivastava D, Gaur S. Lateral closed wedge osteotomy for cubitus varus deformity. *Indian J Orthop.* 2008;42(4):466−470. https://doi.org/10.4103/0019-5413.43397.

14. Kataoka T, Oka K, Miyake J, Omori S, Tanaka H, Murase T. 3-Dimensional prebent plate fixation in corrective osteotomy of malunited upper extremity fractures using a real-sized plastic bone model prepared by preoperative computer simulation. *J Hand Surg Am.* 2013;38(5):909−919. https://doi.org/10.1016/j.jhsa.2013.02.024.

15. Takeyasu Y, Oka K, Miyake J, Kataoka T, Moritomo H, Murase T. Preoperative, computer simulation-based, three-dimensional corrective osteotomy for cubitus varus deformity with use of a custom-designed surgical device. *J Bone Joint Surg Am.* 2013;95(22):e173. https://doi.org/10.2106/JBJS.L.01622.

16. Omori S, Murase T, Kataoka T, et al. Three-dimensional corrective osteotomy using a patient-specific osteotomy guide and bone plate based on a computer simulation system: accuracy analysis in a cadaver study. *Int J Med Robot.* 2014;10(2):196−202. https://doi.org/10.1002/rcs.1530.

17. Storelli DAR, Bauer AS, Lattanza LL, McCarroll HR. The use of computer-aided design and 3-dimensional models in the treatment of forearm malunions in children. *Tech Hand Up Extrem Surg.* 2015;19(1):23−26. https://doi.org/10.1097/BTH.0000000000000070.

18. Miyake J, Murase T, Oka K, Moritomo H, Sugamoto K, Yoshikawa H. Computer-assisted corrective osteotomy for malunited diaphyseal forearm fractures. *J Bone Joint Surg Am.* 2012;94(20):e150. https://doi.org/10.2106/JBJS.K.00829.

19. Oka K, Murase T, Moritomo H, Yoshikawa H. Corrective osteotomy for malunited both bones fractures of the forearm with radial head dislocations using a custom-made surgical guide: two case reports. *J Shoulder Elbow Surg.* 2012;21(10):e1−e8. https://doi.org/10.1016/j.jse.2012.05.035.

20. de Muinck Keizer RJO, Lechner KM, Mulders MAM, Schep NWL, Eygendaal D, Goslings JC. Three-dimensional virtual planning of corrective osteotomies of distal radius malunions: a systematic review and meta-analysis. *Strateg Trauma Limb Reconstr.* 2017;12(2):77−89. https://doi.org/10.1007/s11751-017-0284-8.

21. Stockmans F, Dezillie M, Vanhaecke J. Accuracy of 3D virtual planning of corrective osteotomies of the distal radius. *J Wrist Surg.* 2013;2(4):306−314. https://doi.org/10.1055/s-0033-1359307.

22. Leong NL, Buijze GA, Fu EC, Stockmans F, Jupiter JB. Distal Radius Malunion (DiRaM) collaborative group. Computer-assisted versus non-computer-assisted preoperative planning of corrective osteotomy for extra-articular distal radius malunions: a randomized controlled trial. *BMC Musculoskelet Disord.* 2010;11:282. https://doi.org/10.1186/1471-2474-11-282.

23. Neer CS. Nonunion of the clavicle. *J Am Med Assoc.* 1960;172:1006−1011.

24. Canadian Orthopaedic Trauma Society. Multicenter randomized clinical trial of nonoperative versus operative treatment of acute acromio-clavicular joint dislocation. *J Orthop Trauma.* 2015;29(11):479−487. https://doi.org/10.1097/BOT.0000000000000437.

25. Jeong H-S, Park K-J, Kil K-M, et al. Minimally invasive plate osteosynthesis using 3D printing for shaft fractures of clavicles: technical note. *Arch Orthop Trauma Surg.* 2014;134(11):1551−1555. https://doi.org/10.1007/s00402-014-2075-8.

26. You W, Liu LJ, Chen HX, et al. Application of 3D printing technology on the treatment of complex proximal humeral fractures (Neer3-part and 4-part) in old people. *Orthop Traumatol Surg Res.* 2016;102(7):897−903. https://doi.org/10.1016/j.otsr.2016.06.009.

27. Yang L, Grottkau B, He Z, Ye C. Three dimensional printing technology and materials for treatment of elbow fractures. *Int Orthop.* 2017;41(11):2381−2387. https://doi.org/10.1007/s00264-017-3627-7.

28. Iannuzzi NP, Leopold SS. In brief: the Mason classification of radial head fractures. *Clin Orthop Relat Res.* 2012;470(6): 1799–1802. https://doi.org/10.1007/s11999-012-2319-2.

29. Sheps DM, Kiefer KRL, Boorman RS, et al. The interobserver reliability of classification systems for radial head fractures: the Hotchkiss modification of the Mason classification and the AO classification systems. *Can J Surg.* 2009;52(4):277–282.

30. Guitton TG, Brouwer K, Lindenhovius ALC, et al. Diagnostic accuracy of two-dimensional and three-dimensional imaging and modeling of radial head fractures. *J Hand Microsurg.* 2014;6(1):13–17. https://doi.org/10.1007/s12593-013-0107-1.

31. Fuller SM, Butz DR, Vevang CB, Makhlouf MV. Application of 3-dimensional printing in hand surgery for production of a novel bone reduction clamp. *J Hand Surg Am.* 2014;39(9): 1840–1845. https://doi.org/10.1016/j.jhsa.2014.06.009.

32. Burn MB, Ta A, Gogola GR. Three-dimensional printing of prosthetic hands for children. *J Hand Surg Am.* 2016;41(5): e103–e109. https://doi.org/10.1016/j.jhsa.2016.02.008.

CHAPTER 9

Three-Dimensional Printing Technology in Foot and Ankle Surgery

JAMES R. JASTIFER, MD • PETER A. GUSTAFSON, PHD

INTRODUCTION

Rapid prototyping via three-dimensional (3D) printing of computer-generated datasets is an established concept in the manufacturing industry, having been invented in 1983.[1] In foot and ankle surgery, however, conversion of computerized datasets to printed objects is rapidly increasing as 3D printer technology has advanced. First described in 1997 for the evaluation of intraarticular calcaneal fractures, 3D printing in foot and ankle surgery started slowly but has recently gained momentum as the technology has dispersed.[2] In this original report the 3D-printed models were not found to be statistically superior to software-based 3D reconstructions of the calcaneal fractures. The recent advancements within foot and ankle surgery are an adoption from similar technology in other body parts including patient-specific instrumentation in total joint arthroplasty, procedure rehearsal, patient and medical educational tools, preoperative planning, and patient communication.[3–10] The applications of 3D printing in foot and ankle surgery which are the most useful are clinical scenarios when complex 3D special relationships are most important.

There have been few reports or descriptions in the published literature using 3D printing technology in foot and ankle surgery. Chung et al. used 3D prints of calcaneal fractures for the preoperative planning and for creation of preshaped calcaneal plates.[2] Similarly, Giovinco et al. used CT data for presurgical planning of charcot foot reconstruction.[10] The current authors described the technique and a case report for the correction of a posttraumatic ankle deformity with a corrective osteotomy.[11] A subsequent case report using a custom talar prosthesis based on a mirror image of the contralateral side CT scan was reported.[12] More recently, Smith et al. report an implantable 3D-printed plate for the correction of hallux valgus, which has recently received the FDA approval.[13]

DEFORMITY CORRECTION

There are several causes of bony deformity including acquired deformity from primary or secondary disease processes, traumatic malunion (Case 1), or congenital deformity (Case 2). Regardless of the circumstance, the clinical deformity can be difficult to interpret radiographically. In these situations 3D prints can be useful in quantifying and qualifying the deformity as well as helping plan surgical procedures. Holding and manipulating a 3D print of a bony deformity can be very helpful in understanding the special relationships present. The benefit to the surgeon can be in better understanding the deformity and subsequently planning the trajectory of fixation devices. In these cases the patient can also benefit in a similar way by allowing them to review the deformity with the surgeon and have a better understanding of the treatment plan. In our experience this is tremendously helpful: a more informed patient is a better partner in their clinical care.

CASE 1[11]

Fig. 9.1 demonstrates a patient with chronic ankle pain after an ankle fracture treated nonoperatively. The patient was diagnosed with a medial malleolus nonunion and a fibular malunion (Fig. 9.1A and C). The process of generating 3D prints started with bilateral weight-bearing radiographs and CT scans. CT data were obtained using DICOM format (Digital Imaging and Communications in Medicine) and imported into a software program capable of performing reconstruction algorithms for bone and soft tissue (3D Slicer, www.slicer.org). From the DICOM image, a triangulated 3D surface representation and compatible file (.stl) were created. A series of factors impact the quality of the generated surfaces. The voxelization inherent to DICOM images, along with the resolution and noise of the image grayscale density, and the underlying

3D Printing in Orthopaedic Surgery. https://doi.org/10.1016/B978-0-323-58118-9.00009-9

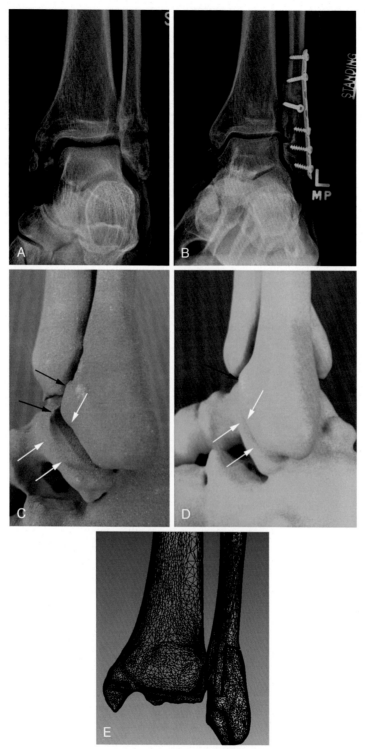

FIG. 9.1 **(A)** Anterior-Posterior (AP) ankle radiograph demonstrating a medial malleolus nonunion and fibular malunion. **(B)** Postoperative radiograph demonstrating correction of fibular malunion after "Z"-shaped osteotomy. **(C)** Preoperative 3D print demonstrating proximal and posterior translation of the distal fibular fragment. **(D)** Contralateral mirrored 3D print. **(E)** "Z"-shaped osteotomy.

anatomical features (fractures, avulsions, adjacent tissue surfaces in direct contact, etc.) can lead to anomalies in the triangulated surfaces representing the tissue volumes. These model imperfections were smoothed using the laplacian smoothing technique within MeshLab (MeshLab, version 1.3.3, www.meshlab.sourceforge.net). For comparison the contralateral CT data were similarly modeled, smoothed, and "mirrored" to demonstrate how the ipsilateral side should look. Both models were printed. A preoperative plan was developed to perform a corrective Z-shaped osteotomy. To further manipulate the models, both were converted into 3D solid models in computer-aided drafting software (FreeCAD, version 0.14, www.freecadweb.org). Subsequently the Z-shaped osteotomy was simulated using Boolean operations as well as translation and rotation of the distal fibular fragment. With reference to the mirrored contralateral side and the necessary manipulations to recreate the ideal anatomy as possible, the deformity magnitude was determined to be 7 degrees of external rotation, 6 mm of loss of fibular length, and 5 mm of posterior translation. The external rotation deformity was found to be corrected with a 3-mm posteriorly based bone wedge. A detailed process for anatomic manipulation with code samples is also described in the study by Gustafson et al. as well as by others.[14,15]

CASE 2

Fig. 9.2 shows the radiographs of a 16-year-old patient with multiple congenital coalitions and a ball and socket ankle joint, as well as a congenital absence of a ray. The patient presented with a painful complex deformity. Segmentation and registration were conducted, and preoperative anatomy was generated as a set of STL surfaces as described in Case 1. Osteotomies were planned to correct the position of the calcaneal tuberosity relative to the talus and the talus relative to the first ray. OpenSCAD was used for the Boolean operations required for simulated osteotomies (http://www.openscad.org/). Preosteotomy and postosteotomy prints were made and reviewed with the patient and his family. The surgery was performed as planned. In this case, 3D printing permitted quantification of intended sizes of the osteotomies including visualization and quantification of the resulting multiplanar corrections. Patient education is a secondary but useful benefit.

JIGS

The purpose of using a jig to guide a surgical cut is to increase reproducibility, accuracy, and efficiency.

A patient-specific cutting jig may provide superior surgical precision, allowing a perfectly fitted jig matched specifically to each patient's bony anatomy, taking the soft tissue considerations out of the picture, which may otherwise provide false landmarks to the surgeon. However, to date, jigs are used in a limited fashion in foot and ankle surgery. They have been limited to this point to ankle arthroplasty. Fig. 9.3 demonstrates a Prophecy navigation guide used with an Infinity total ankle arthroplasty system (Wright Medical Group, Memphis TN). In this case, preoperative imaging is used to create a 3D-printed custom jig for one-time use in the operating room to make the bony cuts for the total ankle arthroplasty. This technology is more commonly used in total knee arthroplasty. The challenge to more widespread adoption of this technology in other foot and ankle–related procedures is the cost of the jig as well as the cost associated with obtaining the extra imaging. To the authors' knowledge there are no studies that support the cost-effectiveness of this technology for this use in terms of improved patient outcomes, although the technology seems promising. Other targets for 3D-printed jigs are for use in osteotomy or fusion procedures to prepare the bony cuts. Unlike for surgical planning, jigs must be made of material that can be sterilized, which is a technology that is not commonly available to community surgeons wishing to do this on their own. The time required to make a patient-specific jig may also not be time-saving given the technical demands of many foot and ankle osteotomies. It has also been argued that creating a jig or guide that is custom made based on imaging data makes the "perfect-fit" jig or guide that takes some of the intraoperative judgment and decision-making by the surgeon out of the picture. This may theoretically make the procedure easier and may allow more difficult procedures to be performed by less experienced surgeons. It is unclear, however, if a patient-specific cutting guide effectively puts more difficult procedures into the hands of those less experienced, easing the technical difficulty of these procedures.

CASE 3

Fig. 9.4 demonstrates a case of intraarticular hardware and heterotopic bone after an ankle open reduction and internal fixation in a young patient with pain after treatment. The 3D print in this case helps the clinician and the patient better understand the position of the hardware and heterotopic bone relative to the joint space as well as the size and location of the heterotopic bone. It also gives the clinician information regarding the reduction of the distal fibular fragment.

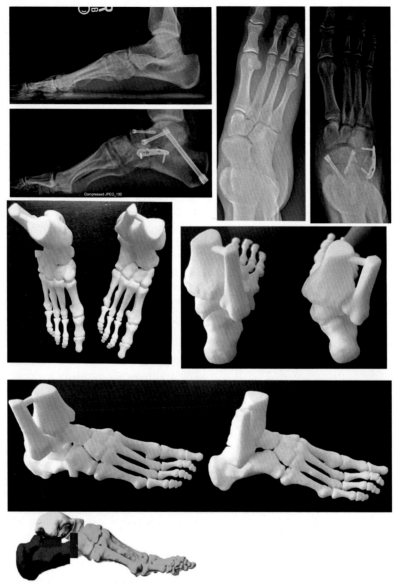

FIG. 9.2 Preoperative and postoperative radiographs and CAD model and 3D prints demonstrating preosteotomy and postosteotomy anatomy. Note that the preoperative deformity is on the right in images of 3D prints. *CAD*, computer-aided design.

3D-PRINTED IMPLANTS

There is great promise in the concept of 3D-printed implants in orthopedics. The complex geometry on the functional unit of bone provides a good example. Take for example an implantable truss system, sold by the company 4WEB Medical (Frisco, TX), Fig. 9.5. This implant concept is a repeating unit of a truss that is custom designed for the patient and surgeon's needs.

In this case the truss design is created to fill a bone defect in a talus with room for the introduction of an intramedullary nail through the implant. This has several important concepts worth pointing out. First, distinction should be made between a custom implant and an "off-the-shelf" implant designed for 3D printing as a manufacturing method. In this case it would be possible to have several "off-the-shelf" sizes of talar

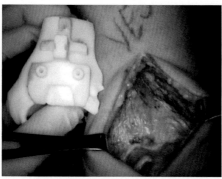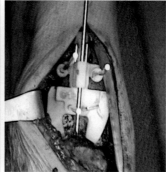

FIG. 9.3 3D-printed jig for use in a Wright Medical Group Prophecy Infinity total ankle arthroplasty. (Figure courtesy of Robert Anderson MD.)

dome replacements with room for an intramedullary nail which would be useful because the truss system in this case provides the benefit of being easily manufactured by 3D printing due to the complex geometry while still allowing 75% open volume to allow for bone graft incorporation.[16] In other words a 3D-printed implant can be beneficial from a manufacturing standpoint without being custom made for a patient due to the ability to manufacture complex geometry with a 3D printer easier than with standard manufacturing methods. There is at least one case report on the use of this technology as a salvage procedure in the case of talar bone loss.[17]

The custom designation of the implant rather than an "off-the-shelf" version has FDA device implications as well. In most cases today when the 3D-printed construct is used as an implant, it is used as a custom device and falls under the FDA's custom device guidelines. These FDA guidance exemption regulations are contained within 520(b) of the FD&C Act. For example, an "off-the-shelf" 3D-printed bone wedge may come in several different sizes and carry the FDA 510(k) clearance, whereas a custom device falls within a separate category.

FOOT AND ANKLE–SPECIFIC 3D PRINTING CONSIDERATIONS

There are several challenges to the application of 3D printing to foot and ankle surgery. In many areas of the body a single large bone may be the target of the application, for example the femur. In this case a CT scan may be easily converted into a surface or solid model because it is the only bone, or surface, of interest. When performed manually or even algorithmically, this may be performed with little time spent by a technician.

Furthermore, it may even be easy to quantify the deformity relative to an axis of interest. For example, relative to the long axis of the femur, a distal femoral deformity may be easily measured.

In the foot or ankle, however, rarely is a single bone or axis the target of interest. Rather, the complex anatomical relationships between bones in the foot are critical to both visualization and function and require additional effort computationally in preparing 3D prints. The sizes of bone are smaller in relationship to the spatial discretization of typical orthopedic imaging, which results in a more coarse surface models that therefore require additional postprocessing to be well suited for 3D printing. Cortices are relatively thin, and the grayscale image density of cancellous bone is difficult to distinguish algorithmically from surrounding soft tissues. Thus 3D segmentation of bony tissue in the foot can take substantial time. Consequently it remains rather uncommon to do preoperative planning for foot and ankle surgery by using 3D printing and digital reconstruction.

Another consideration is the effect of weight-bearing on the deformity and treatment. In most cases CT and MRIs of the foot or ankle are obtained with the patient non–weight-bearing. Most treatment considerations in foot and ankle surgery include the effect that weight-bearing has on the deformity. This includes most deformity conditions about the foot and ankle such as pes planovalgus, pes cavus, and fixed arthritic deformity when adjacent joint changes are of interest. A 3D print of non–weight-bearing studies may not be as clinically useful as that of other areas of the body.

The third challenge in foot and ankle surgery is that many of the common deformity conditions are driven by an imbalance in intrinsic and extrinsic muscle forces in addition to the patient's body weight. This effect, in a

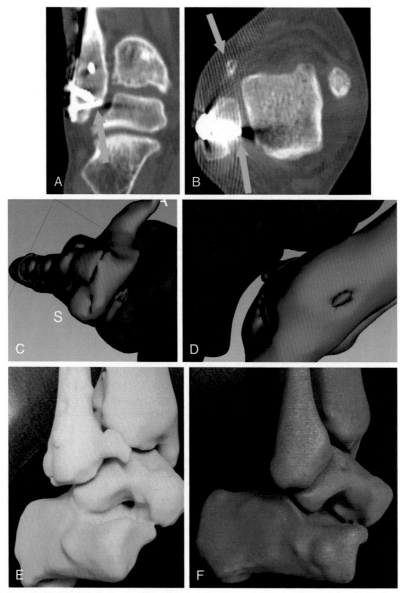

FIG. 9.4 **(A and B)** CT images of a patient with lateral ankle pain after an ORIF. Clinically the concern is for heterotopic bone and intraarticular screw positioning. **(C and D)** Images demonstrate the 3D model of the bone. **(E and F)** Images demonstrate a 3D print of the affected and mirrored contralateral side. *ORIF*, open reduction and internal fixation.

similar way to weight-bearing, should be considered in most complex foot and ankle cases. Tendon pathology and contributing force is difficult to capture with a 3D printer or imaging at this point because of the contrast difference between the bones and the tendons. Although this is an area of future research and development, it is not clear when, for the sake of ease and cost,

it is acceptable to ignore the tendons in the modeling process and when they should be included. How does the tension of the muscles and the downstream effect that muscle tension has on joint position play into the clinical scenario? For example, the clinical information gained in a non—weight-bearing 3D print of a patient with adult-acquired posterior tibial deficiency is

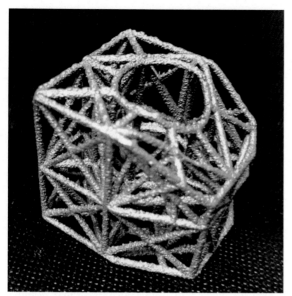

FIG. 9.5 3D-printed implantable cage made by 4WEB Medical (Frisco, Tx).

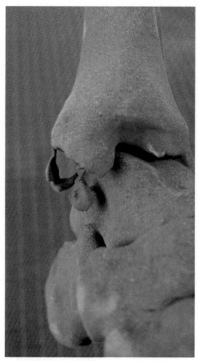

FIG. 9.6 Image of a medial malleolus nonunion 3D print demonstrating the fragile elements necessary to maintain the special relationship between the small bone fragments and the tibial bone.

much different than if that 3D print were obtained with weight-bearing and still different if it were obtained in a heel rise position. There remains a balance between the limits of 3D printing technology and the classic information surgeons use to make routine surgical decisions.

Another challenge in foot and ankle printing is the number of bones in foot and ankle applications. In the knee or hip there are commonly one or two bones of interest. In the foot and ankle there are often multiple bones that are related to the clinical concern. This difference poses a several-pronged challenge. First, from a technical standpoint, creating a single-surface model from a CT scan of the foot for example means combining the talus, calcaneus cuboid, navicular, cuneiforms, and metatarsals together into a single-surface model. At the very least the bones of clinical concern must be combined. This requires one of two things. (1) The bones must be combined into a single surface by smoothing or modifying the patient's anatomy, or (2) beams much be created between each of the bones manually, see Fig. 9.6. This has the potential to add error in the clinical scenario because the anatomy of the patient and the CT scan no longer match the anatomy of the 3D print. This process requires either manual input or a computer algorithm. It is not clear what type of ethical or liability-related implications this decision-making process presents to third parties including companies. Another challenge is that small bone fragments can be difficult to print and maintain

given the small beam elements required to attached them, see Fig. 9.7.

Furthermore, the phalanges are useful for foot and ankle complex visualization purposes but may or may not have influence on surgical planning. Therefore each 3D surface reconstruction must weigh the cost of extraction of these surfaces versus the benefit. The shear number of phalangeal bones, their relative size and relation to the ankle joint, and their position during imaging make the cost/benefit analysis difficult.

Despite the many challenges in the application of this technology, the advancements in recent years have put this technology in the hands of the masses, which means there are many people finding innovative ways to solve these problems. In this light the authors have several recommendations to the readers interested in applying this technology in their practice.

First, there are several FDA-approved 3D-printed implants and companies on the market, and the number of these will likely increase steadily. These companies are obvious partners to work with to provide improved patient care. Second, for deformity or unique cases the techniques commonly used can be performed with a

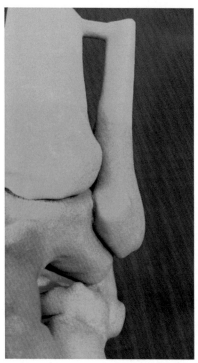

FIG. 9.7 Image of ankle 3D print demonstrating the threshold needed to combine the talus, tibia, and fibula into a single-surface model for printing. Note the beam element connecting the fibula to the talus. Also note that the ankle joint space itself becomes limited to visualization with smoothing.

standard computer, available to most surgeons and engineers. In the event that the surgeon is not proficient with these techniques or technology, we recommend contacting a nearby university with an engineering college. This technology is ubiquitous in these institutions, and most engineering colleges have the ability and generally the willingness to partner on a case-by-case basis with surgeons. Third, in an era of large capital expenditures for electronic medical record and PACS software systems, the technology required for 3D printing on a case-by-case basis is low cost. On the software side, many of the tools are freely available having been developed at universities under open-source licenses and funded through significant federal grant investment. Assuming the continued availability and expansion of those tools, marginal software costs are primarily related to the ongoing training of the software user. The technician and/or engineering time is currently the rate-limiting factor in the expanded use of 3D printing. Model creation time typically ranges

from 30 min to 10 or more hours per model depending on its complexity. Algorithmic development may reduce that cost in the future. The actual 3D printing cost is typically a small portion of the total cost. When done using an on-demand cloud-based service, the price ranges from $50–150 for a plastic model of the foot and ankle bones, depending on the scale. Additional cost may be incurred for other materials such as aluminum or stainless alloys. Another consideration for preoperative planning is that cloud services can take several days to several weeks to deliver the printed model. In-house printing, if available, can typically be done in 12–24 h but can be expected to carry additional material and other overhead costs due to the relative economies of scale.

3D printing also provides unique research opportunities in the foot and ankle setting. The technology has the capability to eliminate many obstacles faced by investigators. Primarily the technology permits the research investigator to print hardware, which would be used as implants, and/or synthetic tissue as specimens, which is otherwise difficult to obtain. While this is an obvious direct benefit of the technology, there are numerous indirect benefits, which must also be considered.

As it regards implant or surgical hardware, the creative investigator has an alternative to purchasing or seeking donation of expensive or specialized and limited-access hardware from the few manufacturers offering surgical products. Manufacturers are understandably leery that their products might be used in unexpected or unapproved ways. They are particularly concerned that their products may be shown inferior to other products. Consequently, some common challenges research studies have faced include the contractual restriction to manufacturers preapproved testing techniques, the manufacture's requirement to be able to review advanced drafts of manuscripts, and the significant delay and cost burden associated with contracts between the investigator and the manufacturer. When constraints are placed on investigator freedom, suboptimal research is a likely outcome. The investigator who can design and rapidly prototype their own hardware for use has freedom to approach research questions unencumbered by the typical risk aversion of the commercial marketplace. As a side benefit the investigator is likely to reduce their conflicts of interest.

Outside of printing hardware, 3D printing may also be used to produce synthetic tissue or other forms of synthetic specimens. Several companies are producing 3D-printed synthetic bones for use in the laboratory, and thus research may be conducted using commercial of-the-shelf specimens in place of difficult-to-obtain human or animal tissue. Perhaps more importantly an investigator can design a pathologic condition into bony or soft tissue and then test (virtually via finite element model or physically via laboratory mechanical testing) that tissue. This is a significant advantage when rare conditions are being researched or when the subjects of that research might otherwise be put at risk as a participant in an unproven trial. Furthermore, as it can reduce or eliminate the use of human tissue and the use of human subjects, 3D printing can therefore reduce or eliminate the facilities cost associated with disinfection, sterilization, or tissue disposal. Likely, the substantial burden of submitting research to institutional review boards in advance of beginning the study

can be reduced. It can further enable much broader multifactorial studies that would be too complex if they involved human subjects. Although these activities are underway in many laboratories around the country, validation of synthetic 3D-printed surrogate tissues remains an ongoing challenge. It is likely that the validity and applicability of these techniques in addition to the desire to have broad consensus on their utility will be debated for years to come.

Given the ability to avoid many of the hidden costs and time commitments which are otherwise an obstacle to research, many research questions that would have been difficult to answer a few years ago may now be easy within reach as the technology has matured and print quality has increased.

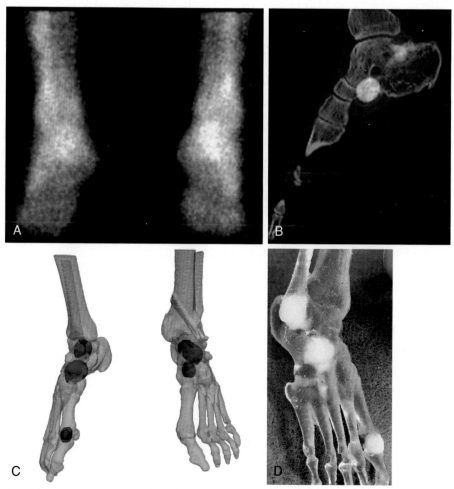

FIG. 9.8 **(A)** 3-phase bone scan. **(B)** SPECT-CT scan. **(C)** 3D model. **(D)** Multicolor 3D print of SPECT-CT scan.

INNOVATION

There are several considerations for future applications of 3D printing in foot and ankle surgery. One of these applications is multicolor printing, Fig. 9.7. This technology holds promise to improve the visualization of the contrast of biological structures such as spectrum-based imaging such as Single Photon Emission Computed Tomography merged with Computed Tomography (SPECT-CT) scans. Several things may improve the use of 3D printing in foot and ankle surgery including the increase in speed of these devices and a decrease in printer cost which will make them more common in clinical practice. Also, automation of the steps involved including software-based automation of the process between obtaining patient data and producing a printable file. This may include special CT/MRI sequences or software-based sequence combination. Although in some cases high-resolution imaging may help, the justification and cost recuperation of these sequences are unknown. To be sure, the future of 3D printing in foot and ankle surgery is bright (Fig. 9.8).

REFERENCES

1. Hull C, Inventor. *Method for Production of Three-dimensional Objects by Stereolithography*. US patent 4,575,330. 1983.
2. Kacl GM, Zanetti M, Amgwerd M, et al. Rapid prototyping (stereolithography) in the management of intra-articular calcaneal fractures. *Eur Radiol.* 1997;7(2):187–191.
3. Hurson C, Tansey A, O'Donnchadha B, Nicholson P, Rice J, McElwain J. Rapid prototyping in the assessment, classification and preoperative planning of acetabular fractures. *Injury.* 2007;38(10):1158–1162.
4. McGurk M, Amis AA, Potamianos P, Goodger NM. Rapid prototyping techniques for anatomical modelling in medicine. *Ann R Coll Surg Engl.* 1997;79(3):169–174.
5. Holubar SD, Hassinger JP, Dozois EJ, et al. Virtual pelvic anatomy and surgery simulator: an innovative tool for teaching pelvic surgical anatomy. *Stud Health Technol Inf.* 2009;142:122–124.
6. Gittard SD, Narayan RJ, Lusk J, et al. Rapid prototyping of scaphoid and lunate bones. *Biotechnol J.* 2009;4(1):129–134.
7. Ciocca L, De Crescenzio F, Fantini M, Scotti R. CAD/CAM and rapid prototyped scaffold construction for bone regenerative medicine and surgical transfer of virtual planning: a pilot study. *Comput Med Imaging Graph.* 2009;33(1):58–62.
8. Windisch G, Salaberger D, Rosmarin W, et al. A model for clubfoot based on micro-CT data. *J Anat.* 2007;210(6):761–766.
9. Guarino J, Tennyson S, McCain G, Bond L, Shea K, King H. Rapid prototyping technology for surgeries of the pediatric spine and pelvis: benefits analysis. *J Pediatr Orthop.* 2007;27(8):955–960.
10. Giovinco NA, Dunn SP, Dowling L, et al. A novel combination of printed 3-dimensional anatomic templates and computer-assisted surgical simulation for virtual preoperative planning in Charcot foot reconstruction. *J Foot Ankle Surg.* 2012;51(3):387–393.
11. Jastifer JR, Gustafson PA. Three-dimensional printing and surgical simulation for preoperative planning of deformity correction in foot and ankle surgery. *J Foot Ankle Surg.* 2017;56(1):191–195.
12. Angthong C. Anatomic total talar prosthesis replacement surgery and ankle arthroplasty: an early case series in Thailand. *Orthop Rev (Pavia).* 2014;6(3):5486.
13. Smith KE, Dupont KM, Safranski DL, et al. Use of 3D printed bone plate in novel technique to surgically correct hallux valgus Deformities. *Tech Orthop.* 2016;31(3):181–189.
14. Gustafson P, Geeslin A, Jastifer J. An open source Reverse engineering Workflow: geometry to Optimization. In: *Paper Presented at: AIAA Science and Technology Forum and Exposition.* 2016.
15. Nocerino E, Remondino F, Uccheddu F, Gallo M, Gerosa G. 3D modelling and rapid prototyping for cardiovascular surgical planning- two case studies. In: *XXIII ISPRS Congress; July 12-19, 2016; Prague, Czech Republic.* 2016.
16. Medical W. https://4webmedical.com/products/osteotomy-truss-system/.
17. Hamid KS, Parekh SG, Adams SB. Salvage of Severe foot and ankle Trauma with a 3D printed scaffold. *Foot Ankle Int.* 2016;37(4):433–439.

CHAPTER 10

3D Printing in Spine Surgery

JOHN BURLESON, MD • CHRISTIAN DIPAOLA, MD

INTRODUCTION

The implantation of spinal instrumentation remains a challenging and critical aspect of spine surgery. The advent and advancement of additive manufacturing technology over the last 30 years has shown promise in aiding surgeons with insertion of spinal instrumentation. Three-dimensional (3D) printing has also gained popularity in the development of novel spinal implants. This new technology could be used to develop personalized implant guides or other patient-specific implantable spinal instrumentation.

Conventional surgical instruments and drill guides are designed to be used many hundreds of times on a variety of patients for multiple procedures. These guides are designed to be durable and simple. The method and skill in which these tools are used however depend wholly on the surgeon and his/her training and experience. Placing pedicle screws by anatomy and feel requires significant skill but the least ancillary equipment. Inserting these screws in the cervical spine or in the setting of complex deformities may increase the risk to neurovascular structures. Placing screws by C-arm fluoroscopy aids the surgeon in visualizing the anatomy that might not be seen with surgical exposure alone. Intraoperative fluoroscopy does increase the radiation to the patient as well as the surgeon, additive over their career. X-ray imaging is not always fail-safe especially in cases of lateral imaging which can be difficult in the cervical-thoracic junction and in patients with a challenging body habitus.

Surgeons can therefore benefit from techniques that do not rely on X-ray imaging intraoperatively. Computerized tomography–guided navigation has gained popularity over the last several years in an attempt to alleviate some of these concerns. It is largely an accurate, albeit expensive, option. The downsides include the reliance on static patient positioning, the high start-up cost of the equipment, and the steep learning curve for the surgeon and staff.

While using navigation, care must be taken while cannulating the pedicle with the probe or drill. The pressure applied to the patient can cause flexing, extending, or twisting of the anatomy and can lead to inaccuracy. Because of the high cost of the equipment, smaller hospitals and practices might not be able to afford computerized navigation.

3D printing, a form of additive manufacturing, has become more popular over the last decade. This technology is not new, but it was previously very expensive to purchase printers and required extensive training to master. Increased interest outside of medicine has driven costs down. Software used with this equipment has also improved in capability and user interface. This has resulted in increased access for nonengineers and hobbyists, some of whom happened to be surgeons.

3D printing technology allows for creation of patient-specific implants and implant guides. These can be printed on an as-needed basis to fit patient-specific anatomy. Off-the-shelf implants can use 3D printing to generate specific surface coatings. These implants could also be printed as needed to cut down on inventory demands. 3D printing of patient-specific drill guides, implants, and surface coatings have already been created throughout the world with a few centers outside of the United States currently leading the way. Even with this new progress, additive manufacturing for use in the operating theater is still in its infancy.

Additive manufacturing (AM) allows for the creation of nearly anything with almost any material imaginable. Although relatively new to medicine in general and spine surgery in particular, this process has been in existence for several decades. Plastic is generally the material of choice. This has been especially true in medicine when AM is used for prototyping, surgical models, and most preoperative planning tools. Most 3D printers use either acrylonitrile butadiene styrene

(ABS), which is used to make Legos®, or polylactic acid (PLA) as their primary plastics. These come on spools with the plastic between 1.75 and 3 mm in diameter. Because of their cheap cost, both plastics are ideal for models used for operative planning. However, ABS and PLA might deform under standard autoclave pressures and temperatures.

Other plastics such as ployetherimide or polyether ether ketone (PEEK) have much higher melting points and cost and are more likely to survive an autoclave without structural damage. Newer plastics such as thermoplastic polyurethane, polyvinyl alcohol (PVA), and high-impact polystyrene (HIPS) allow for a standard printer to create a model with either elasticity or dissolvable plastic. 3D printing in metal is also an option through processes such as selective laser melting (SLM). The machines required to do this are more complex and more expensive but allow for implantable devices to be printed in titanium or similar metals. These machines can also create patient-specific porous coatings, which can be tailored for bony ingrowth.

In this chapter we will focus on three main areas of 3D printing in spine surgery:
1. Patient-specific implant guides
2. Patient-specific implants
3. 3D spine modeling for preoperative planning and education

PATIENT-SPECIFIC IMPLANT GUIDES

This section will include the design and manufacturing of patient-specific spinal implant guides. We will also include instructions in text and tables to help guide surgeons, should they desire to 3D print their own surgical guides.

The topic of 3D-printed implant guides will be divided into four sections:

1.1 Patient-specific implant guides for the cervical spine
1.2 Patient-specific implant guides for the thoracic spine
1.3 Patient-specific implant guides for the lumbar spine
1.4 Future direction of patient-specific implant guides
    3D-printed devices include implants that aid in spinal fixation and instruments that facilitate the surgical procedure. Creating the 3D models of the spine necessary for these designs requires a skill set not possessed by most surgeons. As the technology has improved, many of the more technical coding-like processes have been eliminated to make a more user-friendly experience. This will likely continue to improve as software companies compete, and interest grows.

Patient-specific drill guides of varying design have been demonstrated to be effective throughout the spine. These guides are currently being produced by both device companies and spine surgeons. Sugawara et al. and Kaneyama et al. have investigated several areas of the spine for the implementation of their process. They noted that the thoracic spine frequently presents its own unique problems associated with instrumentation. Dysplastic pedicles, deformity, and other alterations in anatomy can present challenging operations that require long operating times and an increased risk for misplaced spinal instrumentation. Dysplastic pedicles that appear too small on imaging for conventional screw fixation techniques are typically either skipped or fixed with alternative devices such as sublaminar fixation systems. Deformity that could benefit from guidance can also be present in the cervical and lumbar spine. Surgical computerized navigation has been used with some success to address this problem and does allow the surgeon the ability to visualize the start point and angle of screw insertion based on preoperative or intraoperative CT scan. Although this is helpful, it is based on an image that could be rendered inaccurate. If the patient is shifted or if the surgeon pressed down on the patient while probing the pedicle, the navigation accuracy may be affected. Every technique requires the surgeon to use multiple sources of information to assess the safety of inserting instrumentation. Patient-specific screw guide templates (SGTs) can be used as another tool to help mitigate risk in this process.

These guides can be designed and printed either by the surgeon/hospital facility or by the industry. At least one company (Medacta) already offers this commercially.[1] Several surgeons have also performed this, and many have published small case series. The processes vary by surgeon and institution, but the general process remains constant, and the early results are promising.

For the surgeon to begin the process, a preoperative CT scan of the affected area is loaded into multiplanar software (Table 10.1). This is typically loaded as a Digital Imaging and Communications in Medicine (DICOM) file which is the standard medical imaging file type in the United States. That file will then be converted to a stereolithography file by the software. Stereolithography files were originally designed for computer-aided design (CAD) software and are now a standard file format for 3D printing. Once converted to a stereolithography file, the surgeon has the ability

TABLE 10.1

This Table Gives Detailed Instructions for Creating and Printing a Pedicle Screw Drill Guide From a Patient's CT Scan in DICOM Format. This Same Technique Could be Adapted to Placing Screws Anywhere in the Spine

	First Author's Preferred Method for Printing 3D Drill Guides	
1	Download image	Images can be imported from DICOM files directly from most hospital/clinic image-viewing programs or from outside CTs. These files can be uploaded without conversion into many software programs designed to read images.
2	Configure image	My preferred software is Osirix (freeware on Mac, 3DSlicer is a similar program for PC). This "slicer" software allows for reading any type of imaging. Through this software the CT can be reformatted to show structures within a given Hounsfield range. In this case the software is configured to include only cortical bone (the surgeon can decide to include cancellous bone as well). This creates a new CT scan with all desired bone converted to white for 3D rendering, whereas all other structures are converted to black and deleted. The model created here resembles the anatomy of the bone but contains ridges or plateaus limited by the thickness of the CT slices.
3	Export new image	This image is again exported as a stereolithography file.
4	Clean up new image	I open this file in Blender (Mac/PC). Blender is another free program that helps to modify 3D files. Some of this editing can be done in Osirix or 3D slicer, but finer work is done at this stage. These 3D images are essentially made up of many thousands of triangles and a few complex polygons. To make these images more printable, Blender can convert all these into triangles. It can then "smooth" the image by converting each triangle into multiple triangles. One must keep in mind that the more smoothing might result in more esthetic but less accurate models.
5	Create drill guide	The patient-specific drill guide then needs to be created from this model. This is most easily done in 3D slicer but can be performed in many programs. First this model is saved (File 1). The painting tool can be used to add material directly behind the lamina in areas where the drill guide should exist. Small tubes of material (hollow cylinders) are then added to the model to be centered through the pedicle. This new file is then saved under a new name (File 2). Finally the original file (File 1) is then opened in the same working space. The software allows the user to convert any object into a void. This essentially gives the surgeon an eraser in the shape of the vertebrae body. This is lined up over File 2 such that it eliminates all of the original body while leaving the extra material drawn behind the lamina and the tubes sticking out of this material directed toward the pedicles. This file is then saved (File 3). It is very important not to perform any smoothing of this guide after fitting it to the vertebral body digitally.
6	Export new image	This image is again exported as a stereolithography file.
7	Prepare for printing	I use Simplify3D for print preparation. This program is not free ($150) but offers many tools that free programs do not. There are, however, many popular free alternatives such as Repetier or Cura that work well. These programs allow for scaling and orienting of the object over the digital build plate. These programs determine appropriate locations for support material (scaffolding) and allow for helpful structures such as rafts and ooze shields. Rafts help to prevent warping, and ooze shields prevent extra plastic from being extruded when printing with two different plastics. The density of the model and precision of the nozzle can also be tailored at this point. The nozzles and build plate temperatures can also be tailored. When completed, one can preview the print process in the software before exporting to the printer. This allows for circumventing problems without wasting plastic or time.
8	Export to printer	The file can then be saved on an SD card (via an SD card adapter or built-in port) and inserted into the printer. The computer can alternatively be connected directly to the printer. Once the print is initiated, the printer will run on its own until it is finished. Some printers move the build plate down away from the extruders a fraction of a millimeter at a time. Other printers raise the extruders up after each level is completed.

Continued

TABLE 10.1 This Table Gives Detailed Instructions for Creating and Printing a Pedicle Screw Drill Guide From a Patient's CT Scan in DICOM Format. This Same Technique Could be Adapted to Placing Screws Anywhere in the Spine—cont'd		
	First Author's Preferred Method for Printing 3D Drill Guides	
9	Printer specs	I use a FlashForge Creator Pro ($900) to perform my 3D printing. At the time of this publication, home 3D printers run from ~$250 to several thousand dollars. The FlashForge, similar to many modern printers, has 2 nozzles and can alternate between filaments. Although the printers will handle many plastics, I prefer to print in PLA with PVA (dissolvable filament) as part of the support structures. This allows me to place the printed model in water to dissolve away the supports after the model is complete.

DICOM, Digital Imaging and Communications in Medicine.

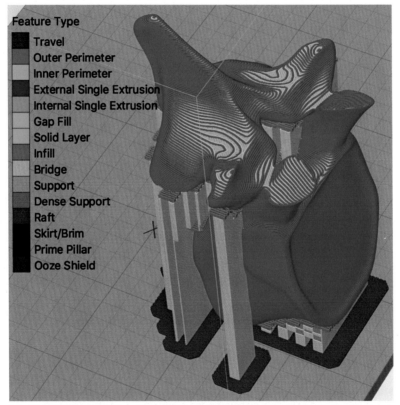

FIG. 10.1 This is a digital image created by "Simplify3D" software. The varying colors demonstrate different print processes. The support material (light gray, dark gray) and raft (purple) facilitate the printing process and are removed from the model after print completion. Image created by the first author.

to modify the CT scan, eliminate soft tissue, and determine which portions of the spine (s)he would like to work with. The surgeon can print out just a spine model, drill guides, or both. Current software, such as Simplify3D, creates support structure known as scaffolding to help facilitate the printing of these complex structures (Fig. 10.1). Scaffolds allow for overhanging pieces of plastic to be printed. Without support structures, there would be nothing for this overhanging plastic to be printed on top of when it comes time to print. This scaffolding can also protect nonvertical cannulations by supporting the "ceiling" of these tunnels.

Rafts, which are flat areas of plastic laid down around the first few layers, help to prevent warping as the plastic cools. Rafts and scaffolding are removed by hand to reveal the finished piece. Many of these pieces of extra plastic break away without difficulty. Cannulated templates or implants with complex mesh patterns can pose a problem as it is difficult to break away internal scaffolding. In situations like this, technical issues such as printing orientation become important. If the drill sleeves are oriented vertically, the printing can take place circumferentially layer by layer as opposed to printing the sleeve on its side. This eliminates the ceiling problem. For drill templates with two drill sleeves, printing in a manner such as to allow both sleeves to be as vertical as possible would likely yield the best results.

Many 3D printers today have multiple nozzles which can allow for printing in two materials. Typically the primary nozzle prints in PLA or ABS, and a second nozzle extrudes PVA or HIPS. Both PVA and HIPS can be used for the scaffolding portion of the print and can then be dissolved away in water (PVA) or D-Limonene (HIPS). This makes for a much cleaner finished product with less postproduction work required. Unfortunately the printing process can take 24+ hours to be completed on large models.

In the case of SGTs the surgeon uses the patient's digital spine model to determine an optimal screw path, start point, length, and size. As described by Sugawara[2], the software is then used to create a piece of plastic only a few millimeters thick which closely approximates the lamina and superior aspect of the spinous process base.[2] This "negative" facilitates a unique fit that should not slip when held in place and should only fit securely when held in the proper location. Small 3-mm holes are digitally created in the plastic to correspond with the start point for the pedicle screws on each side of the spine. This is done for each planned instrumented level. Then a second SGT is created to facilitate drilling of spine. These have the same flat plastic base with an added drill sleeve extending away from the start point in line with the planned screw trajectory in every plane. In this situation the screw length will be predetermined. The drill guide length can be designed to work with standard drill bits, which could allow for the surgeon to "hub" the drill. This could facilitate a quicker operation, similar to the technique used by some for lateral mass screws.[3]

Finally a third set of SGTs are created for each level. These are similar to the drill guides but instead consist of larger tunnels in which the screws themselves fit to ensure they do not deviate from the start point or predrilled path (Fig. 10.2). In this series of articles, the

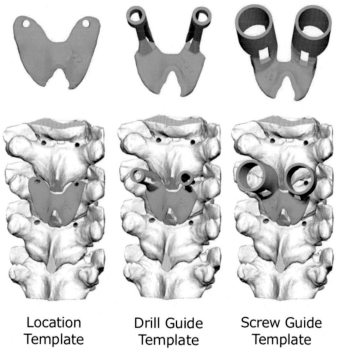

Location Template   Drill Guide Template   Screw Guide Template

FIG. 10.2 Digital representation of three-step screw guide templates (SGTs). The guides are seen in isolation in the above images, and they are positioned on the lamina in the below images. (Printed with permission from Dr. Sugawara.)

guides were held in place with the surgeons' nondominant hand while a burr was used through the start point hole, a drill was used through the drill sleeve, and a pedicle screw was placed through the screw guide. These models could be designed to allow fixation to the lamina with small screws. Although this could be done with a plastic guide, it might be more feasible with metal. Using locking screws in the SGT would help assure a completely stable guidance system.

For Sugawara's studies, two sets of the templates were produced.[2] One was used preoperatively on the spine model, and the second was saved for the operating room (OR) to be used on the patient. This allowed for the surgeon to check for any obvious errors with the template such as pedicular breaches or errors in screw length calculation. This approach could help serve as a quality control measure that could be crucial given the individual nature of these prints. Using personalized guides might help to expand a surgeon's comfort level in challenging scenarios using spinal instrumentation. One example being the potential to avoid dissecting the venous plexus when inserting C1 lateral mass screws.

This entire process is not simple to implement. Establishing a preoperative pathway for 3D modeling requires a team of people working together. All of the guides need to be correctly produced, tested, transported to the ORs, sterilized, and positioned on the correct levels for this to work properly. Some plastics might require special sterilization procedures to avoid deformity of the guide. These guides could also potentially be printed in metal, which would allow them to be sterilized similar to current drill guides. Industry might be able to help implement pathways for SGT creation for surgeons. Although this would require less surgeon involvement, it would certainly require more cost. As of now, the line between device company–led implant creation and surgeon-led operative planning has yet to be clearly defined in this field.

Cervical Spine

Instrumentation of the cervical spine can be fraught with potential complication. The anatomy is smaller than that of other regions of the spine, and neurovascular structures are closer to common and ideal screw trajectories. Lateral mass screws are commonly used in the cervical spine to lessen the risk of injury compared to pedicle screws. Unfortunately, lateral mass screws have only half the pull-out strength of cervical pedicle screws.[4]

Kaneyama attempted a three-step technique to guide cervical pedicle screw placement in C-2. Sugawara originally described this technique for thoracic pedicle screws[2] (Fig. 10.3). In this study his team successfully placed 26 pedicle screws, 12 pars screws, 6 laminar screws, and 4 C1–C2 transarticular screws. Ninety-eight percent (47/48) of the screws were found to have been placed with acceptable parameters.[5] Sugawara then studied C1–C2 fixation with the same SGT guide process. This time they placed C1 lateral mass screws and C2 pedicle or laminar screws. Their 24 C1 lateral mass screws, 20 C2 pedicle screws, and 4 C2 laminar screws were all placed without any cortical breaches.[6] This technique allowed for precise screw placement without necessitating exposure of the C2

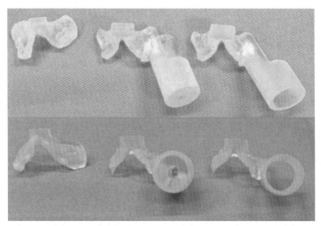

FIG. 10.3 Unilateral three-step screw guide templates (SGTs). The guide on the far left is used to determine a start point with a burr through a small, 3-mm hole. The middle guide is used to guide the drill bit, and the right guide is used to guide the screw during insertion. (Source: Kaneyama.)

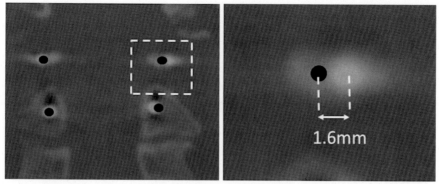

FIG. 10.4 Postoperative coronal CT scan demonstrating the deviation between the planned trajectory of the pedicle screw (*black dot*) versus the actual path of the screw (*larger white dot*). (Printed with permission from Dr. Sugawara.)

nerve root or the venous plexus. Avoiding these dangers could partly address the current surgical complication rate for atlantoaxial fusion which is ~10% with an inhospital mortality of 2.7%.[7] In these authors' hands this new technique resulted in lower blood loss, better accuracy (screw tip deviation averaged 0.7 mm) (Fig. 10.4), and decreased complication rate.

The use of 3D-printed drill guides to place pedicle screws in the subaxial cervical spine has also been studied. The pedicles of C3–C7 are much smaller than the thoracic and lumbar pedicles and are bordered anterolaterally by the vertebral foramen making screw placement challenging. Many surgeons use lateral mass screws for fixation of the subaxial cervical spine for this reason. Navigation has frequently been used to guide the placement of these screws but is subject to failure if the patient's position is altered in any way. This can lead to error in screw positioning, which is frequently unacceptable given the small window between the central canal and vertebral foramen. Insertion of subaxial pedicle screws is rarely performed and not often biomechanically necessary. Risk of injury to the vertebral artery is often not worth the reward of increased biomechanical strength that might not be clinically relevant. However, these authors did use this technique successfully to aid them in placing these screws. The authors created a three-guide system to correctly place 78 of 80 screws safely within the pedicle while the other two had acceptable minor breaches of the pedicle (Fig. 10.5). These authors opted to use 3.5-mm screws and avoid any pedicle with diameters <3.5 mm, whereas other articles preferred to instrument pedicles of smaller sizes with 2.7-mm screws.[4]

Bundoc et al. in the Philippines developed a different technique to solve the same problem. They were able to 3D print models of 5 cadaveric cervical spines. They then inserted K-wires into the pedicles of each vertebral model under direct visualization. Then they applied methylmethacrylate to the lamina encapsulating the base of the K-wire to create their guide. After this hardened, they removed the K-wire and placed the guide onto the actual cadaveric spine and drilled k-wires through the guide. They found a 94% success rate with 3 of 50 screws perforating. Although not as sophisticated as the previously described technique, it yielded similar results. In contrast, multiple articles have demonstrated traditional cervical pedicle screw insertion to be slightly less reliable at 83% –94%. Because of the variation in cervical anatomy, each patient should be individually screened for their eligibility regarding cervical pedicle screw placement. If the surgeon elects to perform this procedure, patient-specific SGTs might improve accuracy.

Thoracic Spine

There are currently fewer published studies involving SGTs of the thoracic spine. In their original article demonstrating the three-guide technique, Sugawara et al. chose to focus on the thoracic spine. They were able to successfully place all thoracic pedicle screws (58 in total) within the pedicular borders.[2] There are studies that show freehand pedicle screw placement in the thoracic spine to have breach rates of 25% –43%. The in-out-in technique, although better than no screw, is associated with ~23% decrease in pedicle screw pull-out strength.[8] Not only were these guided pedicle screws within the pedicle but on postoperative imaging they were found to have screw tips that deviated from their planned course by a mean of 0.89 mm. The authors were also able to reduce their operative time and radiation exposure compared to their prior technique.

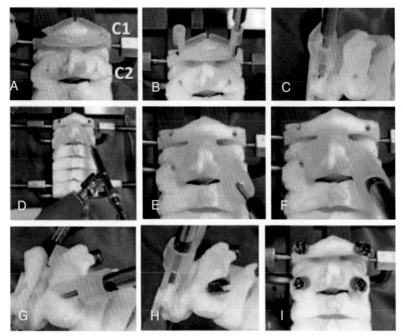

FIG. 10.5 Three-step SGTs being tested on C1–C2 in a cervical model of a patient's spine. This is performed with the first set of templates before being performed in the OR. (J.B. could possibly recreate this (SUGAWARA SPINE 2017).)

Lumbar Spine

The anatomy of the lumbar spine typically allows for a larger margin of error due to pedicular size. The application of drill template technology for traditional lumbar screw placement is debatable for more straight-forward procedures. The added time preoperatively might not result in increased screw placement precision in these cases. This process does require substantial operative planning, and current rates of pedicle breaches in the lumbar spine have been reported as low as 6%. However, there are atypical screw placement options that might benefit from patient-specific guidance.

One such option is the transpedicular transdiscal (TPTD) screw trajectory for three column fusions first introduced by Emery et al.[9] (Fig. 10.6). In this technique it is essential to keep the screws within the pedicle so that they only cross into the more cranial vertebral body after they enter the caudal vertebral body. When performed correctly, this allows the surgeon to approach the spine posteriorly, protect the neural elements, and instrument between the vertebral bodies. This technique was also shown to produce a fusion construct 1.6–1.8x stiffer than a traditional pedicle

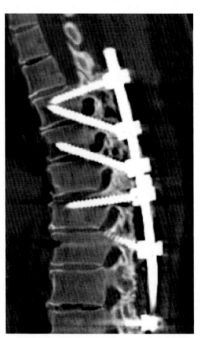

FIG. 10.6 Sagittal CT scans demonstrating transpedicular transdiscal (TPTD) technique at multiple levels combined with the traditional pedicle screw technique. (Printed with permission from Dr. EM Nottmeier.)

screw construct.[10] They also found this construct to have no difference in stiffness compared to posterior instrumentation with interbody fixation. The technical demands of this procedure as well as the use of a computerized navigation system, which comes with equipment costs and extra radiation for the patient, preclude many from adopting this technique. The ability to eliminate the need for navigation while still accurately and precisely placing these TPTD screws could lead to stiffer constructs with less expense.

Shoa et al. tested this by first printing 20 patient spines. They then created patient-specific SGTs with the goal of keeping the pedicle screws in the central axis of the pedicle (medial-lateral) while achieving maximal cranial tilt. They applied the guides to the spine models, drilled for and inserted screws, and then compared their results to their preoperative planned trajectory. They found no statistical difference between their planned trajectory and the location of their screws. Although this TPTD technique has not been demonstrated on patients at this time, SGTs could find viability in the lumbar spine for situations such as this.

Future Direction

Patient-specific SGTs provide a cost-effective alternative for precisely placing posterior spinal instrumentation. Although the advantages are largely positive, there are drawbacks to this new technology. Perhaps the largest of these is the surgical exposure requirement. For the guides to fit properly, all muscle must be removed from the lamina under the SGTs. Minimally invasive surgery including mini incision techniques and tubular retractor system would not be compatible with this technique currently. The time needed to produce the guides is also a limiting factor. The three-guide system took the authors an average of 3 days to produce. This limits their availability for trauma patients.[2,5,6,11]

There are many positive aspects of this budding technology. Small-scale printing can be quite economical. 3D printers with reasonable accuracy are available now starting around $400. The spine models themselves are also quite affordable to produce. One can print an entire cervical model, a set of C2–C6 SGTs for testing on the spine model, and a set of C2–C6 SGTs for the patient for a total of ∼$100. A 10-level thoracic spine fusion costs ∼$250 to template and test. In relation to the cost of the surgery these modeling costs are negligible. Avoiding only one revision surgery due to superior screw placement could pay for hundreds of cases to be performed with SGTs. These could also be printed by industry for the surgeons. Medacta already has an entire system designed to work with their SGTs that they produce for surgeons.[1]

One can imagine future software that might automatically create the templates on uploading of the spine CT scan. This might only require a small amount of tinkering by the surgeon, which could increase the utilization of 3D-printed surgical aids. If the surgeon only needs to confirm positioning of the screws on software and test the guides on a printed model, less computer-savvy surgeons might show interest. Streamlining the process in this way might speed up the production time allowing for use with trauma patients. As 3D printers of varying types become more ubiquitous and the software becomes more user-friendly, adoption of the technology on a large scale might be possible. As this technology is new to most and deviates from the training many surgeons received, it represents a rare opportunity to improve surgical accuracy. We envision this technology has the potential to lead to an evolution in complex spine surgery planning, templating, and execution. With the recent advances in machine learning programming, it is likely that computer programmers could implement deep learning techniques to greatly speed up the template generation process and improve accuracy with each passing case. As with many technologies, small increases in usability could result in dramatically increased adoption in the near future.

PATIENT-SPECIFIC IMPLANTS

This section will include the design and manufacturing of patient-specific spinal implant guides. This is a broad topic that will be divided into six sections:

2.1 Patient-specific cervical spine implants
2.2 Patient-specific thoracic spine implants
2.3 Patient-specific lumbar spine implants
2.4 Surface coatings
2.5 Legal and regulatory considerations
2.6 Future direction

The majority of implants used in the spine are off the shelf and adequate for most patients. One of the major advantages of posterior instrumentation of the spine lies in its modularity that has served surgeons well. Although custom implants are not necessary for most cases, they could prove invaluable to some. For the rare patient who requires more, 3D printers could be used to create patient-specific macro implants as well as carefully designed surface coatings. These implants could provide additional flanges and predesigned screw paths to allow for novel fixation. 3D printing can provide an additional avenue for the creation of these custom implants. Custom implants in the spine could also be tailored to allow for optimal bony ingrowth with patient- or anatomy-specific 3D-printed coatings. This approach has been used for years in other orthopedic situations such as to create custom cages around complex acetabular fractures. Lessons learned in those realms could guide future developments in the spine.

Additive manufacturing allows for the creation of devices that would simply not be possible to produce with traditional methods. Attempting to correct deformity via corpectomy often involves removing the most pathologic segments while the neighboring vertebrae might have slight dysplasia themselves. Because of this, standard interbody devices or cages might not always be ideal. Using available software, a surgeon could determine preoperatively exactly how much lordosis, kyphosis, or coronal angulation the implants need to have (Table 10.2). The implants could also be sized to better match the end plate size for better contact.

Cervical Spine

The use of 3D printing in custom implants in the cervical spine is found throughout the case studies in the literature. Because they are rare, it is uncommon to find an article with more than a few implants. To date, most are implants designed by device companies for the surgeon.

Mobbs et al. described their creation of a corpectomy implant for a C1–C2 chordoma.[12] Their custom implant was designed to replace the C1 and C2 vertebral bodies and fix the basion to the C3 vertebral body (Fig. 10.7). The tumor was resected via a transoral approach, and the custom implant was filled with bone matrix and fixed to the clivus and C3 vertebral body. At 9-month follow-up, flexion and extension radiographs showed no instability, and it was believed to be a fusion (Fig. 10.8). A similar case study was performed by Mao K et al. who demonstrated their ability to 3D print an implant for a patient with a metastatic C1–C4 thyroid papillary carcinoma.[13] They planned on resecting the anterior portion of the C1 ring, making traditional reconstruction options extremely limited. Their implant was made with titanium powder with a large pore size to facilitate bony ingrowth. They printed a total of 32 implants to account for varying resection sizes with the goal being solid fixation into the atlas and vertebral body of C4. The large number of options was particularly useful given the need for an anterior implant that could be fixed into a partially resected C1. Postoperatively the patient improved from a JOA score (Japanese Orthopedic Association scoring system for upper and lower extremity function) of 11/17 to 16/17 and had a stable implant at 1 year.

Thoracic Spine

Wen Jie Choy et al. published their results in the thoracic spine. They printed a custom vertebral body corpectomy implant for a patient with a T9 primary bone tumor causing sagittal and coronal deformity.[14] Their implant was also printed in titanium as a ring complete with porous coated endplates and fixation holes for pedicle screws (Fig. 10.9). This allowed for sagittal and coronal correction as well as planned fixation between a vertebral body implant and the posterior pedicle screw construct not typically available. The surgeons placed the corpectomy cage and fixed it posteriorly with pedicle screws. This created a very rigid 360-degree construct without requiring a plate to keep that cage in place. The surgeons noted a decreased operative time compared with a traditional corpectomy procedure due to the implant being premade (Fig. 10.10). This operative time savings could be critical for patients with tumors who frequently require long cases with potentially high blood loss.

Lumbar Spine

Mobbs et al. 3D printed an L5 interbody implant for a patient suffering from back pain due to his/her L5 superior endplate hemivertebrae causing focal kyphosis.[12] They chose to create this implant in titanium to assure the strength necessary at L4-L5 junction (Fig. 10.11). The implant was designed as a ring structure with a built-in 6 degrees of lordosis. The surface of the metal has a lattice pattern that allows for some ingrowth and creates a modulus similar to bone. This was tested first on a 3D-printed model of the patient's spine and then implanted via a standard anterior approach to the lumbar spine with an anterior plate. Postoperative CT scan demonstrated correction of the lordosis as well as solid fusion (Fig. 10.12). In doing this, they demonstrated a model for predictably correcting relative lumbar kyphosis with extreme accuracy.

Manufacture of custom implants is clearly not a high-volume business. Conventional manufacturing techniques have likely made this less financially feasible due to the time, machinery, and tooling required. However, the process of 3D printing is an ideal manufacturing method to create rapid custom implants. In complex cases involving tumors or deformity this additional technology offers expanded options for reconstruction. These expanded reconstruction options may help save operative time and lead to improved reconstructive stability.

Surface Coating

Creating the optimal pore size of manufactured graft surfaces for bone ingrowth has been an area of interest

TABLE 10.2

This Table Gives Detailed Instructions for Creating and Printing Surgeon-Designed Implants. These Could be Prototype Implants or Implants Designed to be Placed in Patients. (Implants for Patients Would Require the Proper Plastic Such as PEEK etc. as Well as Approval From the Proper Regulatory Groups

		First Author's Preferred Method for Designing & Printing Implants
1	Create design on paper	I typically begin the process by sketching out the planned implant. Drawing the implant from as many perspectives as possible makes 3D design easier.
2	Create digital design	Creation of a 3D model can seem daunting to a novice. It is not necessary to have special training to operate most of this computer-aided design (CAD) software. I prefer TinkerCad for design. This is a free, web-based software package that works on Mac and PC. Digital design is based in the idea of combining polygons to create the object desired. For instance, two spheres could be placed on the end of a cylinder and then "combined" to form one object resembling a dumbbell. Object can also be made to be "void." Making an object a void essentially creates an eraser in the shape of that object. Placing a "void" cylinder through a cube will create a tunnel in the cube once the objects are combined. By using this basic principle many times, surgeons can create complex implant or instrument designs complete with multiple or even moving parts. If the surgeon is creating a patient-specific implant, they can import the patient's anatomy (saved stereolithography file – see Table 3) and use the bony architecture as a void. This basic concept will create an implant that fits perfectly. This process would best be suited for implant prototyping although it would be possible to print an implant in a material like PEEK or titanium that could then be implanted directly.
3	Review design	The design can be viewed from every angle in this CAD software. Device measurements can be tweaked, and pieces can be assembled digitally before printing.
4	Export file	The file is then exported as a stereolithography file.
5	Prepare for printing	I use Simplify3D for print preparation. This program is not free ($150) but offers many tools that free programs do not. There are, however, many popular free alternatives such as Repetier or Cura that work well. These programs allow for scaling and orienting of the object over the digital build plate. These programs determine appropriate locations for support material (scaffolding) and allow for helpful structures such as rafts and ooze shields. Rafts help to prevent warping, and ooze shields prevent extra plastic from being extruded when printing with two different plastics. The density of the model and precision of the nozzle can also be tailored at this point. The nozzles and build plate temperatures can also be tailored. The surgeon can also configure the printer to print one object at a time in instances where the device contains multiple parts. When completed, one can preview the print process in the software before exporting to the printer. This allows for circumventing problems without wasting plastic or time.
6	Export to printer	The file can then be saved on an SD card and inserted into the printer, or the computer can be connected directly to the printer. Once the print is initiated, the printer will run on its own until it is finished. Some printers move the build plate down away from the extruders a fraction of a millimeter at a time. Other printers raise the extruders up after each level is completed.
7	Printer specs	I use a FlashForge Creator Pro ($900) to perform my 3D printing. At the time of this publication, home 3D printers run from ~$250 to several thousand dollars. The FlashForge, like many modern printers, has 2 nozzles and can alternate between filaments. Although the printers will handle many plastics, I prefer to print in PLA with PVA (dissolvable filament) as part of the support structures. This allows me to place the printed model in water to dissolve away the supports after the model is complete.

and continued development in orthopedics for years. Titanium plasma spray (TPS) is an industry standard of surface coatings for bone ingrowth. This process involves spraying titanium onto an otherwise-finished implant. It creates a mean pore size of approximately 140 μm.

Selective laser melting (SLM) is an AM process that can achieve varying pore sizes. Macbarb et al. printed a mean pore size of 290 μm. This very closely approximates that of a cancellous bone.[15,16] 3D-printed surface, unlike TPS, can be tailored to the specific goal of the implant. There is good evidence demonstrating

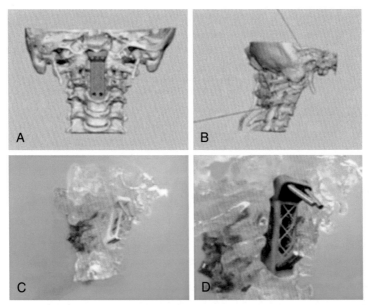

FIG. 10.7 **(A** and **B)** Preoperative digital rendering of occiput to C3 custom interbody implant. **(C** and **D)** Photograph of the implant fixed to a 3D-printed model of the patient's cervical spine.

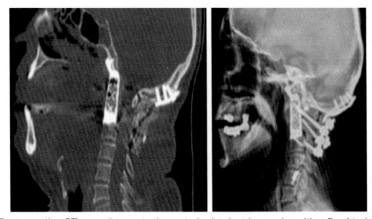

FIG. 10.8 Postoperative CT scan demonstrating anterior implant in good position fixed to basion and C3. Posterior instrumentation was also performed.

that pore sizes between 200 and 400 allow for greater bony ingrowth. The TPS coating process allows for the covering of surfaces with additional metal. It is not used to create the superstructure of implants. The pore size associated with TPS is also not as close to that of the cancellous bone as 3D printing is capable of producing.[17] AM also allows for a lower contact angle between the bone and the implant. This leads to a more hydrophilic surface that facilitates osteoblastic bone generation. This surface has been shown to outperform TPS coating with or without a hydroxyapatite coating by demonstrating increased bony ingrowth and increased cell count through the first 2 weeks after implantation. At 3 weeks the AM interface has also been found to have 43%−48% more calcium production than a TPS coat depending on whether hydroxyapatite was used.[15,16] Theoretically any interbody or corpectomy implant could be capped off with an endplate that has this custom porous coating. Interbody or corpectomy implants 3D printed with an appropriate porosity

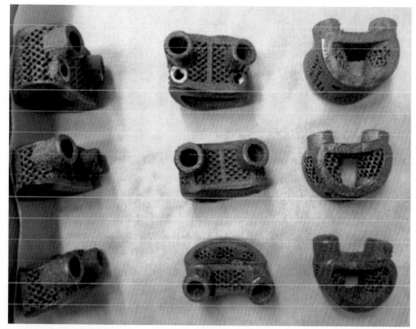

FIG. 10.9 Photograph of nine titanium vertebral models of varying sizes printed for a T9 tumor. Duplicates were also created in case a contamination occurred during the operation.

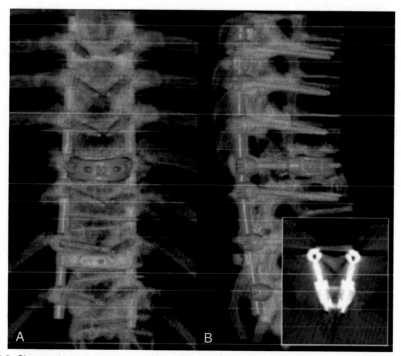

FIG. 10.10 Six-month postoperative colorized CT scan showing alignment of implants with the posterior construct maintaining fixation to the anterior custom implant.

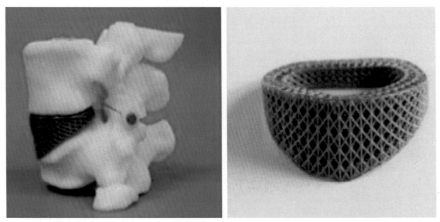

FIG. 10.11 Photograph of the custom-printed titanium mesh interbody cage for L5-L5. Left shows implant positioned in a 3D model of the patient's L4 and L5 vertebral bodies. Right shows the model up close to demonstrate the lattice nature of the implant.

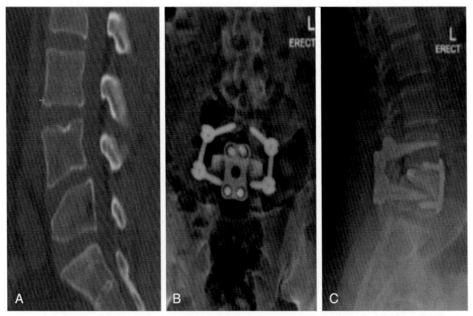

FIG. 10.12 Preoperative and postoperative imaging of the custom-printed titanium interbody implant for L5 hemivertebrae. **(A)** Sagittal CT scan demonstrating preoperative defect superiorly in L5. **(B)** Postoperative X-ray demonstrating anterior and posterior hardware in good position. **(C)** Postoperative lateral X-Ray demonstrating hardware in good position with correction of the defect and the local kyphotic deformity.

(and therefore customizable modulus) would theoretically not only have better bony integration but would likely experience less stress shielding. Off-the-shelf (or non–patient-specific) implants could also be produced with this method. Interbody devices or cages could be produced in standard sizes with custom coatings or varying metal densities throughout.

Legal and Regulatory Considerations

The FDA has recently offered guidance with regard to AM in medicine. The FDA released "Technical Considerations for Additive Manufactured Medical Devices" in December 2017 to address concerns for providers participating in implant and instrumentation design and manufacturing.[18] This guide discusses many topics over 31 pages. A few important points are as follows:

- Patient-specific guides or templates do not qualify as "custom devices" as far as the FDA defines custom. Therefore these devices are not subject to the custom device exemptions.
- Surgeons should be certain of the accuracy demanded of their imaging technology for any given process. If software is used to "smooth" an image and a guide is made from this image, it might not fit real anatomy as well. File conversion can also degrade final product accuracy.
- Many software programs associated with this entire process are internet based or managed by smaller companies. The FDA notes that care must be taken with internet security as private patient information is often involved.
- AM layer by layer frequently results in products that are not anisotropic. Layers can delaminate under stress while orthogonal stress to the build direction might fare better. This should be considered if stress will be imparted on the printed object.
- The process to produce an implant or implant guide must be standardized. The material should be unexpired material used in the correct conditions with the same postprocessing process used every time. Manufacturers must document their procedures and assure the constant achievement of their standard. There are several separate FDA guidelines in place to follow for validation of process.
- If there are any changes to the process used to create these products, the entire process must be revalidated.
- The FDA recommends preforming acceptance activities to test final products. Some options include ultrasound, CT scans, dye penetration, and X-ray. These are not suitable for all materials but can help evaluate for uniformity between prints. Care should be taken to make sure that everything is otherwise kept the same, even small details including location of the print on the build plate.

As surgeons and industry advance their technology, the regulation of patient-specific implants will continue to evolve. Having a framework from the FDA is helpful for individual surgeons who wish to create a 3D printing pathway at their institution. Surgeons interested in 3D printing should seek to be involved at local and national level to help sculpt the regulations in the future as they will undoubtedly become more specific.

Future Direction
Suboptimal access to 3D printing equipment and lack of understanding of clinically relevant applications currently limit the usage of 3D printing in spine surgery. Although prices for the machines required to 3D print on a small scale have dropped significantly, larger machines still remain somewhat expensive. Most private practice surgeons do not own the printers, and many academic surgeons are not using their university's printers. Current lack of familiarity with the software is also an issue. As software improves and these pathways are created, it might be easier to order patient-specific implants based on the surgeon's preferences. Software could be created which allows the surgeon to request a specific lordotic correction, implant height, and/or modulus etc. However, much remains to be determined regarding the regulatory environment of manufacturing implants as the technology becomes more accessible to nontraditional surgical technology developers. Most companies' offerings are still in their infancy in terms of usability and come with a steep learning curve. Mass adoption is likely dependent on either the CAD of implants or the creation of efficient production pathways to avoid unnecessary use of surgeons' time.

3D PRINTING FOR PREOPERATIVE PLANNING AND EDUCATION
As residency work hours have changed in recent years, surgeons at academic institutions are burdened with educating young surgeons with less operative time. Simulated surgery can give trainees more exposure to some of the procedures they might not be able to experience with the current 80-h limit. Simulated surgery might also allow junior residents to gain exposure in a practice setting before they operate on real patients Junior residents stand to gain even more understanding of special anatomy given their limited clinical exposure to complex injuries such as acetabular and calcaneus fractures. The same could be said for residency programs that lack exposure to some injuries or procedures. Nontrauma centers could print models of a rare complex fracture to give the experience to more residents. Residents could learn to do complex spinal procedures, such as osteotomies, on models before performing on patients. This might allow surgeons to feel more comfortable with resident participation during these rarer cases. The models could also be taken into the OR in a sterile bag to aid the surgeons in orienting themselves during surgery. Models that meet this demand are currently quite expensive. 3D printing models as needed could both lower costs and allow surgeons to print models pertaining to the topic being discussed (Table 10.3).

Outside of spine surgery, printing models for medical education has already proven to be helpful.

TABLE 10.3
This Table Gives Detailed Instructions for Creating and Printing a 3D Model of a Patient's Spine From a CT Scan in DICOM Format (the Most Common Format Used in Hospital PACS Systems)

	First Author's Preferred Method for Printing 3D Models	
1	Download image	Images can be imported from DICOM files directly from most hospital/clinic image-viewing programs or from outside CTs. These files can be uploaded without conversion into many software programs designed to read images.
2	Configure image	My preferred software is Osirix (freeware on mac, 3DSlicer is a similar program for PC). This "slicer" software allows for reading any type of imaging. Through this software the CT can be reformatted to show structures within a given Hounsfield range. In this case the software is configured to include only cortical bone (the surgeon can decide to include cancellous bone as well). This creates a new CT scan with all desired bone converted to white for 3D rendering, whereas all other structures are converted to black and deleted. The model created here resembles the anatomy of the bone but contains ridges or plateaus limited by the thickness of the CT slices.
3	Export new image	This new CT scan is then exported as a stereolithography file.
4	Clean up new image	I open this file in Blender. Blender is another free program that helps to modify 3D files. Some of this editing can be done in Osirix or 3D slicer, but finer work is done at this stage. These 3D images are essentially made up of many thousands of triangles and a few complex polygons. To make these images more printable, Blender can convert these all into triangles. It can then "smooth" the image by converting each triangle into multiple triangles. One must keep in mind that the more smoothing might result in more esthetic but less accurate models.
5	Export new image	This image is again exported as a stereolithography file.
6	Prepare for printing	I use Simplify3D for print preparation. This program is not free ($150) but offers many tools that free programs do not. There are, however, many popular free alternatives such as Repetier or Cura that work well. These programs allow for scaling and orienting of the object over the digital build plate. These programs determine appropriate locations for support material (scaffolding) and allow for helpful structures such as rafts and ooze shields. Rafts help to prevent warping, and ooze shields prevent extra plastic from being extruded when printing with two different plastics. The density of the model and precision of the nozzle can also be tailored at this point. The nozzles and build plate temperatures can also be tailored. When completed, one can preview the print process in the software before exporting to the printer. This allows for circumventing problems without wasting plastic or time.
7	Export to printer	The file can then be saved on an SD card (via an SD card adapter or built-in port) and inserted into the printer. The computer can alternatively be connected directly to the printer. Once the print is initiated, the printer will run on its own until it is finished. Some printers move the build plate down away from the extruders a fraction of a millimeter at a time. Other printers raise the extruders up after each level is completed.
8	Printer specs	I use a FlashForge Creator Pro ($900) to perform my 3D printing. At the time of this publication, home 3D printers run from ~ $250 to several thousand dollars. The FlashForge, like many modern printers, has 2 nozzles and can alternate between filaments. Although the printers will handle many plastics, I prefer to print in PLA with PVA (dissolvable filament) as part of the support structures. This allows me to place the printed model in water to dissolve away the supports after the model is complete.

DICOM, Digital Imaging and Communications in Medicine; *PACS*, picture archiving and communication system.

By printing with flexible filament in addition to harder plastics, medical schools have created intubation models for students and residents to use for practice.[19] This created a life-like model with soft tissues analogs as well as bony anatomy. 3D-printed acetabular fractures have also been used to help residents better understand the complex nature and classification of those injuries. Only a small number of the models were printed. They contained enough detail to determine fracture patterns, and the cost was only $100-$200 per model.[20]

3D-printed models have also been evaluated against CT scans and digital reconstructions for their ability to convey anatomical special relationships. These 3D models were found to increase the surgeons' understanding of shape, scale, and anatomy versus digital imaging.[21]

By 3D printing different patient's spines, trainees could gain experience instrumenting patients with all types of anatomy. This could improve their understanding of the spatial relationship between elements of the bony anatomy. It is feasible to create an entire intern/junior resident curriculum around surgical modeling. Taking deformity models into the OR could prove helpful even for the most experienced of surgeons, let alone the residents and fellows. Many surgeons in the United States are already doing this today. Sterile X-ray bags contain 3D-printed models that can be referenced during instrumentation of challenging anatomic locations. Creating training models for education on a large scale might require the endorsement of a device company, orthopedic organization, or research grant but could improve the standardization of orthopedic and neurosurgical resident education.

CONCLUSION

AM in medicine is an emerging field with vast possibility. Although the course of budding technologies is often difficult to predict, 3D printing costs are dropping, software is becoming easier to use, and surgeon familiarity with the concept is increasing. With the growing concern of cost containment in medicine, AM might gain a foothold in areas where technologies such as surgical navigation are currently being used. Some aspects of 3D printing appear to be more ready for mass adoption than others. Drill guides have been shown to be reliable on cadaveric models and are cheap to produce. These could feasibly be produced by surgeons in the near future. Device companies have been producing custom implants for years and are likely to retain that business. 3D printing will allow them to offer surgeons more options.

There is a large amount of excitement around 3D printing in orthopedics, and only time will tell if this will be a passing fad or a major component of our operative processes in the future. Future research will need to include more case studies to expand our understanding of what is possible and randomized trials to ground those possibilities. Through these future studies we will learn whether SGTs, custom implants, 3D-printed surfaces, and preoperative modeling can actually save time and reduce morbidity associated with spine surgery on a large scale. Conventional means

for achieving our goals in surgery will likely continue to be the standard. However, if research shows over time that 3D printing implant guides and implants do improve overall outcomes or decrease cost, spine surgery could look very different over the next few decades.

REFERENCES

1. Putzier M, Strube P, Cecchinato R, Lamartina C, Hoff EK. A new navigational tool for pedicle screw placement in patients with severe scoliosis: a pilot study to prove feasibility, accuracy, and identify operative challenges. *Clin Spine Surg.* 2017;30(4):E439. https://doi.org/10.1097/BSD.0000000000000220.
2. Sugawara T, Higashiyama N, Kaneyama S, et al. Multistep pedicle screw insertion procedure with patient-specific lamina fit-and-lock templates for the thoracic spine: clinical article. *J Neurosurg Spine.* 2013;19(2):185−190. https://doi.org/10.3171/2013.4.SPINE121059.
3. Jeanneret B, Magerl F. Primary posterior fusion C1/2 in odontoid fractures: indications, technique, and results of transarticular screw fixation. *J Spinal Disord.* 1992;5(4): 464−475.
4. Jones EL, Heller JG, Silcox DH, Hutton WC. Cervical pedicle screws versus lateral mass screws. Anatomic feasibility and biomechanical comparison. *Spine.* 1997;22(9): 977−982.
5. Kaneyama S, Sugawara T, Sumi M, Higashiyama N, Takabatake M, Mizoi K. A novel screw guiding method with a screw guide template system for posterior C-2 fixation: clinical article. *J Neurosurg Spine.* 2014;21(2): 231−238. https://doi.org/10.3171/2014.3.SPINE13730.
6. Sugawara T, Higashiyama N, Kaneyama S, Sumi M. Accurate and simple screw insertion procedure with patient-specific screw guide templates for posterior C1-C2 fixation. *Spine.* 2017;42(6):E346. https://doi.org/10.1097/BRS.00000000000001807.
7. Derman PB, Lampe LP, Lyman S, et al. Atlantoaxial fusion: sixteen years of epidemiology, indications, and complications in New York state. *Spine.* 2016;41(20):1586−1592. https://doi.org/10.1097/BRS.0000000000001603.
8. Li N, He D, Xing Y, Lv Y, Tian W. The effect of lateral wall perforation on screw pull-out strength: a cadaveric study. *J Orthop Surg Res.* 2015;10:6. https://doi.org/10.1186/s13018-015-0157-0.
9. Abdu WA, Wilber RG, Emery SE. Pedicular transvertebral screw fixation of the lumbosacral spine in spondylolisthesis. A new technique for stabilization. *Spine.* 1994;19(6): 710−715.
10. Minamide A, Akamaru T, Yoon ST, Tamaki T, Rhee JM, Hutton WC. Transdiscal L5-S1 screws for the fixation of isthmic spondylolisthesis: a biomechanical evaluation. *J Spinal Disord Tech.* 2003;16(2):144−149.
11. Kaneyama S, Sugawara T, Sumi M. Safe and accurate midcervical pedicle screw insertion procedure with the patient-specific screw guide template system. *Spine.* 2015; 40(6):341. https://doi.org/10.1097/BRS.0000000000000772.

12. Mobbs RJ, Coughlan M, Thompson R, Sutterlin CE, Phan K. The utility of 3D printing for surgical planning and patient-specific implant design for complex spinal pathologies: case report. *J Neurosurg Spine.* 2017;26(4): 513–518. https://doi.org/10.3171/2016.9.SPINE16371.

13. Li X, Wang Y, Zhao Y, Liu J, Xiao S, Mao K. Multi level 3D printing implant for reconstruction cervical spine with metastatic papillary thyroid carcinoma. *Spine.* 2017; 42(22):1326–1330. PMID: 28498291.

14. Choy WJ, Mobbs RJ, Wilcox B, Phan S, Phan K, Sutterlin CE. Reconstruction of thoracic spine using a personalized 3D-printed vertebral body in adolescent with T9 primary bone tumor. *World Neurosurg.* 2017;105: 1032. e17. https://doi.org/10.1016/j.wneu.2017.05.133.

15. MacBarb RF, Lindsey DP, Bahney CS, Woods SA, Wolfe ML, Yerby SA. Fortifying the bone-implant interface part 1: an in vitro evaluation of 3D-printed and TPS porous surfaces. *Int J Spine Surg.* 2017;11:15. https:// doi.org/10.14444/4015.

16. MacBarb RF, Lindsey DP, Woods SA, Lalor PA, Gundanna MI, Yerby SA. Fortifying the bone-implant interface part 2: an in vivo evaluation of 3D-printed and TPS-coated triangular implants. *Int J Spine Surg.* 2017;11: 16. https://doi.org/10.14444/4016.

17. Karageorgiou V, Kaplan D. Porosity of 3D biomaterial scaffolds and osteogenesis. *Biomaterials.* 2005;26(27): 5474–5491. https://doi.org/10.1016/j.biomaterials.2005. 02.002.

18. *Technical Considerations for Additive Manufactured Medical Devices.* United States Food and Drug Administration; 2017.

19. Smith ML, Jones JFX. Dual-extrusion 3D printing of anatomical models for education. *Anat Sci Educ.* 2018; 11(1):65–72. https://doi.org/10.1002/ase.1730.

20. Manganaro MS, Morag Y, Weadock WJ, Yablon CM, Gaetke-Udager K, Stein EB. Creating three-dimensional printed models of acetabular fractures for use as educational tools. *Radiographics.* 2017;37(3):871–880. https:// doi.org/10.1148/rg.2017160129.

21. Cromeens BP, Ray WC, Hoehne B, Abayneh F, Adler B, Besner GE. Facilitating surgeon understanding of complex anatomy using a three-dimensional printed model. *J Surg Res.* 2017;216:18–25. https://doi.org/10.1016/ j.jss.2017.04.003.

FURTHER READING

1. Kim B, Hong K, Park K, Park D, Chung Y, Kang S. Customized cranioplasty implants using three-dimensional printers and polymethyl-methacrylate casting. *J Korean Neurosurg Soc.* 2012;52(6):541–546. https://doi.org/10.3340/jkns. 2012.52.6.541.

CHAPTER 11

Pediatric Hip and Acetabulum

BRIAN M. HAUS, MD

Hip preservation surgery encompasses a heterogenous group of procedures aimed at preventing arthritis in young patients with complex femoral and acetabular deformities. Periacetabular osteotomy (PAO) is performed to correct acetabular deficiencies in patients with hip dysplasia and acetabular retroversion. Open surgical dislocation and proximal femoral rotational osteotomies are performed to correct complex deformities of the proximal femur in patients with slipped capital femoral epiphysis (SCFE) and Legg-Calve-Perthes disease. For these procedures, preoperative and intraoperative decision-making is based on assessment and measurements taken from radiographs and intraoperative fluoroscopy. However, despite the importance of radiographs in guiding surgical management, radiographs have limited reliability.[1]

Through computer-aided design, advanced imaging from CT scans can be used to create 3D models of patient anatomy to assist in surgery and to help educate patients preoperatively.[2] Because the success of hip preservation surgery depends on accurate restoration of a congruent joint without impingement or instability,[3-5] 3D modeling and printing offer significant advantages in improving the assessment of patient-specific deformities relative to radiographs.

Preoperative planning for all patients begins with routine pelvic radiographs including anteroposterior (AP), abduction internal rotation, false profile, and bilateral Dunn lateral views. A pelvic CT scan of the pelvis with 3D reformatting is also obtained, including single-slice cuts through the distal femur to assess femoral version. The Digital Imaging and Communications in Medicine data from the 3D CT scan can then be uploaded to commercially available software (Materialise, Leuven, Belgium), (Xilloc, Gilleen, Netherlands) (PolyJet, Stratasys, Eden Praire, MN). The computer modeling software is then used to simulate patient-specific osteotomies of the proximal femur and acetabulum and to virtually reorient the osteotomies around the joint to maximize joint congruity. The dynamic computer interface provides the ability to simulate dynamic motion by facilitating virtual

movement of the femur through expected range of motion before and after the osteotomy. As such, potential impingement and instability can be assessed dynamically, as well as changes in the final range of motion.

Once the osteotomy plans are finalized, a model of the pelvis is 3D printed. The model is then sterilized for use in the surgical field, where it can be placed directly next to the patient. With the 3D model in close proximity, one or more osteotomies are performed, and the rotation and orientation of the planned correction is mimicked on the patient. Currently, custom-printed cutting guides are not used because of the overlying iliopsoas muscle and hip capsule make access to the ischium and pubis difficult. Fluoroscopic images are taken in standard fashion to confirm ideal correction after the osteotomy, and if there is agreement, the osteotomy is stabilized on the patient.

Because of our experience with the reliability of the 3D-printed models in predicting a surgical plan, we now use them for preoperative planning for all complex hip and acetabular osteotomies. Three cases are briefly summarized in the following to illustrate their use in surgical planning in patients with hip dysplasia, SCFE, and Perthes Disease.

HIP DYSPLASIA

Adolescent patients with hip dysplasia have poor anterior and lateral acetabular coverage of the femoral head. The etiology of the undercoverage can be associated with multiple deformities about the hip including acetabular dysplasia, excessive acetabular anteversion or retroversion, excessive lateralization of the femoral head in the joint, or excessive anteversion of the femoral neck. Symptomatic patients are candidates for acetabular correction with a periacetabular osteotomy (PAO), a procedure that allows reorientation of the acetabulum to improve femoral head coverage after four osteotomy cuts are made.

Accordingly, the goals of a PAO are to increase anterior and lateral femoral head coverage while correcting

3D Printing in Orthopaedic Surgery. https://doi.org/10.1016/B978-0-323-58118-9.00011-7

the acetabular version and to medialize the joint space while maximizing joint congruity. These goals are achieved by using traditional radiographs and intraoperative fluoroscopy to correct deficient hip dysplasia measurements to normalized hip measurements. The goal of a PAO is therefore to normalize the lateral center edge angle (LCEA; normal >25 degrees), the femoral head extrusion index (FHEI; normal >79), the medial joint space (normal < 10 mm) measured on the AP view, and the anterior center edge angle (ACEA; normal >20 degrees) measured on the false profile view (Fig. 11.1). The anteversion of the acetabulum is corrected so that the relationship of the projection of the crossover of the anterior and posterior wall lies over the superolateral femoral head on the AP view when the coccyx is 2 cm from the pubic symphysis and the obturator foramen are symmetric (Fig. 11.1).

One of the challenges of treating hip dysplasia using traditional radiographs is identifying the proper amount and orientation of acetabular correction with a PAO. Because radiographs and intraoperative fluoroscopy have been shown to have limited reliability in measuring LCEA, ACEA, and acetabular anteversion,[1] the amount and orientation of the correction performed during surgery may be inappropriate. Undercorrection of the acetabulum may cause persistent instability, and overcorrection can create impingement. As both scenarios can cause poor outcomes,[3–5] it is essential to achieve the proper amount of correction in each plane for every patient. Additionally, it can be difficult preoperatively to determine whether or not an acetabular-sided osteotomy alone is sufficient enough to achieve adequate femoral head coverage and medialization of the joint or whether or not a femoral-sided correction is also needed to achieve these goals. Computer modeling and 3D-printed models offer an effective strategy to plan for these challenges preoperatively.

With this technology, it is possible to use the 3D computer modeling to more accurately predict the appropriate amount of correction for each patient. Each of the deficient hip measurements can first be measured, and the PAO can then be modeled to correct them to normal values. The 3D computer modeling allows the acetabulum to be dynamically rotated in multiple planes similar to what is accomplished during surgery to improve anterior and lateral coverage and acetabular anteversion (Fig. 11.2). Once the version, the LCEA, and the ACEA are normalized, the FHEI and medial joint space can be measured to determine if there is adequate medialization of the joint space and femoral head coverage. If the medial joint space

remains greater than 10 mm and/or there is an FHEI of greater than 79 degrees after a modeled PAO, then a femoral varus intertrochanteric osteotomy (ITO) can be modeled to help medialize the joint and improve femoral head coverage (Fig. 11.3C). Use in the sterile field is especially advantageous as the distance and orientation of the acetabular correction on the model can be directly compared to the patient's intraoperative correction (Fig. 11.4).

A case example of a 16-year-old female with a painful bilateral, right greater than left, hip dysplasia is presented. She was diagnosed with bilateral developmental dysplasia of the hip (DDH) at 13 months and underwent bilateral adductor tenotomy, closed reduction, and spica casting. She later developed worsening right hip pain at age 14 and became wheelchair bound. Her examination demonstrated bilateral hip pain with flexion/internal rotation and extension. Her range of motion showed bilateral femoral anteversion with 80 degrees of prone internal rotation. Her radiographs and CT scan demonstrated severe bilateral hip dysplasia with excessive lateralization of the joint and markedly inadequate lateral and anterior coverage of the femoral head (Fig. 11.2). Additionally, her CT scan showed femoral anteversion of 35 degrees. An MRI showed a labral tear on the right, but not the left hip.

Using computer modeling, the 3D pelvis was placed in the standard position for assessing acetabular version and femoral coverage on radiographs—an AP position with the obturator foramen symmetric and the coccyx 2 cm from the public symphysis. A simulated PAO was first performed on the left to determine if adequate correction and maintenance of joint congruity could be achieved with an acetabular-sided correction alone.[3] (Fig. 11.3A and B). The four osteotomy cuts of the PAO were then simulated and the acetabulum rotated to normalize the LCEA, ACEA, FHEI, acetabular version, lateralized hip center, and joint congruency. The PAO was then similarly modeled on the right hip. When this was attempted, it was determined that although the LCEA and ACEA were corrected to 32 and 25 degrees, respectively, the hip center remained greater than 10 mm lateralized[6] (Fig. 11.3C). Given this, the decision was made to improve femoral head medialization, joint congruity, and femoral head coverage by performing a concomitant femoral-sided correction with a varus derotational ITO (Fig. 11.3C). Computer modeling allowed derotation of 15 degrees and coronal (varus) correction of 20 degrees, from 150 to 135 degrees. Once this was attained, a PAO was again modeled to achieve a congruent joint with an LCEA and an ACEA greater than 30 degrees, a medialized hip center of

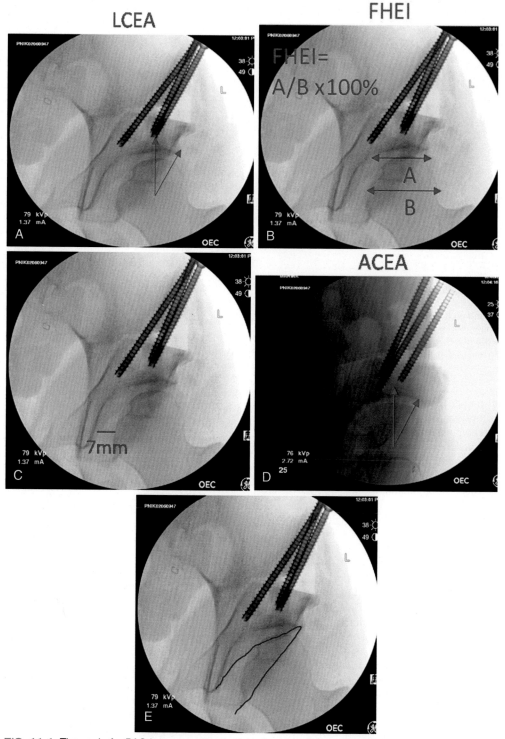

FIG. 11.1 The goal of a PAO is to normalize the lateral center edge angle (LCEA) to less than 25 degrees (11.1A), the femoral head extrusion index (FHEI) to greater than 79 (11.1B), and the medial joint space to less than 10 mm (11.1C), as measured on the AP view. On the false profile view, the goal is to correct the anterior center edge angle (ACEA) to greater than 20 degrees (11.1D). The anteversion of the acetabulum is corrected so that the relationship of the projection of the crossover of the anterior and posterior wall lies over the superolateral femoral headon the AP view when the coccyx is 2 cm from the pubic symphysis and the obturator foramen are symmetric (11.1E).

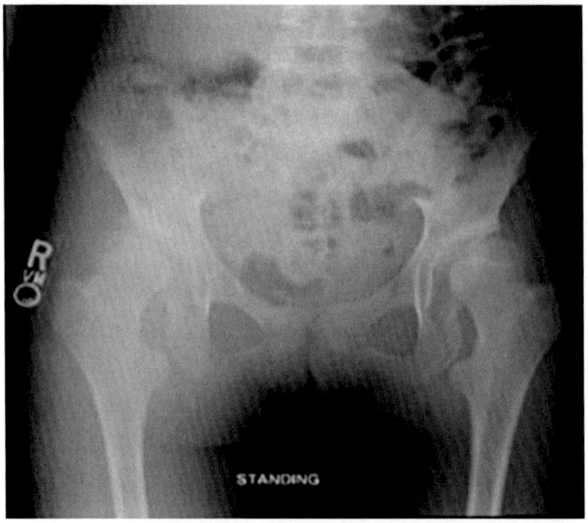

FIG. 11.2 **Hip Dysplasia.** The patient was a 16-year-old female with bilateral hip dysplasia with right hip LCEA of −5 degrees and an ACEA of −2 degrees, an FHEI of 48 and lateralized hip center of 16 mm, and a left hip LCEA of 2 degrees, ACEA of 5 degrees, an FHEI of 55 and lateralized hip center of 5 mm, with bilateral femoral neck shaft angles of 145 degrees.

5 mm, and proper acetabular anteversion without crossover or impingement (Fig. 11.3C). Once the simulated PAO was completed, the distance and orientation from the displaced acetabulum to the adjacent ilium were measured in multiple planes to determine the degree of correction for later use on the patient. A 3D model was then printed and sterilized for use (Fig. 11.4A and B).

Her hip surgeries were staged, with the right side performed first. Because of her labral tear, she first underwent a right hip arthroscopy and labral repair. An ITO was then performed before the PAO. The ITO was performed as planned, adding in 15 degrees of varus and 15 degrees of derotation. Using the same technique described by Ganz[3], the periacetabular osteotomy was then performed. With the acetabulum adequately mobilized, the 3D-printed model was placed next to the patient and the acetabulum was medialized, rotated, and anteverted using the model as a guide. The orientation and distance of the acetabulum relative to the ilium was then matched to the model (Fig. 11.4C). One year later, after recovering from the PAO on the right, she had a PAO on her left side. As planned by the computer modeling, an acetabular-only-sided correction was performed, and the PAO achieved an LCEA of 32 degrees, an ACEA of 25 degrees, and an FHEI of 82 degrees with the medial joint space at 5 mm (Fig. 11.5).

SLIPPED CAPITAL FEMORAL EPIPHYSIS

Patients with SCFE are treated with in situ fixation to prevent further slippage of the physis relative to the femoral neck. Although the physis is stabilized with surgery, patients maintain a residual prominence of the femoral head-neck metaphysis which can cause femoroacetabular impingement. In addition to impingement, the metaphyseal prominence can also cause acetabular inclusion, during which the deformity pathologically enters the joint with hip flexion and causes tears of the labrum and cartilage. Owing to the complexity of the 3D anatomy of the proximal femoral metaphysis, it can be difficult to determine which surgical option is best for each patient. Options for management include traditional methods such as flexion valgus internal rotation osteotomy or a Southwick[8]/Imhauser[7]-type osteotomy, which aims to restore anatomy by redirecting the metaphyseal prominence away from the joint to prevent impingement, but not resecting it. More modern techniques, such as an open surgical dislocation or hip arthroscopy and femoroplasty, aim to decrease impingement and inclusion by resecting the prominence, but not redirecting it. Because the ideal treatment for post-SCFE deformity is not well established, it can be difficult to determine which procedure, or combination of procedures, is best used to restore the proximal femoral morphology and eliminate impingement for patients with varied deformities. Radiographs and static CT scans offer limited information in understanding the dynamic pathoanatomy of a deformity. An advantage of computer modeling is that it offers the capability of applying 3D visualization and dynamic modeling to SCFE deformity with different techniques applied preoperatively. From this, it can be determined that patients with mild anterolateral dynamic impingement could be treated with an arthroscopic femoroplasty, whereas those with more global dynamic impingement may require a more invasive open surgical dislocation to perform the femoroplasty. Similarly, for others it can be determined that their dynamic deformity is best treated with a sliding flexion valgus internal rotation osteotomy, in conjunction with an antecedent femoroplasty performed via hip arthroscopy. In this way, computer modeling allows deformity-specific dynamic correction individualized for each patient with SCFE. Once the planned 3D-printed model is printed out, it is helpful to perform dynamic flexion, abduction, and internal rotation to evaluate the accuracy of the preoperative plan. In addition, the availability of the model on the sterile field facilitates direct visualization of the orientation of

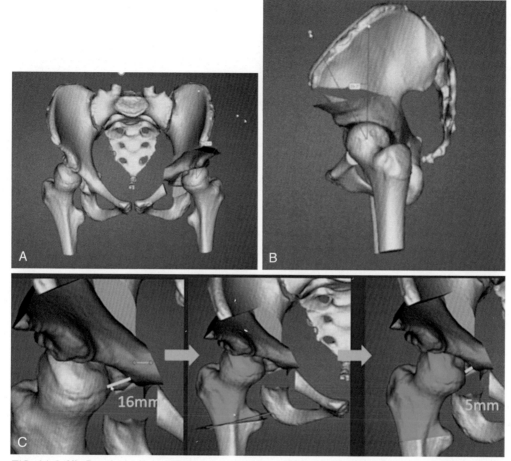

FIG. 11.3 **Hip Dysplasia. (A** and **B)** 3D computer modeling allowed simulation of patient-specific correction with a proximal femoral ITO and a PAO to achieve a congruent joint with an LCEA and an ACEA of greater than 30 degrees, a medialized hip center of 5 mm, and a femoral neck angle of 135 degrees on the left. **(C)** On the right, when an acetabular-only-sided correction was simulated with a PAO, the joint remained lateralized more than 10 mm. A femoral varus internal rotation ITO was then simulated to help medialize the joint and improve joint congruity.

proximal and distal fragments of the femur while completing the flexion/valgus osteotomy.

A case example of a 13-year-old female who presented with a chief complaint of bilateral hip pain, right greater than left, is presented. At age 9 she underwent left in situ pinning for SCFE, and then at age 10 she had the same procedure on the right. She had the screws removed 1 year later. Unfortunately her pain worsened, and she developed a limp 2 years later. Her examination showed limited flexion to 90 degrees, abduction to 15 degrees, and external rotation of −10 degrees. She had pain with flexion/internal rotation and flexion/abduction. Her radiographs showed severe

post-SCFE deformity with coxa vara and a large metaphyseal Cam deformity. Her CT scan showed femoral neck retroversion of −20 degrees (Fig. 11.6). An MR arthrogram showed a labral tear with chondrolabral separation.

For preoperative planning we aimed to eliminate the impingement and inclusion of the deformity and to correct the femoral retroversion. We first used 3D modeling to determine the morphology of the metaphyseal CAM deformity in dynamic flexion, rotation, and abduction. From this modeling we determined that the CAM deformity was focally anterior and anterolateral and could be addressed with hip arthroscopy,

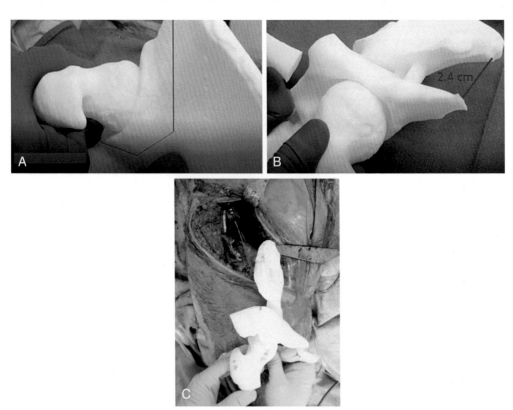

FIG. 11.4 **Hip Dysplasia. (A–C)** Use in the sterile field allowed for direct comparison of the distance and orientation of the acetabular correction on the model to the patient's intraoperative correction.

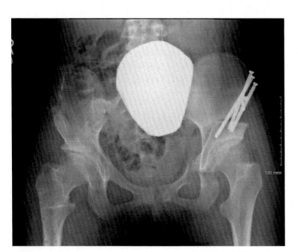

FIG. 11.5 **Hip Dysplasia.** Final radiographs confirm normalization of the LCEA, ACEA, FHEI, and medial joint space after emulating on the patient the same the preoperative plan from 3D models with left PAO and right PAO and ITO.

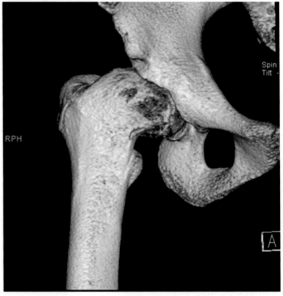

FIG. 11.6 **Slipped Capital Femoral Epiphysis.** The patient was a 13-year-old female with post-SCFE deformity with coxa vara, a metaphyseal CAM deformity, and femoral neck retroversion of −20 degrees.

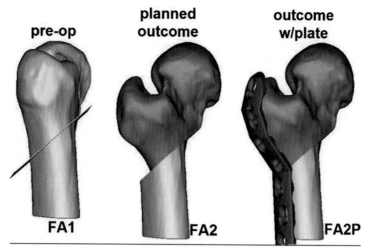

pre-op **planned outcome** **outcome w/plate**

FA1 **FA2** **FA2P**

FIG. 11.7 **Slipped Capital Femoral Epiphysis.** 3D computer modeling allowed patient-specific correction by dynamically simulating an osteochondroplasty by hip arthoscopy followed by a sliding flexion valgus osteotomy to eliminate proximal femoral impingement and inclusion.

rather than a more invasive open surgical dislocation that is used for more global deformities. Once this was performed, the computer modeling was then used to model the appropriate amount of correction in multiple planes by simulating an intertrochanteric flexion-valgus internal rotation osteotomy and then testing for improved flexion, rotation, and abduction. Multiple variations were modeled including various[7,8] sliding osteotomies[9] to determine the best correction to limit impingement and restore anatomy. A deformity-specific sliding oblique osteotomy demonstrated the best correction, and a computer-generated, simulated plate was applied (Fig. 11.7). From this, a printed 3D model with a simulated plate was printed with the same specifications (Fig. 11.8). The actual surgical plate was then bent preoperatively to match the contour of the 3D model and sterilized for surgery.

At the time of surgery an arthroscopic femoroplasty and labral repair were performed. Then the sterilized model was used as a guide to mark the oblique osteotomy along the lateral aspect of the proximal femur just distal to the lesser trochanter. The distal segment was then laterally mobilized, flexed, and internally rotated to match the 3D model. It was stabilized using the prebent 8-hole plate (Fig. 11.8). Preoperative range of motion was flexion to 90 degrees, with no internal rotation. After the correction we were able to flex her to 110 degrees and internally rotate 30 degrees (Fig. 11.9).

AVASCULAR NECROSIS/PERTHES WITH HIP DYSPLASIA

Because femoral deformities associated with Perthes or avascular necrosis (AVN) are among the most complex of the adolescent hip disorders to treat, 3D computer modeling offers perhaps the greatest potential benefit in improving deformity-specific preoperative planning. One challenge in performing an accurate femoroplasty and relative head-neck lengthening via a surgical dislocation is understanding how to remove enough bone to eliminate intraarticular and extraarticular impingement without removing too much bone and creating instability. Preoperative dynamic simulation in flexion, abduction, and rotation using computer modeling helps to predict how to best balance these opposing surgical goals. With concomitant acetabular dysplasia, there is an even greater risk of creating instability, and a pelvic osteotomy is often also required. However, in the setting of an irregularly shaped head, changing the orientation of the acetabulum to improve coverage may create a less congruent joint, increased contact stresses, and possibly increased risk of progression to osteoarthritis. With dynamic computer modeling the potential for a congruent joint with varied surgical modifications can be modeled. The printed 3D models from this preoperative planning improves intraoperative decision-making because the final printed product is life-sized, and therefore the extent of the femoroplasty and orientation of the PAO can be emulated on the patient.

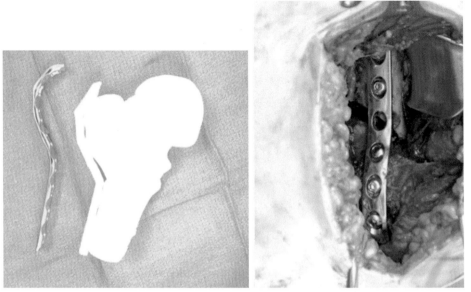

FIG. 11.8 **Slipped Capital Femoral Epiphysis.** Intraoperative use allowed for direct comparison of the orientation of the femoral osteotomy and plate fixation on the model with the patient's intraoperative correction.

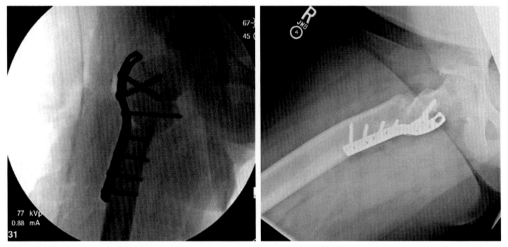

FIG. 11.9 **Slipped Capital Femoral Epiphysis.** Final radiographs confirm elimination of the metaphyseal prominence and impingement after execution of the preoperative plan on the patient.

A case example of a 15-year-old female with a history of left-sided DDH is presented (Fig. 11.10). She was treated with a closed reduction and spica at 6 months of age. She subsequently developed AVN/Perthes-type deformity of the femoral head, which was treated conservatively. She was later referred to our clinic after she developed a year of progressive hip pain and a limp.

Her examination demonstrated left-sided flexion to 110 degrees and internal rotation to 30 degrees, but limited and severely painful external rotation and abduction to 10 degrees. She had a Trendelenburg gait and abductor fatigue. Her radiographs demonstrated severe acetabular hip dysplasia with an ovoid femoral head, a shortened femoral neck, and trochanteric overgrowth.

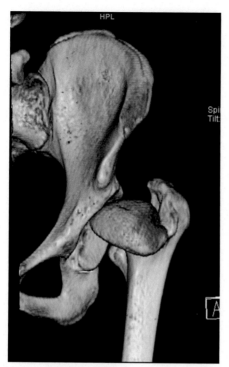

FIG. 11.10 Avascular Necrosis/Perthes with Hip Dysplasia. The patient was a 15-year-old female with instability and joint incongruity associated with a history of hip dysplasia and avascular necrosis.

Flexion and abduction radiographs demonstrated CAM-type femoroacetabular impingement and trochanteric extraarticular impingement (Fig. 11.3A). MR arthrogram demonstrated acetabular chondrolabral separation.

3D computer modeling was performed to determine if a stable and congruent joint could be achieved by performing an open surgical dislocation and relative head neck lengthening followed by a PAO. First, impingement was simulated by dynamically flexing, abducting, and rotating the hip (Fig. 11.11B). The morphology of the CAM lesion at the head-neck junction was identified, and an adequate femoroplasty was simulated to eliminate intraarticular impingement. Then a trochanteric osteotomy and relative head neck lengthening were simulated to eliminate extraarticular impingement. After these corrections a PAO was modeled with simulated anterior, lateral, and version corrections (Fig. 11.11C). The 3D modeling simulation also predicted that undercorrection of the pelvic osteotomy would cause instability, whereas overcorrection would cause incongruity of the joint and impingement (Fig. 11.12). Once the acetabular fragment was virtually

mobilized into a position that provided a stable, congruent joint with adequate coverage but without impingement, the 3D model was printed for use in the operating room (Fig. 11.11D).

At the time of surgery a surgical hip dislocation was performed, and the 3D model was used intraoperatively to guide the extent of the femoroplasty and relative head neck lengthening. The model was used to avoid excessive resection, thereby preventing instability or AVN. Subsequently the PAO was performed, and the 3D model was placed next to the patient to guide the proper correction of the acetabular fragment by matching the distance and orientation of the proximal fragment relative to the distal fragment between the model and the patient (Fig. 11.11E). The final range of motion demonstrated 120 degrees of flexion, 50 degrees of internal/external rotation, and 45 degrees of abduction (Figs. 11.13 and 11.14).

Comparison of Planned and Executed Osteotomies

We recently investigated whether 3D modeling and intraoperatively printed models reliably create a reproducible surgical plan to obtain predetermined parameters of correction[9]. In a series of 10 patients undergoing PAO, we demonstrated that there was no significant difference between measurements of LCEA, ACEA, and FHEI taken on the 3D-modeled hips and on postcorrection radiographs of the patients (data submitted for publication). In addition to demonstrating the reliability of this technique, we also determined that the 3D models reliably predict whether or not a concomitant femoral osteotomy is needed to achieve adequate femoral coverage and medialization of the joint. The study demonstrates the nascent advantages of the technology and demonstrates the ability for 3D modeling and printing to accurately predict postoperative hip coverage parameters in PAO (Fig. 11.15).

DISCUSSION

The complexity of hip preservation surgery demands significant preoperative planning given the diversity of treatment options. Computer modeling and 3D printing provide a tangible portrayal of patient anatomy as well as facilitating simulated reconstructions and instrumentation to best determine the surgical technique. The use of these models, when sterilized on the field, helps to verify the anatomy and provide a patient-specific guide. As the indications for hip preservation surgery evolve, so should the technologies used to perform them. Computer modeling and 3D printers have the

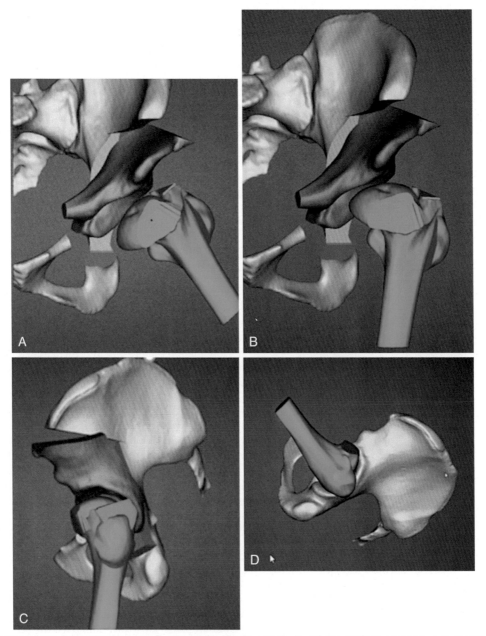

FIG. 11.11 **Avascular Necrosis/Perthes with Hip Dysplasia. (A–D)** The PAO was simulated to improve anterior and lateral coverage and joint stability while maintaining acetabular anteversion and maximizing joint congruency in all ranges of motion. Dynamic flexion, abduction, and rotation was simulated to guide the extent of the head neck osteochondroplasty and the relative head neck lengthening with the goal of eliminating inclusion and intraarticular and extraarticular impingement, as well as maximizing range of motion.

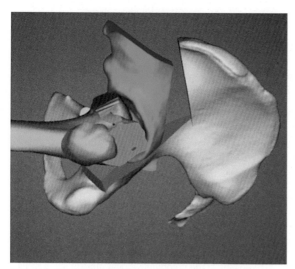

FIG. 11.12 **Avascular Necrosis/Perthes with Hip Dysplasia.** Overcoverage is simulated with computer modeling to show worsening joint congruency and increased impingement.

potential of evolving the indications of hip preservation surgical techniques by providing 3D dynamic modeling, patient-specific correction, and accessibility in the sterile field.

Although the aforementioned case examples demonstrate the nascent advantages of this technology, there are several limitations to the widespread use of the 3D models. Further studies need to be conducted to better understand the reliability of making acetabular measurements from the 3D computer model in comparison to well-established measurements on radiographs. Additionally, how well these models are size matched to the patient needs to be further investigated, as well as how any variability would affect the evaluation and measurements of the acetabulum and the femur. Finally, these studies need to be performed on an adequate number of patients to achieve statistical significance. Nevertheless, given the advantages we have witnessed to date, we believe these techniques will eventually be shown to decrease the steep learning curve of these procedures and improve patient outcomes.

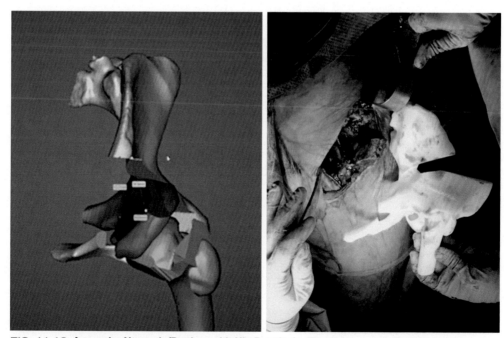

FIG. 11.13 **Avascular Necrosis/Perthes with Hip Dysplasia.** The distance and orientation of the acetabular correction on the model can be directly compared to the patient's intraoperative correction to complete the preoperative plan.

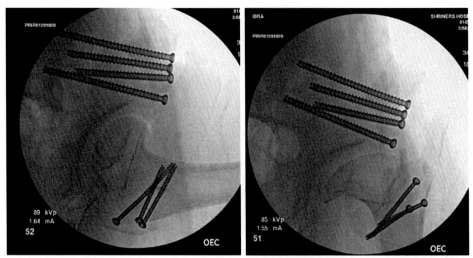

FIG. 11.14 **Avascular Necrosis/Perthes with Hip Dysplasia.** By following the preoperative plan, the patient underwent an open surgical dislocation, osteochondroplasty, relative head neck lengthening, trochanteric distalization, followed by a PAO. Final fluoroscopic views showing improved acetabular coverage in the setting of improved joint congruity with elimination of impingement.

Patients	Pre-op LCEA	Pre-op ACEA	Pre-op FHEI	3D Model LCEA	3D Model ACEA	3D Model FHEI	Post-op LCEA	Post-op ACEA	Post-op FHEI
Patient 1	40°	45°	100	32°	27°	80	26°	30°	83
Patient 2	-9°	-13°	46	32°	25°	85	31°	30°	80
Patient 3	12°	-4°	64	30°	27°	86	30°	29°	82
Patient 4	-10°	-9°	48	31°	30°	82	30°	29°	83
Patient 5	-16°	0°	47	30°	25°	85	28°	31°	83
Patient 6	-4°	-5°	50	29°	27°	84	29°	23°	90
Patient 7	-12°	-18°	46	26°	25°	85	28°	24°	80
Patient 8	8°	-10°	51	30°	25°	87	27°	25°	90
Patient 9	4°	14°	52	32°	35°	86	27°	30°	90
Patient 10	4°	-6°	49	30°	29°	85	27°	34°	83

FIG. 11.15 A table showing comparison of preoperative and postoperative LCEA, ACEA, and FHEI in 10 patients who underwent PAO using 3D modeling and printing. The 3D modeling—simulated LCEA was, on average, within 2 degrees (range 0—6) of postoperative LCEA. The 3D modeling—simulated ACEA was within a mean of 3 degrees (range 1—6) of postoperative ACEA. The 3D modeling—simulated FHEI was within a mean of 4 degrees (range 1—6) of postoperative FHEI.

REFERENCES

1. Clohisy JC, Carlisle JC, Trousdale R, et al. Radiographic evaluation of the hip has limited reliability. *Clin Orthop Relat Res.* 2009;467:666—675.
2. Eltorai AE, Nguyen E, Daniels AH. Three-dimensional printing in orthopedic surgery. *Orthopedics.* 2015;38(11):684—687.
3. Siebenrock KA, Scholl E, Lottenbach M, Ganz R. Bernese periacetabular osteotomy. *Clin Orthop Relat Res.* 1999;363:9—20. https://doi.org/10.1097/00003086-199906000-00003.
4. Steppacher SD, Tannast M, Ganz R, Siebenrock KA. Mean 20-year followup of Bernese periacetabular osteotomy. *Clin Orthop Relat Res.* 2008;466:1633—1644.
5. Matheney T, Kim YJ, Zurakowski D, Matero C, Millis M. Intermediate to long-term results following the bernese periacetabular osteotomy and predictors of clinical outcome: surgical technique. *J Bone Joint Surg Am.* 2010;92(suppl 1 pt. 2):115—129. https://doi.org/10.2106/JBJS.J.00646.
6. Clohisy JC, Carlisle JC, Beaule PE, et al. A systematic approach to the plain radiographic evaluation of the young adult hip. *J Bone Joint Surg Am.* 2008;90(suppl 4):47—66.

7. Imhauser G. Pathogenesis and therapy of hip dislocation in youth. *Z Orthop Ihre Grenzgeb*. 1956;88:3–41.
8. Southwick WO. Osteotomy through the lesser trochanter for slipped capital femoral epiphysis. *J Bone Joint Surg*. 1967;49A:807–835.
9. Monazzam S, Calafi A, Leshikar H, Haus BM. 3D modeling with intraoperative 3D printed models predict postoperative hip coverage parameters in periacetabular osteotomy (PAO). In: *Presented at AAOS 2018 Annual Meeting, March 6, 2018, Submitted to Hip International*. December 2017.

CHAPTER 12

Pediatric Spine and Extremity

LAWRENCE I. KARLIN, MD • ANDREA S. BAUER, MD

INTRODUCTION

Patient-specific anatomic models produced through three-dimensional (3D) printing are especially helpful for the accurate analysis required for planning and performing orthopedic surgery in the pediatric population. Although there is a dramatic size difference between children, a greater challenge to sufficient understanding of the anatomy is the analysis of the highly variable and unpredictable developmental and congenital deformities. In these cases the models are a single study that provides true to size visualization of the anatomy from all perspectives and offers the opportunity to simulate surgical procedures. We have used these models in spinal and extremity surgery when confronted with complex deformities. They are used preoperatively for the planning of osteotomies, the determination of instrumentation size and placement, the customization of implants, and the creation of guides for use during surgery. In the operating room, they are used as a reference for instrumentation implantation and have minimized or eliminated the need for intraoperative imaging or additional dissection for improved visualization. Less time is spent on intraoperative decision-making.

COMPLEX SPINAL DEFORMITIES ASSOCIATED WITH MYELOMENINGOCELE

Our experience with 3D models in the planning and performance of spinal deformity surgery in children with myelomeningocele serves as an ideal example of the benefits of this technique. These deformities arguably pose the greatest challenge of spinal deformity surgery. In addition to the medical comorbidities, there are unique technical obstacles: the bony elements are, to a variable and unpredictable degree, both dysraphic and dysplastic, the deformities can be developmental, congenital, or a combination of the two, and the overlying soft tissue is deficient. While third generation instrumentation has addressed the difficulty of treating the dysraphic spine, the complication rates for failure of

fixation, instrumentation prominence and soft tissue ulceration, and pseudarthrosis in the era of segmental instrumentation are reported as high as 89% and are certainly related to pathologic anatomy.[1–10] The goal is to anticipate these problems and take measures to avoid them. For this purpose, 3D models are invaluable because they provide an instantaneous depiction of all the anatomic relationships needed to determine the appropriate strategies.

The models clearly demonstrate congenital deformities that are not easily appreciated on standard two-dimensional imaging and allow for the planning of osteotomies or resections required to obtain sufficient spinal mobility. The models display the segmental anatomy so that instrumentation can be placed to maximize the purchase at each level. At the same time, they clearly demonstrate the intersegmental relationships to allow, where possible, the positioning of the entry points and orientation of the anchors to provide low profile instrumentation which is oriented harmoniously to minimize the stresses placed during rod placement or deformity corrective maneuvers. To provide stable constructs with minimal prominence, the surgeons are able to choose from standard techniques, modify those techniques, or innovate new techniques. Since the models are an accurate representation of the size of the spinal elements, the size of the hooks or pedicle screws can be determined, and in many cases the rods contoured prior to the surgery. A time-consuming intraoperative process is avoided. The following cases performed on children with myelomeningocele provide examples of ways in which 3D models improved our surgical outcomes.

Neuromuscular and Congenital Scoliosis

This young girl had a rapidly progressive scoliosis (Fig. 12.1A). The 3D model clearly showed an unsegmented bar that was not appreciated on the official interpretations of the plain radiographs or computed tomography (CT) scans at the apex of the deformity

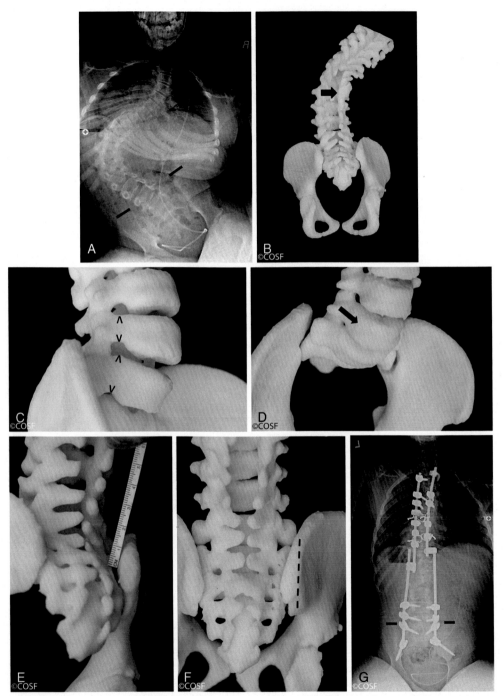

FIG. 12.1 This 11 year old skeletally immature girl with myelomeningocele has rapidly progressive scoliosis and pelvic obliquity. (A) The sitting upright a/p radiograph. (B) An unsegmented bar at the apex of the deformity (arrow). (C,D) The lumbar and sacral pedicles are sufficiently large to allow the surgeon to vary the entry points and orientations of the screws to maintain low profile instrumentation. (E,F) The pelvic relationships permit a low profile construct without the need for the bulk of a transverse connector. (G) The co-linear alignment of the anchors in each limb of the deformity allows the surgeon to easily engage each rod. The deformity is corrected with a cantilever technique after the stresses produced by the manipulation have been distributed over multiple segments. (Reprinted with permission Wolters Kluwer Health, Inc.)

(Fig. 12.1B). The bone stock in the lumbar, sacral, and iliac area was sufficient for conventional lumbosacral fixation using first sacral (S1) pedicle and iliac screws[11,12] (Fig. 12.1C and D). In myelomeningocele patients the sacral deficiency and iliac anatomy usually preclude the use of the sacral alar iliac technique.[13] Based on an analysis of the lumbar pedicle heights, widths, and angulations, as well as the sacral and iliac dimensions and relationships, a stable and nonprominent instrumentation sequence was designed. The S1 area was sufficiently covered by the iliac crest to protect an S1 pedicle screw (Fig. 12.1E). By making a vertical cut in the ilium and countersinking its entry, the iliac

screw was similarly low profile (Fig. 12.1F). The lumbar and S1 pedicles were of sufficient size and angulation to permit enough variation in the pedicle screw placement to create a colinear orientation which allowed us to easily engage the precontoured rods without stress on the individual anchors or the use of bulky transverse connectors (Fig. 12.1G).

Congenital Kyphosis

This 7-year-old child had recurrent ulceration over the gibbus and poor sitting balance (Fig. 12.2A). A growth preserving procedure was planned. The deformity was corrected by several pedicle subtraction osteotomies

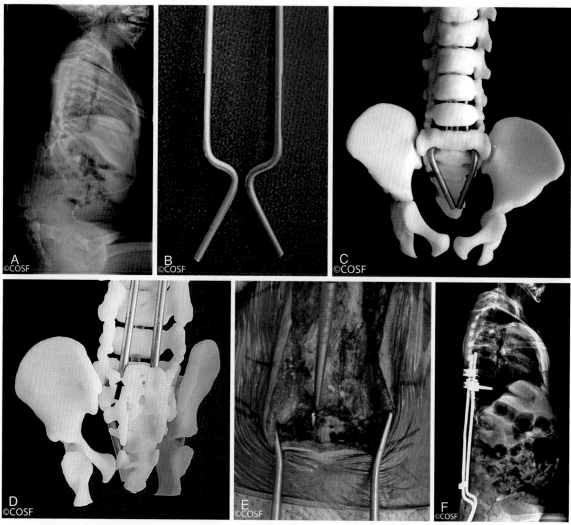

FIG. 12.2 Congential kyphosis. (A)The sitting upright lateral radiograph. (B,C) The implants are custom contoured on the models. (D,E) An anatomic irregularity (arrow) noted on the model was used as a reference for the S1 neural foramen. The same irregularity was verified at the time of surgery. (F) The lateral radiograph after surgery. (reprinted with permission, Wolters Kluwer Health, Inc.)

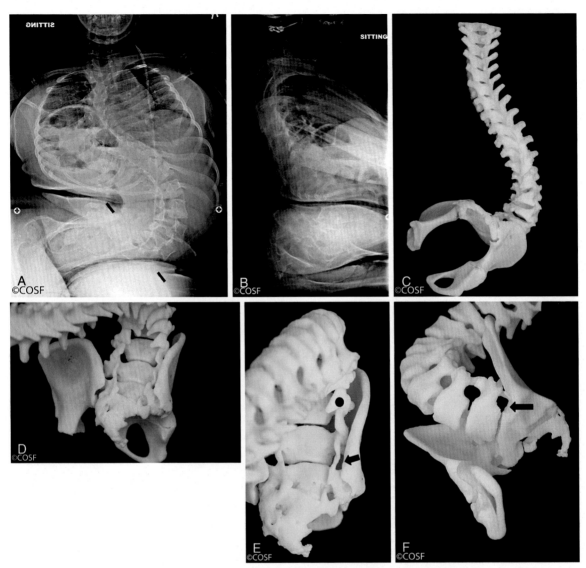

FIG. 12.3 A 13 year old girl with dramatic rotatory deformity and pelvic asymmetry. (A,B) The sitting upright radiographs. (C,D)The 3-D model demonstrates the rotational deformity and asymmetry of the pelvis. The right ilium is markedly rotated and the ischium is near the midline. (E,F) The most secure anatomic area for the right pelvic anchors were the S1 pedicle and the S2 neural foramen. A sacral construct of pedicle screw and lamina hook was innovated. The hook size was measured on the model prior to the surgery.

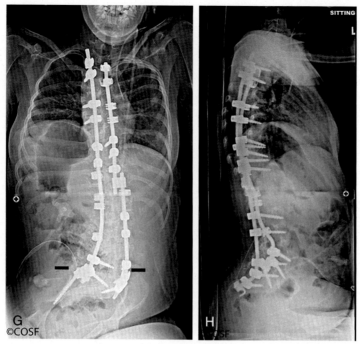

FIG. 12.3 cont'd.

performed with preservation of the vertebral end plates and stabilized with the Warner-Fackler instrumentation technique.[14] Devised for use in paraplegic myelomeningocele patients with congenital kyphosis, this method provides low profile fixation with posterior spinal rods contoured to pass through the S1 neural foramina and lie against the anterior aspect of the sacrum. To minimize the chance of injury to the pelvic structures that cannot be visualized in this posterior approach, the rods were contoured on the model prior to the surgery (Fig. 12.2B–D). At the time of the procedure, the rod ends were cut and the edges filed. The irregularities in the sacrum noted on the model were true to the intraoperative findings and served as landmarks for the predetermined entry points; dissection within the canal was minimized (Fig. 12.2E).

Neuromuscular Scoliosis and Pelvic Anomaly

EE is 13-years-old and has a severe scoliosis, marked pelvic obliquity, and seating imbalance (Fig. 12.3A and B). The extent of the asymmetric deformity within the pelvis itself was only appreciated on the 3D model. The right ilium is thin and angled greater than 90 degrees to the sacrum precluding the standard forms of pelvic fixation (Fig. 12.3C and D). The sacral anatomy permits an S1 screw (Fig. 12.3E). While the width and

angulation of the S2 pedicle prevented a second screw, the bone stock at the S2 neural foramen was sufficient for a lamina hook (Fig. 12.3F). These two anchor points provided adequate fixation for a lateral cantilever manipulation and permitted correction of the pelvic obliquity (Fig. 12.3G and H).

Congenital Kyphosis and Scoliosis

A boy aged 14 ½ years with a history of seating intolerance presented with an unusual deformity pattern; the angular kyphotic deformity was more cephalad than usual and was associated with a coronal translation (Fig. 12.4A and B). The model clearly showed a hemivertebrae at the apex of the gibbus and multiple levels of failure of segmentation within the lordotic cephalic limb of the thoracic deformity (Fig. 12.4C and D). This knowledge permitted the planning of an asymmetric apical vertebral resection and the accommodation of the thoracic lordosis. Additionally the gradual lessening of the extent of the lumbar dysraphism in the more caudal elements necessitated a more midline placement of the lumbar pedicle screws. These were oriented to engage the iliac screws without the use of a transverse connector. To avoid prominent instrumentation at the area of the gibbus and maintain a linear relationship of the upper and lower rods, a more midline

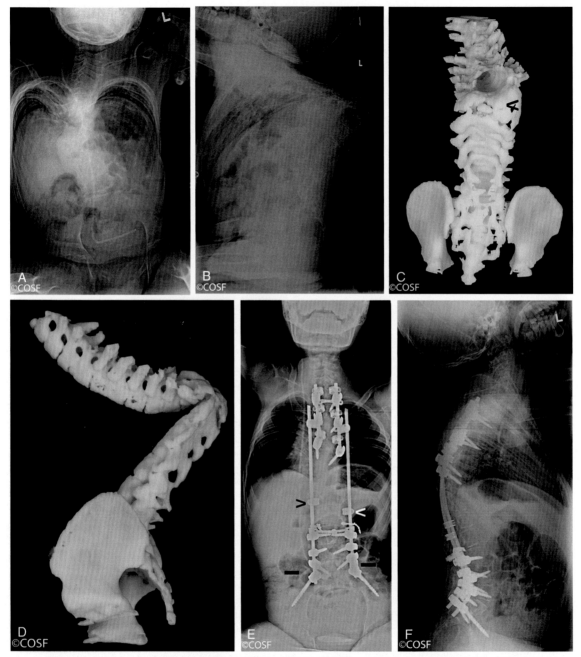

FIG. 12.4 Congenital kyphosis and congenital scoliosis. (A,B)The upright radiographs demonstrate the unusual combination of deformities. (C,D)The 3-D model shows the hemivertebra at the apex of the gibbus (arrow). Note that the posterior elements become less dysraphic toward the lumbosacral area. (E,F) Fixation designed for sub-laminar fixation were used for purchase around the strongest segmental element, the pedicle (arrows). In this position within the spinal canal the rods were low profile and collinear with the upper construct. (Reprinted with permission, Wolters Kluwer Health, Inc.)

fixation technique was innovated. A polyester tape and metallic anchor implant designed for sublaminar placement was used in an off-label technique. The anchors were placed through neural foramina with nonfunctioning nerve roots and around the excellent bone stock of the pedicles providing a low profile anchor that protected the more caudal screws from pull-out (Fig. 12.4E and F).

Congenital Kyphosis Following Neonatal Kyphectomy

A neonatal kyphectomy was performed at the time of sac closure in this young boy. He is now 5-years-old, weighs 12.5 kg, lacks sitting balance, and has recurrent skin ulceration over his gibbus (Fig. 12.5A and B). The last ulceration required a rotation flap. A growth preserving construct was planned using a single level kyphectomy, and an extraperiosteal approach was planned for the placement of the thoracic sublaminar cables. Here again the anatomy did not permit a standard pelvic fixation technique. The sacrum did not provide sufficient support for the stresses of S1 presacral fixation alone, but the ilium seemed to have excellent bone stock (Fig. 12.5C and D). The caudal fixation consisted of iliac screws with supplemental anchorage through the second sacral neural foramina. Prior to surgery, the presacral portion of the rod was contoured on the model and designed to hug the undersurface of the sacrum (Fig. 12.5E and F).

THE USE OF CUSTOM THREE-DIMENSIONAL PRINTED GUIDES FOR PEDIATRIC UPPER EXTREMITY OSTEOTOMIES

Deformities of the forearm can be difficult to appreciate in all planes, making analysis and correction of these deformities challenging. Uniplanar angulation and translation of the radius and ulna can be measured on plain radiographs, but rotational deformity can only be estimated on two-dimensional imaging. Common techniques are to look for the bicipital tuberosity to be approximately 180 degrees from the radial styloid on an anteroposterior radiograph of the forearm, as well as for the cortices above and below the fracture site to be the same width.[15,16] Although there are several osteotomy techniques based on plain radiographs in the literature, these require intraoperative decision-making which can become quite complicated in cases of multiplanar deformities or those that affect critical areas such as the distal radioulnar joint (DRUJ).[17,18]

3D imaging, such as CT scanning and computer modeling enable much clearer visualization of rotational deformities.

Indications/Contraindications

The indications for the use of 3D printed guides in the upper extremity are limited to complex or difficult unilateral deformities and not less involved deformities that can be corrected by single uniplanar osteotomies. The authors have found this technique to be most effective for pediatric forearm malunions, especially those which lead to incongruity and instability of the DRUJ. Complex distal radial malunions, although rare in the pediatric population, are also very amenable to this technique. In the planning process, the affected side is mirrored onto the normal contralateral side to plan the correction. Although age-matched control scans can be used instead, this makes treatment of Madelung's and other bilateral conditions less amenable to this technique.

Planning and Surgical Technique

There are several ways in which computer modeling and 3D printing can be integrated into the correction of forearm deformities. These generally begin with a bilateral forearm CT done in a standardized position, such that the images of the affected arm can be mirrored onto the images of the normal arm. Once the CT scan is completed, commercial software products can be used to build 3D models, including Synthes PreOPlan (Depuy Synthes, West Chester, PA), Materialise OrthoView (Materialise, Plymouth, MI), and BrainLab TraumaCad (BrainLab, Westchester, IL). These 3D models can be visualized on the computer or translated to a physical model using a 3D printer (Fig. 12.6). For some cases, simply viewing the computer image or physical model can help the surgeon understand the deformity and allow more efficient preoperative planning. For more complex cases, the computer model can be used to virtually plan the osteotomies, and 3D printed patient-specific drill guides and cutting guides can be created to use intraoperatively. These guides are available in the United States through Materialise, an additive manufacturing company. It should be noted that although these guides are FDA-approved for use in children, the guides must be created and used within a short period of time after the CT scan to ensure appropriate fit on the growing skeleton. Finally, the technology exists to 3D print custom plates for individual patients, but this is not currently approved for use in the United States.

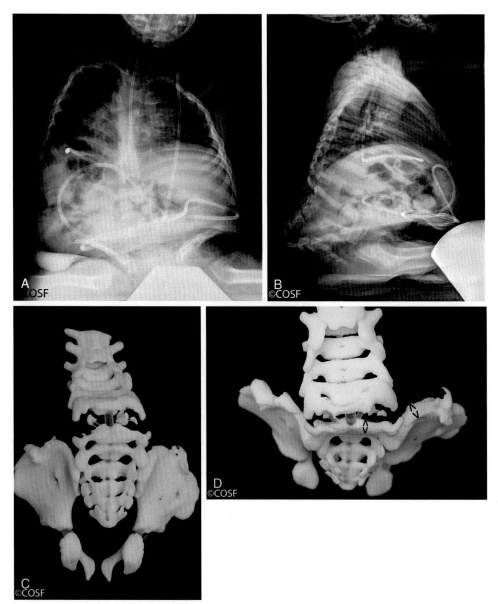

FIG. 12.5 Myelomeningocele congenital kyphosis. (A,B) A 12.5 kg 5 year old boy with recurrent skin ulceration. (C,D) Vertebral remnants of the neonatal kyphectomy are seen on the A/P model. The ilium provides more bone stock than the sacrum (arrows).

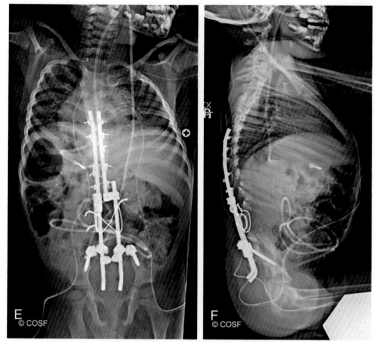

FIG. 12.5 cont'd. (E,F) Pelvic fixation utilized the ilia. Prior to surgery the rods were contoured on the 3-D models to enter the S2 neural foramina and rest flush against the adjacent sacrum.

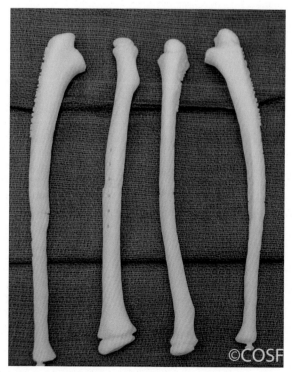

FIG. 12.6 CT generated model of forearm translated to a physical model using a 3-D printer.

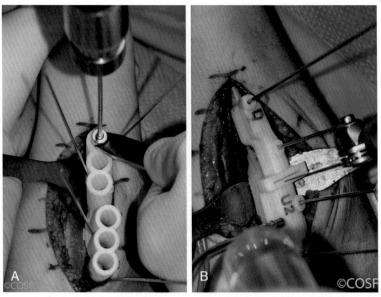

FIG. 12.7 The intraoperative use of the drill (A) and cutting guides (B).

The process begins with a bilateral CT scan. Data from the CT scan are uploaded, and the surgeon works with an engineer to plan the osteotomies and select the appropriate plate via web conferencing. Once the surgical plan is finalized, which may take several web conferences and/or email exchanges, the engineer creates the appropriate cutting and drill guides which are then shipped to the hospital for sterilization. Fig. 12.7A and B demonstrate intraoperative use of a drill guide and cutting guide, respectively.

Case Example: DRUJ Instability After Pediatric Forearm Malunion

A 13-year-old boy fell off his bicycle onto an outstretched left arm. There was no initial treatment, and 6 months later he presented with a forearm deformity, supination limited to 45 degrees and instability at the DRUJ (Fig. 12.8). Bilateral CT scan of the forearms was performed, and a 3D model was created which demonstrated the large deformity quite clearly (Fig. 12.9). Based on this model, a double osteotomy in the radius was created, with the plan to fix both osteotomies simultaneously using the Synthes LCP Dia-Meta volar distal radius plate (Fig. 12.10). Patient-specific cutting and drill guides were created using a 3D printer to use at the time of surgery, based on the planned osteotomies and the

digital specifications of the plate (Fig. 12.11). At 1 year after surgery, the patient had full forearm rotation with a stable DRUJ and no pain (Fig. 12.12).

CURRENT CLINICAL LITERATURE

The studies of 3D printed models used in clinical orthopedics are recent, and within these there are few studies that deal specifically with the pediatric population. In the adult literature, there are a number of reports on the experience of the use of patient-specific guides for the placement of pedicle screws. Improved accuracy has been documented for screws placed at C1 and C2,[17,18] the mid-cervical area,[19] and the thoracic spine.[20]

In spinal surgery performed in the pediatric population, accuracy of instrumentation and outcomes has been reported. In a series of 126 patients with posterior corrective surgery for Lenke I adolescent idiopathic scoliosis, Yang et al. compared the results when free hand pedicle placement was performed with and without the use of 3D printed models. Those with models had statistically significant diminished blood loss, shorter operative times, and fewer blood transfusions. There was a lower rate of screw misplacement in curvatures greater than 50 degrees.[21]

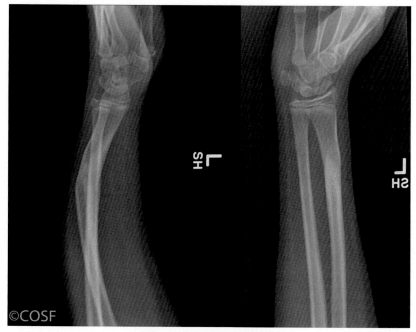

FIG. 12.8 Forearm deformity.

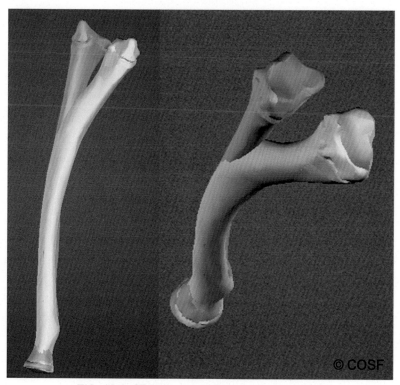

FIG. 12.9 CT generated model of forearm deformity.

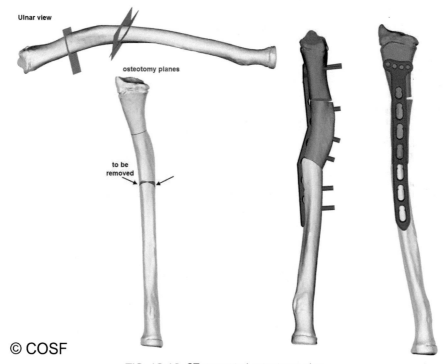

FIG. 12.10 CT generated osteotomy plan.

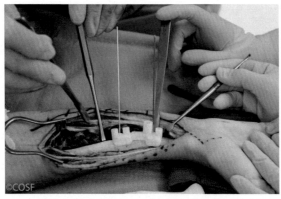

FIG. 12.11 Intra-operative use of drill guide.

In the surgical treatment of congenital scoliosis with pedicle screw fixation, Wu et al. reported a lower incidence of screw misplacement and less operative time with the use of rapid prototyping technique.[22] Karlin et al. performed a retrospective study of the role of personalized 3D printed models for the treatment of spinal deformity in children with myelomeningocele. Subjective and objective comparisons were made between seven patients in whom 3D models were used and 10 patients with similar deformities in whom models were not used. The authors felt that the models improved the planning for low-profile secure instrumentation. While the small and variable patient sample precluded statistical analysis, those patients with 3D models had greater deformity correction and less fluoroscopy time.[23] In tumor surgery, Xu et al. reported the successful use of a personalized 3D-printed vertebral body for reconstructive

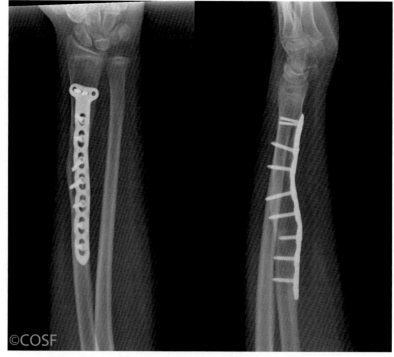

FIG. 12.12 Radiograph performed 1 year after corrective surgery.

surgery after C2 resection for Ewing sarcoma in a 12-year-old boy.[24]

Bauer et al. studied preoperative computer simulation and patient-specific guides used for the surgical correction of forearm deformity in children. In this retrospective review of 19 forearm malunions the average forearm rotation improved form 85–138 degrees. DRUJ instability was corrected in all cases.[25]

Experience with the use of patient-specific 3D-printed models for use in the planning and performance of orthopedic surgery in children is limited. Early studies and our experience are encouraging, but further studies are needed to establish that the technique produces sufficient improvement in outcomes to support the added effort and expense.

REFERENCES

1. Altiok H, Finlayson C, Hassni S, Sturm P. Kyphectomy in children with myelomeningocele. *Clin Orthop Relat Res.* 2011;469:1272–1278.
2. Banta JV. Combined anterior and posterior fusion for spinal deformity in myelomeningocele. *Spine.* 1990;15:946–952.
3. Comstock SA, Cook PC, Leahey JL, El-Hawary R, Hyndman JC. Posterior kyphectomy for myelomeningocele with anterior placement fixation: a retrospective review. *Clin Orthop Relat Res.* 2011;469:1265–1271.
4. Geiger F, Parsch D, Carstens C. Complications of scoliosis surgery in children with myelomeningocele. *Eur Spine J.* 1999;8:22–26.
5. Ko AL, Song K, Ellenbogen, Avellino AM. Retrospective review of multilevel spinal fusion combined with spinal cord transection for treatment of kyphoscoliosis in pediatric myelomeningocele patients. *Spine.* 2007;32:2493–2501.
6. Mazur J, Menelaus MB, Dickens DR, Doig WG. Efficacy of surgical management for scoliosis in myelomeningocele: correction of deformity and alteration of functional status. *J Pediatr Orthop.* 1986;6:568–575.
7. Niall DM, Dowling FE, Fogarty EE, Moore DP, Goldberg C. Kyphectomy in children with myelomeningocele: a long-term outcome study. *J Pediatr Orthop.* 2004;24:37–44.
8. Parsch D, Geiger F, Brocai DR, Lang RD, Carstens C. Surgical management of paralytic scoliosis in myelomeningocele. *J Pediatr Orthop.* 2001;10:10–17.
9. Rogers WB, Williams MS, Schwend RM, Emans JE. Spinal deformity in myelodysplasia: correction with posterior pedicle screw instrumentation. *Spine.* 1997;22:2435–2443.

10. Ward WT, Wenger DR, Roach JW. Surgical correction of myelomeningocele scoliosis: a critical appraisal of various spinal instrumentations systems. *J Pediatr Orthop.* 1989;9: 262–268.

11. Kuklo TR, Bridwell KW, Lewis SJ, Baldus C, Blanke K, Iffrig TM. Minimum 2-year analysis of sacropelvic fixation and L5-S1 fusion using S1 and iliac screws. *Spine.* 2001;26: 1976–1983.

12. Peele NW, Lenke LG, Bridwell KH, Sides B. Comparison of pelvic fixation techniques in neuromuscular spinal deformity correction: Galveston rod versus iliac and lumbosacral screws. *Spine.* 2006;31:2392–2398.

13. Sponseller PD, Zimerman RM, Ko PS, Pull Ter Gunne AF, Mohamed AS, Chang TL, et al. Low profile pelvic fixation with the sacral alar iliac technique in the pediatric population improves results at two-year minimum follow-up. *Spine.* 2010;35:1887–1892.

14. Warner WC, Fackler CD. Comparison of two techniques in treatment of lumbar kyphosis in myelodysplasia. *J Pediatr Orthop.* 1993;13:704–708.

15. Evans EM. Rotational deformity in the treatment of fractures of both bones of the forearm. *J Bone Joint Surg.* 1945;27A:373–379.

16. Creasman C, Zaleske DJ, Ehrlich MG. Analyzing forearm fractures in children: the more subtle signs of impending problems. *Clin Orthop.* 1984;118:40–53.

17. Price CT, Knapp DR. Osteotomy for malunited forearm shaft fractures in children. *J Pediatr Orthop.* 2006;26(2): 193–196.

18. VanGeenen RC, Besselaar PP. Outcome after corrective osteotomy for malimited fractures of the forearm sustained in childhood. *J Bone Joint Surg Br.* 2007;89(2): 236–239.

19. Sugawara T, Higashiyama N, Kaneyama S, Sumi M. Accurate and simple screw insertion procedure with patient-specific screw guide templates for posterior C1-2 fixation. *Spine.* 2017;42:E340–E346.

20. Kaneyama S, Sugawara T, Sumi M, Higashiyama N, Takabatake M, Mizoi K. A novel screw guiding method with a screw guide template system for posterior C-2 fixation: clinical article. *J Neurosurg Spine.* 2014;21: 23–1238.

21. Kaneyama S, Sugawara T, Sumi M. Safe and accurate mid-cervical pedicle screw insertion procedure with the patient-specific screw guide template system. *Spine.* 2015;40: E341–348.

22. Sugawara T, Higashiyama N, Kaneyama S, Takabatake M, Watanabe N, Fujouchida D, et al. Multistep pedicle screw insertion procedure with patient-specific lamina fit-and-lock templates for the thoracic spine. *J Neurosurg Spine.* 2013;19:185–190.

23. Yang M, Li C, Li Y, Zhao Y, Wei X, Zhang G, et al. Application of 3D rapid prototyping technology in posterior corrective surgery for Lenke I adolescent idiopathic scoliosis patients. *Medicine (Baltimore).* 2015;94:e582.

24. Wu ZX, Huang LY, Sang HX, Ma ZS, Wan SY, Cui G, et al. Accuracy and safety assessment of pedicle screw placement using rapid prototype technique in severe congenital scoliosis. *J Spinal Disord Tech.* 2011;24:444–450.

25. Karlin L, Weinstock P, Hedequist D, Prabhu SP. The surgical treatment of spinal deformity in children with myelomeningocele: the role of personalized three-dimensional printed models. *J Pediatr Orthop B.* 2017;26: 375–382.

26. Xu N, Wei F, Liu X, Jiang L, et al. Reconstruction of the upper cervical spine using a personalized 3D-printed vertebral body in an adolescent with Ewing sarcoma. *Spine.* 2016;41:E50–54.

27. Bauer AS, Storelli DAR, Sibbel SE, McCarroll HR, Lattanza LL. Preoperative computer simulation and patient-specific guides are safe and effective to correct forearm deformity in children. *J Pediatr Orthop.* 2017;37: 504–510.

CHAPTER 13

3D Printing in Orthopedics—Upper Extremity Arthroplasty

DEEPAK M. CHERIACHAN, MD • MATTHEW DIPAOLA, MD •
JOSEPH P. IANNOTTI, MD, PHD • ERIC T. RICCHETTI, MD

INTRODUCTION

The use of shoulder arthroplasty in the United States grew by 2.5-fold in the decade from 1990 to 2000.[1] The reverse shoulder arthroplasty (RSA) was approved by the FDA for use in the United States in November 2003, further accelerating the rate of growth of utilization of shoulder replacements in this country. Since that time indications for RSA have expanded to a spectrum of glenohumeral pathologies, including glenohumeral arthritis, irreparable rotator cuff tears, failed conventional total shoulder arthroplasty (TSA), rheumatoid arthritis, proximal humerus fractures, malunions, and proximal humerus tumors. An aging population coupled with a higher future revision burden will continue to fuel the growth of shoulder arthroplasty procedures into the future.

Both anatomic TSA and RSA can provide excellent function with survivorship exceeding 85% at 10 years.[2,3] Despite advances in glenoid preparation and component design, positioning of the glenoid in TSA and the glenosphere in RSA remains a potential challenge. Issues relating to the glenoid component are a common cause for poor function or revision surgery.

In TSA, glenoid loosening remains the most frequent cause of late implant failure.[4] While late failure of the rotator cuff may accelerate glenoid loosening, malpositioning of the glenoid component, a factor under the direct control of the operating surgeon, may also lead to late glenoid loosening particularly in shoulders with more severe pathology.[5]

Glenosphere malpositioning in RSA has been associated with a variety of complications, including bony impingement, scapular notching, dislocation, component loosening, and early mechanical failure. Scapula notching is perhaps the most well-studied complication of RSA and has a reported prevalence of 0—96% depending on implant positioning and design. Notching occurs when repeated impingement of the humeral cup against the scapular neck during arm adduction and/or rotation of the humerus leads to progressive wear of the inferior neck of the scapula. A cascade of events may ensue potentially resulting in polyethylene wear, osteolysis about the glenohumeral joint, and implant loosening, making notching a concern. Recent studies suggest that scapular notching can negatively impact clinical function.[6] Multiple studies have shown that glenosphere position relative to the scapula directly influences the incidence of notching.[7–12]

Reasons for malpositioning of the glenoid component or glenosphere include inaccurate assessment of the pathologic anatomy,[5] incorrect choice of implant and/or positioning of the implant to correct pathology,[13] and inaccurate execution of the preoperative plan at the time of surgery.[13,14] Two-dimensional (2D) CT of the shoulder initially improved the assessment of glenoid pathology over plain radiographs. The use of three-dimensional (3D) CT is now becoming more common, as it has been shown to more accurately represent pathologic anatomy of a diseased shoulder than 2D CT.[15]

To improve the choice of both the implant and implant position in shoulder arthroplasty, surgeons are now increasingly using preoperative planning with 3D CT imaging and virtual implants for digital templating. Patient-specific instrumentation (PSI) offers further improvement in the surgeons' ability to execute the preoperative plan. PSI helps the surgeon transfer information from the preoperative planning software to the surgical site, and currently includes single use and reusable instruments, as well as tools for intraoperative computer-aided navigation.

This chapter is divided into five sections. The first section discusses the principles behind the ideal shoulder arthroplasty implant placement, with a focus on the

3D Printing in Orthopaedic Surgery. https://doi.org/10.1016/B978-0-323-58118-9.00013-0

use of 3D planning to determine the optimal placement of the glenoid component to achieve a maximum correction of pathology, backside seating, and preservation of subchondral bone in TSA and maximum impingement free range of motion and stability while avoiding notching in RSA. Different design features that assist in special circumstances are also discussed. The second section will discuss the use of 3D planning in the assessment of variations in scapular anatomy and glenoid bone loss and how this affects surgical decision-making. This section highlights the utility of the glenoid vault model to assist with implant placement. The third section will discuss the use of 3D printed patient specific guides and their use in achieving ideal implant position. This section reviews the current literature on PSI and will discuss the commercially available systems for 3D templating and PSI. The fourth section will discuss the emerging use of 3D printed implants in shoulder arthoplasty and the fifth section will review the application of 3D planning in the elbow.

PRINCIPLES IN IMPLANT PLACEMENT
Anatomic Total Shoulder Arthroplasty

In the setting of anatomic TSA for a patient with an intact rotator cuff the most important parameters to consider when implanting the glenoid component are glenoid retroversion, inclination, and bone loss. With the exception of patients with developmental glenoid dysplasia, we believe that the desired implant and level of correction should replicate premorbid version, inclination, and joint line position as closely as possible. Studies assessing premorbid or nonpathologic glenoid anatomy have shown that retroversion typically falls within a range of 6–8 degrees and superior inclination ranges from 4 to 12 degrees.[16–20]

Both clinical and biomechanical data have shown increased risk for glenoid component loosening with placement of the glenoid in retroversion.[21–23] Ho et al.[22] reviewed 66 total shoulder arthroplasties with an all polyethylene press-fit pegged glenoid component and showed that glenoid component placement in greater than 15 degrees of retroversion was associated with increased osteolysis around the central peg. Farron et al.[21] performed a finite element analysis of glenoid components inserted in varying degrees of retroversion. They showed that increasing glenoid retroversion induced a posterior displacement of the glenohumeral contact point during rotation which significantly increased stress in the cement mantle and glenoid bone with an exponential increase in micromotion at the bone-cement interface (to a maximum of 706%)

with retroversion beyond 10 degrees. Superior tilt has also been shown to be associated with secondary rotator cuff dysfunction with superior subluxation at midterm follow-up although a threshold cut-off has not been defined.[24] Hopkins et al.[23] also showed in a finite element analysis that inclination errors had the highest potential for mechanical failure of the cement mantle, with shear forces being more detrimental than axial forces.

Primary glenohumeral osteoarthritis is often associated with posterior glenoid wear, and techniques to correct retroversion include asymmetrical reaming, bone grafting, and the use of augmented glenoid components. Reaming of the anterior glenoid (high side) may be able to correct mild to moderate amounts of retroversion (≤ 15 degrees, ≤ 5 mm). But with greater deformity there is an increased risk of reducing bone stock and medializing the joint line with eccentric reaming and potentially causing implant perforation of the glenoid vault medially. Significant glenoid reaming can also result in component loosening secondary to loss of subchondral bone support, which is thought to be critical to long-term stability of the glenoid component.[25,26] Several studies have shown that asymmetrical reaming can correct to a limit of 15 degrees version before peg perforation of the glenoid vault occurs.[27,28] Bone grafting with internal fixation is an option for greater degrees of bone loss and retroversion but is a technically demanding procedure with mixed clinical results.[29–31] It has traditionally been considered in cases involving more than 1 cm of posterior bone loss, and the surgeon can use the cut humeral head, iliac crest autograft, or allograft depending on the severity of deformity and bone loss. However, graft integration and resorption are always concerns.

Given the technical difficulty with bone grafting and the limitations of asymmetric reaming, augmented glenoid components offer an attractive alternative to correction of more severe deformity and glenoid retroversion. Current implant options available include the DePuy StepTech (DePuy, Warsaw, IN, USA), which offers implants with a posterior step of 3, 5, and 7 mm; the Exactech Equinoxe (Exactech, Gainesville, FL, USA), which offers a fully wedged posterior augment in 8 and 16 degrees options; and the Tornier Aequalis Perform + (Bloomington, MN, USA), which offers a half wedge posterior augment in 15, 25, and 35 degrees options. These implants can allow for correction of version without medialization of the joint line. Reduction in the amount of bone removal and decreased medialization of the joint line allows for improved balance and tension of the rotator cuff muscles acting across the joint. Recent studies have shown promising short-term results with the use of augmented glenoid components with improvement in pain, range of motion, shoulder scores, and good seating of the component at 2–3 year follow-up with improvement of glenoid retroversion.[32–34]

Reverse Total Shoulder Arthroplasty

The position and orientation of the glenosphere in RSA directly influences glenohumeral range of motion, stability, implant impingement, and scapular notching. Scapular notching signifies impingement of the humeral cup against the scapular neck during arm adduction and/or rotation of the humerus. Ideally, the glenosphere should be placed in a location that maximizes impingement free range of motion and stability while avoiding notching. Gutierrez et al. developed a computational model to assess the hierarchy of surgical factors that affect motion after RSA. That study identified increased glenosphere lateral offset and inferior translation as the two most important factors to maximize abduction. They found that an increased varus humeral-neck shaft angle was also associated with superior abduction.[7]

Multiple studies, using a glenosphere with a medial center of rotation (COR), have shown that inferior placement of the glenosphere results in increased range of motion and reduced scapular notching.[8,9,12] Ideally, the glenoid baseplate should be placed in the location that will allow the glenosphere to slightly overhang the glenoid rim inferiorly. Baseplate position must also account for the dimensions of the glenoid vault so that the central peg of the baseplate has stable fixation in bone. Different manufacturers offer different baseplate and glenosphere design features to facilitate inferior offset of the glenosphere, while still providing good fixation in bone. Eccentricity built into the baseplate or glenosphere is a common design feature to achieve these goals. A baseplate that has a central compression screw is another design feature to improve baseplate fixation, with increased compression between the baseplate and glenoid bony surface.

Superior-inferior tilt (inclination) is defined relative to the coronal axis of the scapula. The glenosphere should be positioned in neutral or slightly inferior tilt to maximize range of motion.[8,35–37] This may be more challenging with superior bone loss, as commonly seen in rotator cuff tear arthropathy, and may require use of a bone graft or augmented component to achieve this goal. Anterior-posterior tilt (version) is defined relative to the transverse axis of the scapula. The optimal amount of implant version is less well understood. Several

authors have defined the "ideal" glenosphere version as 0° relative to the transverse axis of the scapula;[35,36] however, we believe that correction to premorbid version and joint line is optimal, as with anatomic TSA. This allows for correction to the patients physiologic version, which would result in less frequent over correction of pathologic retroversion, less overreaming, and less medialization of the joint line when compared to correcting to 0°, allowing for improved balance of soft tissues across the prosthetic glenohumeral joint. When there is minimal glenoid bone loss, the surgeon may use the plane of the glenoid fossa as a reference to place the baseplate in the correct amount of version. However, this becomes increasingly difficult with more significant glenoid bone loss and retroversion. Retroverted glenoids with posterior bone loss may require significant anterior reaming or use of a posterior bone graft or augmented component to achieve the premorbid version and joint line.

The ideal medial-lateral glenosphere offset is an area of active debate. Grammont's design places the COR medial to the glenoid baseplate and includes a humeral component with a valgus neck-shaft angle around 155 degrees. When compared to historical designs that preceded the Grammont, these features decreased shear stress across the glenoid baseplate allowing for better stability and contributed to its adoption as the first reliable RSA design. Medialization of the COR does come with some downsides. Long-term studies have shown that designs with a traditional medial COR have been associated with reduced range of motion and increased scapular notching.

Alternative designs lateralize the COR and include a humeral component with a more anatomic neck shaft angle.[7,8] Werner et al.[38] performed 3D computer templating to show a significant increase in impingement free range of motion with a 135 degrees humeral neck shaft angle and glenoid lateralization (Fig. 13.1). Range of motion improved in adduction, extension, and external rotation at the side; however, there was a slight decrease in abduction. Similarly, Erickson et al.[39] found a lower rate of scapular notching in RSA with a humeral neck shaft angle of 135 degrees (2.83%) versus 155-degrees (16.80%). While early lateralized designs suffered from fixation issues, technological advances in baseplate fixation such as locking screws, a central compression screw, and porous ingrowth coating appear to have been successful in reducing the high failure rate associated with early lateralized designs.

A variety of manufacturers now offer options to adjust the amount of lateral offset of the glenosphere. The Zimmer Trabecular Metal Reverse Shoulder System

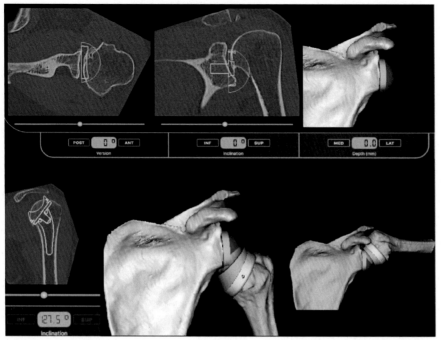

FIG. 13.1 Three-dimensional computed tomography planning of a 135 degrees humeral neck shaft angle humeral component, with the glenoid baseplate inserted flush with the inferior rim of the glenoid. In simulated abduction, bone-to-implant impingement was present at the superior edge of the glenoid. (Reprinted with permission from Elsevier from Werner BS, Hudek R, Burkhart KJ, Gohlke F. The influence of three-dimensional planning on decision-making in total shoulder arthroplasty. *J Shoulder Elbow Surg*. August 2017; 26(8):1477−1483.)

is a Grammont style system that offers 2.5 and 4.5 mm width baseplates, which can be used to compensate for central glenoid bone loss or mild joint line medialization. The Exactech Equinoxe offers baseplates with superior or posterior augments for these common areas of bone loss. The DJO AltiVate reverse system offers a wide range of glenosphere designs that lateralize the COR from 2 to 10 mm. The Tornier Aequalis offers a lateralized glenosphere and also offers half- and full-wedge implants in 15 and 35 degrees and lateralized augmented baseplates of 3 and 6 mm using porous titanium designed for bone ingrowth. Newer asymmetric humeral polyethylene liner designs also act to lateralize the humerus and improve impingement free range of motion and reduce the rate of notching.

Permeswaran et al.[40] investigated the effect of humeral polyethylene liner rotation on subluxation and impingement using 3D virtual templating. All subluxation due to impingement occurred during external rotation and extension; however, 90 degrees anterior rotation of the thicker inferior aspect of the asymmetric liner resulted in 0 mm of subluxation and no impingement in external rotation whereas 90 degrees of posterior rotation resulted in 8.8 mm of subluxation and impingement at 16 degrees of external rotation. 3D imaging with preoperative planning and templating can help maximize impingement-free range-of-motion and function with any implant design by defining the optimal location for the implant relative to the patient's specific anatomy.

Two-Dimensional versus Three-Dimensional CT Imaging

3D CT imaging and implant templating provide superior accuracy over 2D CT imaging for quantifying glenoid bone loss and guiding surgical decision-making.[14,15,41,42] 3D CT enables the surgeon to define the planes of the glenoid and scapula. This allows more precise measurement of glenoid version and inclination and eliminates measurement error due to the plane of image acquisition (gantry angle). The measurement of glenoid version using 2D CT scans is inaccurate in the presence of as little as 1 degree of out of plane imaging.[43]

Hoenecke et al.[44] compared the measurement of glenoid version and maximum wear of the glenoid surface with respect to the scapula plane on both 2D axial CT scans and 3D CT reconstruction models. They showed that the original CT scans were almost never perpendicular to the scapular body. They also showed that the point of maximum wear was missed on 2D scans in 52% of cases and that absolute error in version measured on the 2D CT slice passing through the tip of the coracoid was 5.6 degrees, while in 20% of cases, the error was more than 10 degrees. Additionally, Bokor et al.[45] showed that minor rotation of the scapula of 15 degrees can alter the accuracy of glenoid version by up to 10 degrees. Inaccuracy in the assessment of bony pathology can create problems at the time of surgery potentially resulting in a change of surgical plan. In a study of 50 patients undergoing TSA comparing preoperative assessment on 2D CT versus 3D CT planning software, Werner et al.[42] reported seven (14%) patients had a change in the choice of implant based on 3D planning. Scalise et al.[15] compared the assessment of the zone of glenoid bone loss, glenoid version, and glenoid component fit among four experienced shoulder surgeons and showed that the use of 3D CT reconstructions improved interrater reliability. Additionally, they showed that there was a significantly higher ability to determine potential glenoid vault perforation compared to 2D CT.

Use of 3D Planning in the Assessment of Glenoid Pathology and Virtual Implant Templating

The use of 3D planning software allows the surgeon to better assess the degrees of bone loss and subtle variations in glenoid morphology. The ability to reformat the axis of the CT to the scapular plane allows the surgeon to visualize bone loss in three dimensions and to manipulate and rotate the images to attain a better understanding of glenoid pathology. In a patient with acquired bone loss resulting from wear of the glenoid fossa or developmental bone deficiency due to dysplasia, positioning of the glenoid component during surgery in the correct location and orientation can be challenging without the use of preoperative planning tools, and even in the hands of experience surgeons, there is a wide range of error.

Preoperative 3D planning and virtual implant templating begins with obtaining a high-quality CT scan of the proximal humerus and entire scapula, including the medial border, using slices of 1 mm or less in thickness. The Digital Imaging and Communications in Medicine images are imported into a software program for 3D reconstruction. The exact methods of 3D reconstruction and measurement of bony anatomy in 3D can vary across different software programs, but the scapular plane is generally used as a reference. The plane of the scapula can be defined by marking the inferior angle of the scapula, the center of the glenoid, and the trigonum of the scapula (confluence of the body and spine at the medial border of the scapula). The plane of the glenoid can then be defined by marking three points on the face of the glenoid. Care must be taken to avoid placing markers on peripherally projecting osteophytes, which can result in an error of measured version. The 2D images are then reformatted based on the plane of the scapula, allowing the degree of version and inclination of the glenoid to be measured. Some types of 3D planning software will automatically identify anatomical points to recreate the plane of the scapula and glenoid providing measured version and inclination; however, this does not allow the surgeon to determine what constitutes true glenoid bone loss as opposed to peripheral osteophytes to ensure accurate measurements. The 2D orthogonal images are also used for cross-referencing during templating. The surgeon can best understand the pattern of bony erosion by visualizing the 3D reconstruction of the glenoid and scapula, particularly by rotating the scapula to obtain multiple viewing perspectives. 3D imaging also provides useful information about the surface anatomy of the glenoid. Surface irregularities such as indentations and osteophytes seen on 3D images can be used as intraoperative landmarks for placing standard or patient-specific pin guides in the correct superior-inferior and anterior-posterior location. These surface features are also helpful for determining the proper rotational orientation of certain patient-specific pin guides.

Virtual templating allows the surgeon to simulate different glenoid components on a 3D reconstruction of the patient's scapula. This helps the surgeon to determine which implant best produces the desired glenoid version, inclination, and joint line position, while maintaining good back-side contact (Fig. 13.2A−K). With the exception of patients with developmental glenoid dysplasia, we believe that the desired implant and level of correction should replicate premorbid version, inclination, and joint line position as closely as possible. This premorbid anatomy may be difficult to determine in the pathologic glenoid with significant bone loss or deformity; however, the 3D glenoid vault model of the normal glenoid vault has been shown to be a highly consistent and conserved shape across individuals that is predictive of premorbid glenoid

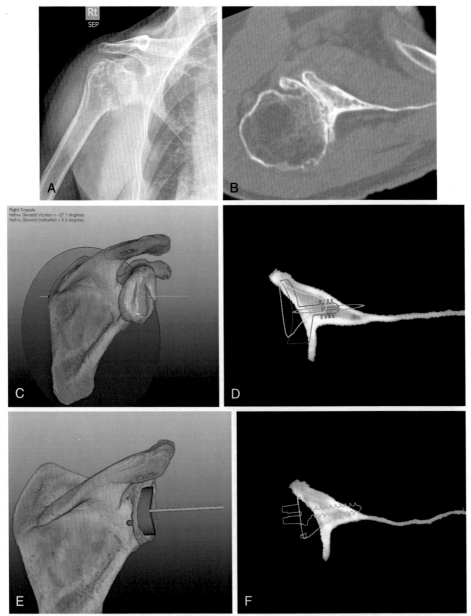

FIG. 13.2 Illustrative case of three-dimensional (3D) templating using OrthoVis preoperative planning software from Custom Orthopaedic Solutions (Cleveland, Ohio). **(A)** Preoperative anteroposterior (AP) X-ray demonstrating severe glenohumeral osteoarthritis. **(B)** Preoperative axial CT cut showing a B3 Glenoid with posterior humeral head subluxation and overlay of the glenoid vault model (blue) illustrating pathologic joint line medialization due to posterior and central glenoid bone loss. **(C)** Preoperative 3D CT image showing the position of the glenoid vault model (blue) in 3D, again demonstrating the area of posterior and central glenoid bone loss. Three points on the glenoid and scapula are selected to determine the planes of the glenoid (green) and scapula (blue). The software uses this information to automatically calculate glenoid version (−27.1 degrees) and inclination (0.3 degrees) in 3D. **(D and E)** Templating with a posterior augmented glenoid component, demonstrating persistent joint line medialization relative to the vault model on the axial image **(D)** even when the maximum posterior augment is used (7 mm posterior step). Peg perforations of the superior and posterior peripheral pegs are also seen on the 3D CT view **(E)** when templating with this implant. **(F–I)** Templating with a reverse total shoulder arthroplasty. Glenoid baseplate position on the axial image **(F)** demonstrates correction to the premorbid joint line and version relative to the vault model.

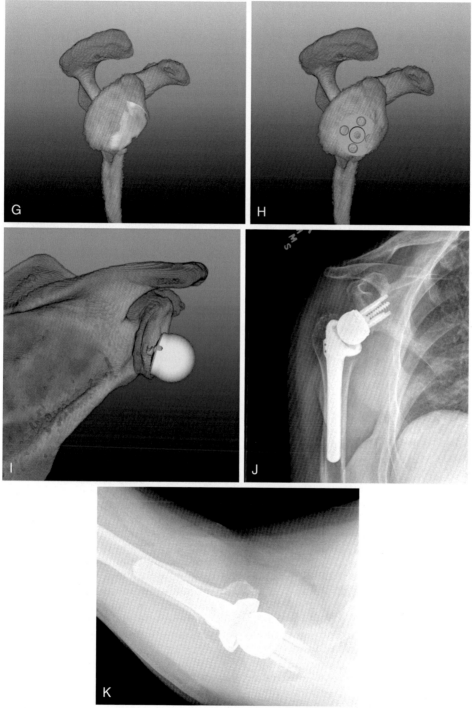

FIG. 13.2 cont'd.

The baseplate is seen to have approximately 50% backside contact with simulated reaming on the 3D CT view **(G** and **H)**, and the areas with lack of backside contact can be seen on the axial image and 3D CT view **(F** and **H)**. The region of the baseplate without backside contact can be addressed with glenoid bone grafting. **(J** and **K)** Postoperative AP and axillary radiographs demonstrating execution of the preoperative plan with a reverse total shoulder arthoplasty and posterior glenoid bone grafting using autograft from the resected humeral head.

version, inclination, and joint line position in the pathologic glenoid.[17–20] This model can, therefore, be used with 3D planning to estimate native glenoid version, inclination, and joint line position in the setting of glenoid bone loss and help with determining optimal glenoid implant position.

Sizing and placing the vault model requires adjustments in three planes. In the axial and sagittal planes the vault is aligned with the inner cortical margin of the anterior wall of the glenoid, and in the coronal plane the vault is aligned with the inner cortical margin of the superior wall at the suprascapular notch. When the vault model is positioned correctly, its medial portion will closely follow the preserved 3D internal architecture of the patient's medial glenoid. In pathologic shoulders the lateral portion of the vault model represents the anatomy of the premorbid glenoid and defines where bone loss has occurred.

The vault model is a helpful tool for determining surgical strategy and implant placement in both TSA and RSA. It is the authors' practice to place the TSA glenoid component in the medial-lateral location, version, and inclination represented by the vault model. The RSA baseplate can also be placed in the version and joint line position represented by the vault model, while neutral or slightly inferior inclination is chosen. Bone loss, depending on its severity, may be addressed by asymmetric or high side reaming, use of an augmented glenoid component, bone grafting the glenoid, or selecting an implant system with a lateral-ized glenosphere design or augmented baseplate to achieve optimal implant placement (Fig. 13.2A–K).

Once the desired implant and its location are chosen, the software calculates the location and orientation of the central guide pin. The surgeon notes the specific placement of the guide pin relative to the local anatomy of the glenoid fossa, including a biconcave line when present and small indentations or osteophytes on the periphery, as well as the trajectory of the pin relative to the glenoid surface at that location. The surgeon should be aware that in glenoids with acquired bone loss, posterior erosion and significant osteophyte formation may skew the ideal location of the guide pin on the surface of the glenoid because the center of the glenoid vault does not always correspond to the center of the arthritic glenoid surface. 3D planning also helps locate the guide pin when the instrumentation includes a drill guide that is the size and shape of the eventual glenoid component. In this situation, the surgeon should reference an en face view of the implant on the 3D preoperative plan and note the position of the implant relative to bony landmarks and the rim of the glenoid. The surgeon then places the drill guide in the same location as the implant on 3D preoperative plan to aid accurate pin placement.

After preoperatively placing the implant, some software allows the surgeon to perform simulated reaming to plan reaming depth and location. Reaming of the glenoid surface should preserve the subchondral bone. In TSA after reaming, the surgeon can assess the amount of bone removal required to provide good backside contact of the glenoid component. If there is concern of violation of subchondral bone support or perforation of the glenoid pegs, the surgeon can also trial the use of augmented implants to minimize bone loss and maximize implant support (Fig. 13.2A–K). In RSA the surgeon confirms that the baseplate is placed sufficiently inferior on the glenoid. If it is not, the implant is repositioned and these steps are repeated. Occasionally the guide pin may need to be positioned slightly anterior or posterior to the center of the glenoid in order to ensure that the central peg/screw of the baseplate is contained within the glenoid vault.

Eccentric glenosphere and baseplate designs offer additional flexibility to choose a contained location for the central peg/screw while positioning the glenosphere in the desired location. When the vault is too shallow to contain the central peg in any location, bone grafting may be required. The width of the bone graft can be calculated by determining how much bone loss has occurred relative to the vault model. Klein et al., has also described the use of the alternate glenoid centerline to increase the amount of fixation in bone when advanced posterior bone loss is present. The alternate centerline directs the center screw or peg of the baseplate along the axis of the scapular spine from the center of the glenoid to the junction of the scapular spine as it joins the body of the scapula.[46] The alternate centerline has negative consequences because it places the implant in approximately 30 degrees of anteversion. This will compromise rotational motion of the arm and create impingement with the coracoid.

Virtual templating has been shown to improve the accuracy of guide pin position and orientation using standard instrumentation. Iannotti et al. compared standard and PSI with 3D templating to standard instrumentation with 2D imaging in placing the guide pin for anatomic TSA in nine bone models from patients with a variety of patterns of glenohumeral arthritis. They found that 3D templating with standard instrumentation improved the accuracy of pin position by 4.5 ± 1.0 degrees in version, 3.3 ± 1.3 degrees in inclination, and 0.4 ± 0.2 mm in location.[14] The authors followed this study with a randomized clinical trial of 46 patients undergoing anatomic TSA. They again demonstrated that 3D templating with standard instrumentation or PSI was superior to standard instrumentation with 2D imaging. 3D templating significantly improved the accuracy of implant placement to within 5 degrees of desired inclination or 10 degrees of version.[41]

Patient-Specific Guides

Once the location and orientation of the glenoid implant and guide pin are templated in the 3D planning software, it is desirable to replicate that position at the time of surgery. PSI has been demonstrated to help achieve that goal, and its effect may be greater in more pathologic glenoids. PSI provides a method to accurately transfer information from the preoperative 3D planning software to the surgical site. The simplest method of PSI is through use of standard instrumentation used in a patient-specific way based upon the 3D preoperative plan. More advanced PSI involves creating a custom guide based on a 3D preoperative plan that references the patient's glenoid to place the guide pin in the desired location, version, and inclination.

There are two categories of commercially available PSI. The first type includes a disposable, single-use instrument generated from the preoperative plan and placed into a 3D printed instrument. Many of these systems also provide a 3D model of the patient's glenoid as a reference during surgery. The second category uses a reusable instrument that may be adjusted to define the location of the guide pin in relation to glenoid anatomy. Preoperative planning software for these instruments also allows implant templating. After the components have been virtually positioned, the software generates instructions for configuring the guide using a reusable and adjustable base. Alternatively, the guide can be configured by using a 3D printed model of the glenoid having contained within it the location and orientation of the guide pin that was determined on the preoperative planning software.

Currently, four manufacturers offer PSI for shoulder arthroplasty. DJO, Tornier, and Zimmer-Biomet offer single use PSI, and Arthrex offers patient-specific reusable instrumentation. All manufacturers provide software that allows the surgeon to template their implants on a 3D CT reconstruction of the patient's scapula.

The DJO Matchpoint system includes software that allows the surgeon to manipulate a reformatted 3D model of the scapula derived from thin-cut CT images. Landmarks on the glenoid and scapula are selected to generate a coordinate system for measuring glenoid version and inclination. The surgeon is then able to perform virtual surgery by simulating placement of the glenoid guide pin, reaming, and templating. Once a surgical plan is confirmed, this information is used to fabricate a patient-specific pin guide that references the surface of the glenoid and coracoid. This guide is used to place the guide pin, which determines the orientation of the glenoid component or baseplate. A 3D bone model of the patient's glenoid is also provided.

The Zimmer system includes similar software but allows complete implant templating. The surgeon is able to virtually ream the glenoid, place baseplate screws, and trial different size glenospheres in order to generate a surgical plan. This information is then used to fabricate a 3D bone model of the patient's glenoid and multiple patient specific guides. The guides include a pin guide to direct baseplate location, a ream guide to direct the depth of reaming, a roll guide to control rotation of the implant, and a drill guide that is placed over the baseplate to control the direction and length of the screws (Fig. 13.3).

The Biomet system includes software that allows the surgeon to virtually template the glenoid baseplate on a 3D reconstruction of the glenoid and scapula. This information is used to manufacture a 3D printed bone model and a guide that includes drill cylinders for both anatomic and RSA.

The Tornier PSI system is available for use with the Aequalis PerFORM + shoulder system featuring anatomic and RSA. The provided BLUEPRINT software is unique in that it allows the surgeon to create a 3D reconstruction from the patient's CT and perform virtual implantation without the need for a company engineer. It also allows for virtual simulation of range of motion to assess for bony impingement with RSA implants. The software includes algorithms for determining the glenoid version, inclination, and radius of curvature of the articular surface. These algorithms allow calculation of version and inclination even if the original CT scan does not include the entire scapula. After virtual templating, the software determines the ideal guide pin entry point and trajectory. The surgeon then selects four different points on the edge of the glenoid that will establish the position of the PSI guide feet. The surgeon must select one point on the posterior rim of the glenoid and three points on the anterior rim. The manufacturer provides a 3D bone model, along with the patient-specific guide. Because the guide does not have a large contact area with the articular surface, it is very important to pay attention to rotational alignment when placing it on the glenoid.

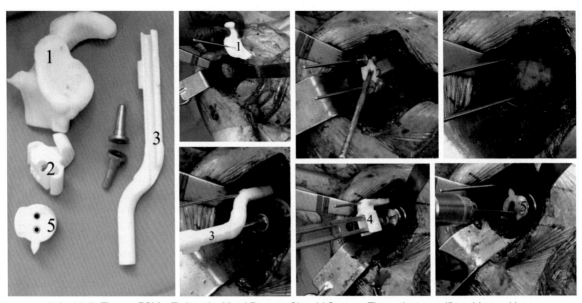

FIG. 13.3 Zimmer PSI for Trabecular Metal Reverse Glenoid System. The patient-specific guides and bone model are shown (Left). The bone model (1) is generated from a three-dimensional (3D) reconstruction of the patient's glenoid and comes with two predrilled holes showing guide pin locations and an engraved outline of the pin guide to help the surgeon orient the guide on the patient's glenoid. The pin guide (2) is placed flush on the glenoid with the hook referencing the anterosuperior quadrant. The guide is then secured with two 2.5 mm pins. A 6 mm cannulated drill bit is placed over the inferior pin to create a pilot hole for the glenoid reamer. The cannulated reamer is then placed over the inferior pin and the ream guide (3) is attached to the superior pin. After reaming, the inferior pin is removed and the pilot hole is overdrilled with a 7.5 mm drill bit to accommodate the baseplate post (not shown). The baseplate is then inserted with the roll guide (4) attached to the insertion handle and superior pin. The screw guide (5) is placed in the cavity of the baseplate with the arrow pointing towards the superior pin. After drilling pilot holes for the two baseplate screws, the guide is removed and a depth gauge is used to confirm screw length. (Reprinted with permission from Thieme from Donohue KW, Ricchetti ET, Eltelbany AS, et al. Patient-specific instruments and implants in reverse shoulder arthroplasty. In: Dines D, Dines J, Edwards TB, eds. *Reverse Shoulder Arthroplasty: A Practical Approach*. 1st ed. Thieme; 2017:201.)

The Arthrex VIP system is licensed through Custom Orthopaedic Solutions (Cleveland, Ohio). The software functions are similar to that of the Zimmer system. The surgeon uploads the CT images to the company, which produces a preliminary surgical plan based upon the surgeon's general preferences. The surgeon then reviews, modifies, and approves the final surgical plan. The instrumentation set has all of the component parts for the reusable PSI. Instructions for setting the reusable PSI from a model of the glenoid and guide pin are sent to the surgeon (Fig. 13.4). The PSI is assembled and adjusted at the time of surgery by setting it to a 3D bone model of the glenoid containing a guide pin in the planned guide pin trajectory or by setting it to an adjustable base device that sets the legs of the reusable PSI in the correct position to achieve the planned guide pin position when the PSI is placed on the

patient's glenoid (Fig. 13.5). After use, the instruments can be sterilized for reuse.

Multiple studies have investigated the accuracy of single-use PSI in reverse and anatomic shoulder arthroplasty. In a multisurgeon cadaveric study by Throckmorton et al.[47], 70 shoulders with radiographically confirmed osteoarthritis were randomized to PSI or standard instrumentation for anatomic and reverse TSA. In anatomic TSA, PSI was found to improve mean deviation in version from 8 to 5 degrees and inclination from 7 to 3 degrees. The difference between PSI and standard instrumentation did not reach statistical significance in reverse TSA; however, multivariate analysis for the entire cohort (anatomic TSA and reverse TSA) found that patient-specific guides significantly improved accuracy and reduced the incidence of component malposition. The greatest benefit of PSI was seen in glenoids

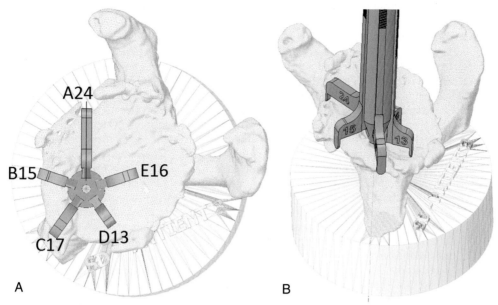

FIG. 13.4 Intelligent Reusable Instrument (IRI) surgical plan. **(A** and **B)** Instructions for calibrating the patient-specific IRI are generated from the preoperative planning software after selecting implant version, inclination, and roll. The IRI utilizes five interchangeable feet that may be adjusted to match the surface anatomy of the glenoid. This allows the guide pin to be inserted in the desired location and orientation from the preoperative plan.

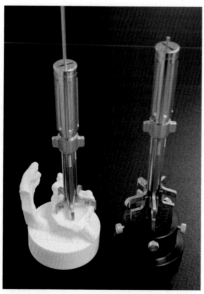

FIG. 13.5 Intelligent Reusable Instrument (IRI) with setting of the legs of the PSI using a three-dimensional (3D) bone model of the patient's glenoid (left image) or using an adjustable base device (right image).

with >10 degrees of retroversion. The authors found no relationship between surgeon experience in shoulder arthroplasty and accuracy with the use of standard instrumentation or PSI. In another cadaveric study, Levy et al.[48] used 3D planning software and PSI to place an RSA baseplate in 14 shoulders. The location and trajectory of the guide pin was then evaluated with 3D CT imaging and compared with the preoperative plan. The authors demonstrated accuracy in version of 2.6 ± 1.7 degrees, inferior tilt of 1.2 ± 1.2 degrees, and starting point location 1.2 ± 0.7 mm. Walch et al.[49] performed a similar cadaveric study using 3D planning software and PSI for anatomic TSA in 18 shoulders. Guide pin placement was also evaluated by 3D CT imaging and found to have a similar level of accuracy. Average deviation from the preoperative plan measured 1.64 ± 1.01 degrees in version, 1.42 ± 1.37 degrees in inclination, and 1.05 ± 0.31 mm in starting point location.

While these cadaveric studies show promising results, the ability to optimally use a PSI in vivo to accurately place a glenoid component can be complicated due to surgical exposure. Inadequate surgical exposure due to joint contractures, poor soft tissue releases, and body habitus can compromise correct seating of the intraoperative PSI guides and ultimately may decrease the accuracy of guide pin and glenoid component placement.

Hendel et al.[13] performed the first randomized controlled clinical trial comparing standard instrumentation and 2D planning to PSI and 3D templating in 31 patients undergoing anatomic TSA. PSI and 3D templating reduced mean deviation in version from 6.9 to 4.3 degrees, and in inclination from 11.6 to 2.9 degrees. The authors found that PSI had the greatest benefit in patients with glenoid retroversion in excess of 15 degrees. In this group, the average deviation in implant position from the preoperative plan improved from 10 to 1.2 degrees. PSI had no difference in patients with retroversion <7 degrees. This is consistent with the findings of Throckmorton et al. that suggested increased benefit of PSI in patients with more severe glenoid deformity. 3D templating and PSI also significantly improved selection of the optimal glenoid implant and reduced the frequency of implant malposition. Gauci et al.[50] used 3D templating and a custom patient-specific alignment guide to place the guide pin in 17 patients undergoing TSA. The authors compared the accuracy of implant placement on postoperative 3D CT reconstructions with their preoperative plan. The mean difference in entry point was 0.1 ± 1.4 in the anteroposterior plane and 0.8 ± 1.3 mm in the superoinferior plane. The mean difference in orientation was 3.4 ± 5.1 degree for version and 1.8 ± 5.3 degrees for inclination. In a similar study, Dallalana et al.[51] demonstrated high accuracy with PSI in vivo in 20 patients who underwent shoulder arthroplasty (10 TSA and 10 RSA) with the aid of a CT-based PSI system. Postoperative CT scans showed a mean deviation from plan of 1.8 ± 1.9 degrees in glenoid version and of 1.3 ± 1.0 degrees in inclination. The mean deviation in position on the glenoid face was 0.5 ± 0.3 in the anteroposterior plane and 0.8 ± 0.5 mm in the superoinferior plane. Mulligan et al.[52] compared the use of PSI in revision shoulder arthroplasty in 50 patients and showed improved accuracy of the PSI guide compared to standard instrumentation. They found average deviation in version from anatomic was 8 degrees with traditional techniques and 5 degrees with the targeting guide. They showed a particular benefit in cases of revision to TSA where deviation was 10 degrees with the traditional technique and 3 degrees with the targeting guide.

Reusable PSI may offer cost advantages because it does not require fabrication of a custom guide. The previously mentioned 3D templating studies by Iannotti et al.[14,41] also examined the effectiveness of a patient-specific reusable guide (Intelligent Reusable Instrument IRI) to assist with guide pin placement (Fig. 13.6). In the sawbones study the authors found that standard instrumentation with 2D imaging

produced a mean deviation from planned component position of 11.1 ± 7.3 degrees in version, 10.7 ± 5.8 degrees in inclination, and 2.9 ± 1.6 mm in position. The authors reported an undercorrection of version and inclination in almost all cases. The use of 3D imaging with standard instrumentation improved the mean deviation from plan to 6.7 ± 5.9 degrees in version, 9.3 ± 5.6 degrees in inclination, and 2.4 ± 1.3 mm in location. 3D templating with the reusable PSI improved the mean deviation from plan even further to 3.1 ± 2.6 degrees in version, 2.8 ± 2.1 degree in inclination, and 1.2 ± 0.7 mm in location. They reproduced this finding in a randomized controlled trial of 46 patients undergoing anatomic TSA.[41] In that study, patients were randomized to either 3D templating with a patient-specific intelligent reusable instrument or 3D templating with standard instrumentation. These groups were compared to a historical control group using 2D imaging with standard instrumentation. The authors found that both 3D templating with PSI and 3D templating with standard instrumentation significantly improved the accuracy of glenoid placement. The average deviation from the intended implant position measured 4.0 ± 1.0 degrees in version and 3.1 ± 1.0 degrees in inclination for the PSI group, 4.3 ± 1.2 degrees in version and 4.1 ± 1.4 degrees in inclination for the 3D templating with standard instrumentation group, and 6.9 ± 2.1 degrees in version and 11.1 ± 2.9 degrees in inclination for the 2D imaging with standard instrumentation group.

Lewis et al.[53] performed a similar study that examined the use of a reusable 6-pin array guide on bone models from nine patients with varying amounts of glenohumeral arthritis. The authors compared pin placement with PSI and 3D templating to two groups where the pin was placed by a freehand technique without instrumentation. In the groups without instrumentation, the surgeon either used no imaging or was assisted by a 3D preoperative plan. The authors found that PSI with 3D templating significantly reduced version errors (3 ± 2 degrees), when compared to the freehand technique with 3D planning (8 ± 6 degrees) and without imaging (9 ± 7 degrees). PSI with 3D templating also significantly decreased inclination errors (3 ± 2 degrees), when compared to the freehand technique without imaging (9 ± 6 degrees). The generalizability of this study is limited by the lack of a control arm using standard instrumentation.

It is important for the surgeon to familiarize themselves with the details of the particular commercially available PSI and preoperative planning software that he or she is using. The surgeon should know if the PSI was created from bony anatomy (CT scan) or from

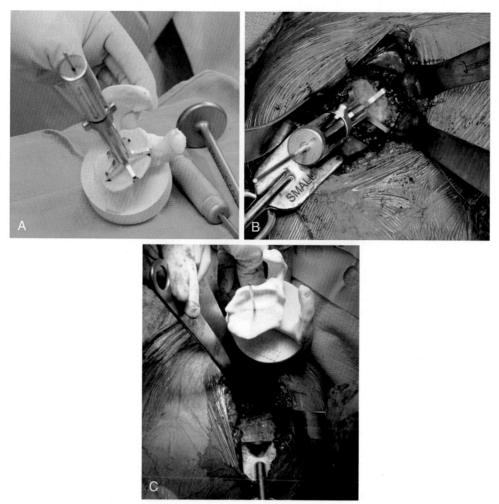

FIG. 13.6 Intelligent Reusable Instrument (IRI) during intraoperative use. The patient-specific IRI guide is placed onto a three-dimensional (3D) bone model of the patient's glenoid. The bone model is manufactured with a drill hole that positions the guide pin in the location and orientation determined by the preoperative plan **(A)**. The surgeon notes the location and length of the IRI guide feet on the bone model and secures them in this position, then transfers the IRI guide to the same position on the patient's own glenoid for guide pin placement **(B)**. The guide pin is then inserted and the surgeon can confirm the guide pin's position and orientation in the patient's glenoid as correct by comparing it to the position on the bone model **(C)**.

bony and cartilaginous anatomy (MRI). If the PSI was created from bony anatomy using a CT scan, the surgeon needs to carefully remove any remaining cartilage, fibrous tissue and labrum from the glenoid fossa, as is commonly seen on the unworn surface of biconcave glenoids. Osteophytes should be left intact at this point because PSIs most often are created from images that include the osteophytes. This ensures that the PSI rests on the landmarks it was intended to rest on, improving the fit of the device. For PSIs that have some components that rest on the base of the coracoid for reference, the labrum and periosteum need to be meticulously removed so that the PSI again rests solely on bone. The surgeon should reference images from the preoperative plan to ensure that the PSI is in the correct location, and the surgeon should also ensure that the PSI mates perfectly with the glenoid as intended. Once the PSI is correctly placed and stable, the guide pin is then inserted. Its position and placement should be compared to the preoperative plan and any adjustments should be made before proceeding with further glenoid instrumentation according to manufacturer recommendations.

After placing the guide pin, the surgeon must still control both the depth of reaming and also maintain reaming in the trajectory of the guide pin. Bending of the central guide pin with the reamer can occur resulting in the implant being in a different position than the guide pin. The surgeon must also control the roll or rotation of the implant, which means the rotation of the pegs or keel of the glenoid component in anatomic arthroplasty and the rotation of the baseplate screw holes in reverse TSA. Careful preoperative planning and intraoperative referencing of the plan will assist in this step and minimize the chance of unplanned component perforation. The Zimmer PSI system uses multiple guides to aid in controlling these variables in this part of the procedure.

It is important for any user of PSIs to remember that the PSI does not define the optimum implant placement. Rather, it only provides the ability to accurately reproduce the planned position of the implant. The surgeon must still use judgment in deciding what implant to use and where to place it for each patient. These parameters are determined preoperatively by the surgeon. And there is still debate about ideal implant position that only long-term clinical follow-up studies will ultimately resolve.

Intraoperative navigation has also been utilized to improve the accuracy of glenoid placement in both anatomic TSA and RSA. It can allow for accurate execution of the preoperative plan intraoperatively without the creation of a patient-specific guide. A metaanalysis by Sadoghi et al on five studies performing intraoperative navigation in shoulder arthroplasty.[54] showed an improvement in weighted mean version of navigated shoulders of 4.4 degrees retroversion vs. 10.6 degrees for standard instrumentation. They also reported a reduction in screw perforation with navigation. However, despite the improvement in accuracy, clinical studies have raised potential technical difficulties with navigation. Edwards et al.[55], reporting on a case series of 27 patients, noted that the accuracy of the system was

2.6 degrees and that additional operative time was initially 20–30 min but improved to approximately 10 min with experience. In the only prospective randomized clinical trial, Kircher et al.[56] compared standard instrumentation to navigation in TSA in 20 patients and found that standard instrumentation improved retroversion from 14.4 to 10.9 degrees and navigation improved retroversion from 15.4 to 3.7 degrees but that navigation was aborted due to technical problems in 37.5% of patients and that operative time was 31.5 min longer in the navigation group. ExactechGPS is an intraoperative navigation system, which can be used with the Exactech Equinoxe shoulder system. It allows for real-time assessment of retroversion and inclination, as well as reaming and drilling depth to improve placement of both the glenoid component or baseplate and screws.

3D Printed Implants in Shoulder Arthoplasty

Dealing with complex glenoid deformity is one of the most challenging aspects of shoulder arthroplasty. These deformities can be present secondary to severe primary degenerative or congenital pathology, and it can also be seen secondary to bone loss in the setting of revision surgery. Large defects or cavitary lesions result in a lack of bony support for the glenoid component, limiting treatment options and affecting clinical results. Custom-made implants may hold promise for dealing with bone loss in these complex cases.

Zimmer Biomet has released an FDA-approved patient-specific vault reconstruction system for RSA in patients with severe soft-tissue deficiency and glenoid bone loss.[57] The prosthesis is made using CAD/CAM (computer-aided design/computer-aided manufacturing) reconstructions based on the patient's 3D CT reconstructions (Fig. 13.7). Preoperative planning also allows for the planning, placement, size, and trajectory of the implant screws to gain the best glenoid fixation. The implant fills bone voids with a porous plasma spray–coated titanium, which allows for biological fixation and can potentially account for bone loss up to 50 mm × 50 mm × 35 mm. Chammaa et al.[58] reported on another CAD/CAM custom-made prosthesis in the United Kingdom in which 37 patients with severe bone loss were treated with the CAD-CAM TSR (Stanmore Implants Worldwide, Elstree, UK). The prosthesis is custom made using preoperative 3D CT reconstructions and resembles a total hip prosthesis with five components including a large hydroxyapatite-coated titanium glenoid shell, with slots for screw fixation into the scapula and titanium fixation screws, followed by a polyethylene liner and a cobalt-chrome humeral stem with a 28 or 32 mm-sized humeral

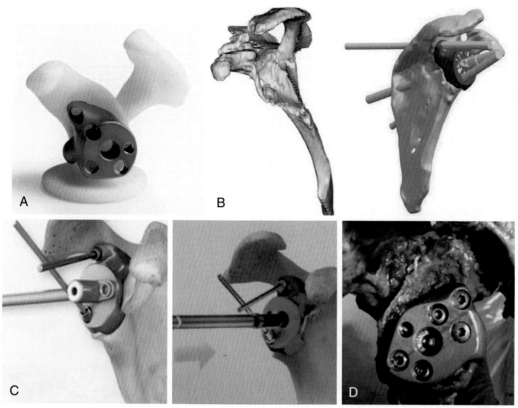

FIG. 13.7 Demonstration of the Zimmer Biomet Vault Reconstruction System Implant. **(A)** Implant positioned on pathologic glenoid bone model. **(B)** Three-dimensional (3D) CT reconstruction images demonstrating severe glenoid pathology with proposed custom glenoid component position and screw trajectory. **(C)** Implant positioned on glenoid and secured with temporary pin fixation through predetermined screw holes. The central screw hole can then be drilled once the implant is securely positioned. **(D)** Implant fixed with central 6.5 mm compression screw and predetermined peripheral screws. (**(A, C,** and **D)** Reprinted with permission from Zimmer Biomet Inc. **(B)** Reprinted with permission from Frontline Medical Communications from Dines DM, Gulotta L, Craig EV, Dines JS. Novel solution for massive glenoid defects in shoulder arthroplasty: a patient-specific glenoid vault reconstruction system. *Am J Orthop.* March/April 2017;46(2):104–108.)

head. At a mean follow-up of 5 years, the study showed a significant improvement in mean pain level with activity from 9.2 ± 1.7 to 2.4 ± 2.9 and improvement in the Oxford Shoulder Score from 11 ± 8 points to 27 ± 11 points. Complications requiring reoperation occurred in nine patients (24%).

3D printed custom implants offer potential hope in the management of severe glenoid bone loss in the setting of primary or revision shoulder arthroplasty. Additional clinical outcome studies are needed to define their effectiveness and role.

Application of 3D Planning in Elbow Arthritis

The use of 3D CT scanning and planning has been applied to the elbow, although there is comparatively very little literature regarding this. In the setting of

elbow osteoarthritis, osteophytes from reactive bone and cartilage formation cause impingement, secondary restriction in range of motion, and eventually joint contracture. Commonly, static 2D CT scans are used for the assessment of impingement locations in the elbow joint. Dynamic assessment of impingement using 3D CT models can be used to virtually simulate range of motion to detect impingement locations for preoperative planning in debridement arthroplasty of the elbow.[59–62] Nishiwaki et al.[60] performed CT scans in 30 patients with osteoarthritis of the elbow to generate 3D models. They assessed the volume of impinging bone with varying flexion angles. They were able to show increasing volumes of bony impingement between the coronoid process and coronoid fossa with increasing flexion angles and increasing bony

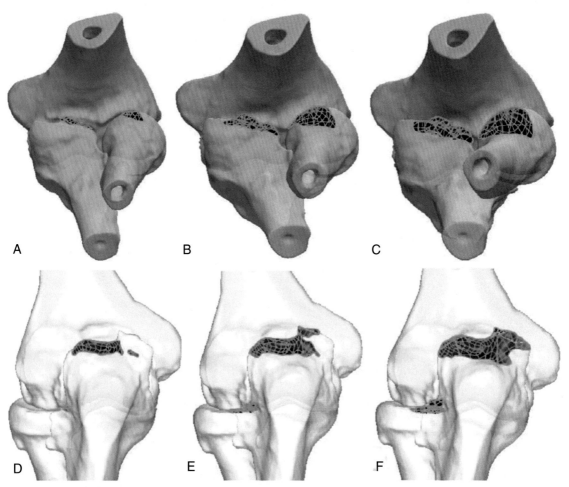

FIG. 13.8 Computational semitransparent models of an elbow with extensive osteophytes showing the overlapping bony regions (indicated by red mesh) which impinge during simulated range-of-motion. Anterior views at elbow flexion angles of (A) 120 degrees, (B) 130 degrees, and (C) 140 degrees. Posterior views at elbow flexion angles of **(D)** 20 degrees, **(E)** 10 degrees, and **(F)** 0 degrees. (Reprinted with permission from Elsevier from Nishiwaki M, Willing R, Johnson JA, King GJ, Athwal GS. Identifying the location and volume of bony impingement in elbow osteoarthritis by 3-dimensional computational modeling. *J Hand Surg*. July 2013; 38(7):1370–1376.)

impingement between the radial head and radial fossa with increasing extension angles (Fig. 13.8). They also identified unique areas of impingement between the radial head and posterior capitulary osteophyte using the virtual models. Both Miyake et al.[59] and Yamamoto et al.[62] showed clinical improvement in range of motion and elbow function scores with the application of 3D planning to clinical cases. However the limitation to both of their studies was a lack of a control arm to assess if 3D planning increased the gain of range of motion due to debridement of impingement lesions. Further comparative studies are needed to assess the

true value of 3D planning in outcomes for debridement arthroplasty of the elbow. Owing to the larger market share, shoulder 3D printing technology has become more widespread in use compared to elbow technology thus far. However, we expect the technology will have further applications to elbow arthroplasty in the future.

CONCLUSION

Both anatomic and reverse total shoulder replacement provide successful results for patients with degenerative conditions of the shoulder. Failure of the glenoid component is a common cause for revision in both types of shoulder arthroplasty. Although many factors influence the duration and function of a prosthetic shoulder, one factor that the surgeon can control is the position of the glenoid component. 3D planning software, PSI and custom prosthesis are now available to surgeons to improve the accuracy of implant positioning, particularly in the setting of severe deformity and bone loss. Long-term studies will ultimately be needed to show what effect this new technology will have on the survival and clinical function of shoulder arthroplasty.

REFERENCES

1. Kim SH, Wise BL, Zhang Y, Szabo RM. Increasing incidence of shoulder arthroplasty in the United States. *J Bone Jt Surg Am.* 2011;93(24):2249–2254. https://doi.org/10.2106/JBJS.J.01994 [published Online First: Epub Date].

2. Bacle G, Nove-Josserand L, Garaud P, Walch G. Long-term outcomes of reverse total shoulder arthroplasty: a follow-up of a previous study. *J Bone Jt Surg Am.* 2017;99(6): 454–461. https://doi.org/10.2106/JBJS.16.00223 [published Online First: Epub Date].

3. Norris TR, Iannotti JP. Functional outcome after shoulder arthroplasty for primary osteoarthritis: a multicenter study. *J Shoulder Elbow Surg.* 2002;11(2):130–135.

4. Papadonikolakis A, Neradilek MB, Matsen FA. Failure of the glenoid component in anatomic total shoulder arthroplasty: a systematic review of the English-language literature between 2006 and 2012. *J Bone Jt Surg Am.* 2013;95(24): 2205–2212. https://doi.org/10.2106/JBJS.L.00552 [published Online First: Epub Date].

5. Iannotti JP, Greeson C, Downing D, Sabesan V, Bryan JA. Effect of glenoid deformity on glenoid component placement in primary shoulder arthroplasty. *J Shoulder Elbow Surg.* 2012;21(1):48–55. https://doi.org/10.1016/j.jse.2011.02.011 [published Online First: Epub Date].

6. Mollon B, Mahure SA, Roche CP, Zuckerman JD. Impact of scapular notching on clinical outcomes after reverse total shoulder arthroplasty: an analysis of 476 shoulders. *J Shoulder Elbow Surg.* 2017;26(7):1253–1261. https://doi.org/10.1016/j.jse.2016.11.043 [published Online First: Epub Date].

7. Gutiérrez S, Comiskey CA, Luo ZP, Pupello DR, Frankle MA. Range of impingement-free abduction and adduction deficit after reverse shoulder arthroplasty. Hierarchy of surgical and implant-design-related factors. *J Bone Jt Surg Am.* 2008; 90(12):2606–2615. https://doi.org/10.2106/JBJS.H.00012 [published Online First: Epub Date].

8. Li X, Knutson Z, Choi D, et al. Effects of glenosphere positioning on impingement-free internal and external rotation after reverse total shoulder arthroplasty. *J Shoulder Elbow Surg.* 2013;22(6):807–813. https://doi.org/10.1016/j.jse.2012.07.013 [published Online First: Epub Date].

9. Nyffeler RW, Werner CM, Gerber C. Biomechanical relevance of glenoid component positioning in the reverse Delta III total shoulder prosthesis. *J Shoulder Elbow Surg.* 2005;14(5):524–528. https://doi.org/10.1016/j.jse.2004.09.010 [published Online First: Epub Date].

10. Paisley KC, Kraeutler MJ, Lazarus MD, Ramsey ML, Williams GR, Smith MJ. Relationship of scapular neck length to scapular notching after reverse total shoulder arthroplasty by use of plain radiographs. *J Shoulder Elbow Surg.* 2014; 23(6):882–887. https://doi.org/10.1016/j.jse.2013.09.003 [published Online First: Epub Date].

11. Poon PC, Chou J, Young SW, Astley T. A comparison of concentric and eccentric glenospheres in reverse shoulder arthroplasty: a randomized controlled trial. *J Bone Jt Surg Am.* 2014;96(16):e138. https://doi.org/10.2106/JBJS.M.00941 [published Online First: Epub Date].

12. Simovitch RW, Zumstein MA, Lohri E, Helmy N, Gerber C. Predictors of scapular notching in patients managed with the Delta III reverse total shoulder replacement. *J Bone Jt Surg Am.* 2007;89(3):588–600. https://doi.org/10.2106/JBJS.F.00226 [published Online First: Epub Date].

13. Hendel MD, Bryan JA, Barsoum WK, et al. Comparison of patient-specific instruments with standard surgical instruments in determining glenoid component position: a randomized prospective clinical trial. *J Bone Jt Surg Am.* 2012;94(23):2167–2175. https://doi.org/10.2106/JBJS.K.01209 [published Online First: Epub Date].

14. Iannotti J, Baker J, Rodriguez E, et al. Three-dimensional preoperative planning software and a novel information transfer technology improve glenoid component positioning. *J Bone Jt Surg Am.* 2014;96(9):e71. https://doi.org/10.2106/JBJS.L.01346 [published Online First: Epub Date].

15. Scalise JJ, Codsi MJ, Bryan J, Brems JJ, Iannotti JP. The influence of three-dimensional computed tomography images of the shoulder in preoperative planning for total shoulder arthroplasty. *J Bone Jt Surg Am.* 2008;90(11): 2438–2445. https://doi.org/10.2106/JBJS.G.01341 [published Online First: Epub Date].

16. Churchill RS, Brems JJ, Kotschi H. Glenoid size, inclination, and version: an anatomic study. *J Shoulder Elbow Surg.* 2001;10(4):327–332. https://doi.org/10.1067/mse.2001.115269 [published Online First: Epub Date].

17. Codsi MJ, Bennetts C, Gordiev K, et al. Normal glenoid vault anatomy and validation of a novel glenoid implant shape. *J Shoulder Elbow Surg.* 2008;17(3):471–478. https://doi.org/10.1016/j.jse.2007.08.010 [published Online First: Epub Date].

18. Ganapathi A, McCarron JA, Chen X, Iannotti JP. Predicting normal glenoid version from the pathologic scapula: a comparison of 4 methods in 2- and 3-dimensional models. *J Shoulder Elbow Surg.* 2011;20(2):234–244. https://doi.org/10.1016/j.jse.2010.05.024 [published Online First: Epub Date].

19. Ricchetti ET, Hendel MD, Collins DN, Iannotti JP. Is premorbid glenoid anatomy altered in patients with glenohumeral osteoarthritis? *Clin Orthop Relat Res.* 2013; 471(9):2932–2939. https://doi.org/10.1007/s11999-013-3069-5 [published Online First: Epub Date].

20. Scalise JJ, Codsi MJ, Bryan J, Iannotti JP. The three-dimensional glenoid vault model can estimate normal glenoid version in osteoarthritis. *J Shoulder Elbow Surg.* 2008;17(3):487–491. https://doi.org/10.1016/j.jse.2007.09.006 [published Online First: Epub Date].

21. Farron A, Terrier A, Büchler P. Risks of loosening of a prosthetic glenoid implanted in retroversion. *J Shoulder Elbow Surg.* 2006;15(4):521–526. https://doi.org/10.1016/j.jse.2005.10.003 [published Online First: Epub Date].

22. Ho JC, Sabesan VJ, Iannotti JP. Glenoid component retroversion is associated with osteolysis. *J Bone Jt Surg Am.* 2013;95(12):e82. https://doi.org/10.2106/JBJS.L.00336 [published Online First: Epub Date].

23. Hopkins AR, Hansen UN, Amis AA, Emery R. The effects of glenoid component alignment variations on cement mantle stresses in total shoulder arthroplasty. *J Shoulder Elbow Surg.* 2004;13(6):668–675. https://doi.org/10.1016/S10582746 04001399 [published Online First: Epub Date].

24. Young AA, Walch G, Pape G, Gohlke F, Favard L. Secondary rotator cuff dysfunction following total shoulder arthroplasty for primary glenohumeral osteoarthritis: results of a multicenter study with more than five years of follow-up. *J Bone Jt Surg Am.* 2012;94(8):685–693. https://doi.org/10.2106/JBJS.J.00727 [published Online First: Epub Date].

25. Haines JF, Trail IA, Nuttall D, Birch A, Barrow A. The results of arthroplasty in osteoarthritis of the shoulder. *J Bone Jt Surg Br.* 2006;88(4):496–501. https://doi.org/10.1302/0301-620X.88B4.16604 [published Online First: Epub Date].

26. Walch G, Young AA, Melis B, Gazielly D, Loew M, Boileau P. Results of a convex-back cemented keeled glenoid component in primary osteoarthritis: multicenter study with a follow-up greater than 5 years. *J Shoulder Elbow Surg.* 2011;20(3):385–394. https://doi.org/10.1016/j.jse.2010.07.011 [published Online First: Epub Date].

27. Clavert P, Millett PJ, Warner JJ. Glenoid resurfacing: what are the limits to asymmetric reaming for posterior erosion? *J Shoulder Elbow Surg.* 2007;16(6):843–848. https://doi.org/10.1016/j.jse.2007.03.015 [published Online First: Epub Date].

28. Nowak DD, Bahu MJ, Gardner TR, et al. Simulation of surgical glenoid resurfacing using three-dimensional computed tomography of the arthritic glenohumeral joint: the amount of glenoid retroversion that can be corrected. *J Shoulder Elbow Surg.* 2009;18(5):680–688. https://doi.org/10.1016/j.jse.2009.03.019 [published Online First: Epub Date].

29. Hill JM, Norris TR. Long-term results of total shoulder arthroplasty following bone-grafting of the glenoid. *J Bone Jt Surg Am.* 2001;83-A(6):877–883.

30. Nicholson GP, Cvetanovich GL, Rao AJ, O'Donnell P. Posterior glenoid bone grafting in total shoulder arthroplasty for osteoarthritis with severe posterior glenoid wear. *J Shoulder Elbow Surg.* 2017;26(10):1844–1853. https://doi.org/10.1016/j.jse.2017.03.016 [published Online First: Epub Date].

31. Sabesan V, Callanan M, Ho J, Iannotti JP. Clinical and radiographic outcomes of total shoulder arthroplasty with bone graft for osteoarthritis with severe glenoid bone loss. *J Bone Jt Surg Am.* 2013;95(14):1290–1296. https://doi.org/10.2106/JBJS.L.00097 [published Online First: Epub Date].

32. Favorito PJ, Freed RJ, Passanise AM, Brown MJ. Total shoulder arthroplasty for glenohumeral arthritis associated with posterior glenoid bone loss: results of an all-polyethylene, posteriorly augmented glenoid component. *J Shoulder Elbow Surg.* 2016;25(10):1681–1689. https://doi.org/10.1016/j.jse.2016.02.020 [published Online First: Epub Date].

33. Stephens SP, Spencer EE, Wirth MA. Radiographic results of augmented all-polyethylene glenoids in the presence of posterior glenoid bone loss during total shoulder arthroplasty. *J Shoulder Elbow Surg.* 2017;26(5):798–803. https://doi.org/10.1016/j.jse.2016.09.053 [published Online First: Epub Date].

34. Wright TW, Grey SG, Roche CP, Wright L, Flurin PH, Zuckerman JD. Preliminary results of a posterior augmented glenoid compared to an all polyethylene standard glenoid in anatomic total shoulder arthroplasty. *Bull Hosp Jt Dis.* 2013;2015(73 suppl 1):S79–S85.

35. Verborgt O, De Smedt T, Vanhees M, Clockaerts S, Parizel PM, Van Glabbeek F. Accuracy of placement of the glenoid component in reversed shoulder arthroplasty with and without navigation. *J Shoulder Elbow Surg.* 2011;20(1):21–26. https://doi.org/10.1016/j.jse.2010.07.014 [published Online First: Epub Date].

36. Randelli P, Randelli F, Arrigoni P, et al. Optimal glenoid component inclination in reverse shoulder arthroplasty. How to improve implant stability. *Musculoskelet Surg.* 2014;98(suppl 1):15–18. https://doi.org/10.1007/s12306-014-0324-1 [published Online First: Epub Date].

37. Heylen S, Van Haver A, Vuylsteke K, Declercq G, Verborgt O. Patient-specific instrument guidance of glenoid component implantation reduces inclination variability in total and reverse shoulder arthroplasty. *J Shoulder Elbow Surg.* 2016;25(2):186–192. https://doi.org/10.1016/j.jse.2015.07.024 [published Online First: Epub Date].

38. Werner BS, Chaoui J, Walch G. The influence of humeral neck shaft angle and glenoid lateralization on range of motion in reverse shoulder arthroplasty. *J Shoulder Elbow Surg.* 2017;26(10):1726–1731. https://doi.org/10.1016/j.jse.2017.03.032 [published Online First: Epub Date].

39. Erickson BJ, Frank RM, Harris JD, Mall N, Romeo AA. The influence of humeral head inclination in reverse total shoulder arthroplasty: a systematic review. *J Shoulder Elbow Surg.* 2015;24(6):988–993. https://doi.org/10.1016/j.jse.2015.01.001 [published Online First: Epub Date].

40. Permeswaran VN, Caceres A, Goetz JE, Anderson DD, Hettrich CM. The effect of glenoid component version and humeral polyethylene liner rotation on subluxation and impingement in reverse shoulder arthroplasty. *J Shoulder Elbow Surg.* 2017;26(10):1718–1725. https://doi.org/10.1016/j.jse.2017.03.027 [published Online First: Epub Date].

41. Iannotti JP, Weiner S, Rodriguez E, et al. Three-dimensional imaging and templating improve glenoid implant positioning. *J Bone Jt Surg Am.* 2015;97(8):651–658. https://doi.org/10.2106/JBJS.N.00493 [published Online First: Epub Date].

42. Werner BS, Hudek R, Burkhart KJ, Gohlke F. The influence of three-dimensional planning on decision-making in total shoulder arthroplasty. *J Shoulder Elbow Surg.* 2017;26(8):1477–1483. https://doi.org/10.1016/j.jse.2017.01.006 [published Online First: Epub Date].

43. Bryce CD, Davison AC, Lewis GS, Wang L, Flemming DJ, Armstrong AD. Two-dimensional glenoid version measurements vary with coronal and sagittal scapular rotation. *J Bone Jt Surg Am.* 2010;92(3):692–699. https://doi.org/10.2106/JBJS.I.00177 [published Online First: Epub Date].

44. Hoenecke HR, Hermida JC, Flores-Hernandez C, D'Lima DD. Accuracy of CT-based measurements of glenoid version for total shoulder arthroplasty. *J Shoulder Elbow Surg.* 2010;19(2):166–171. https://doi.org/10.1016/j.jse.2009.08.009 [published Online First: Epub Date].

45. Bokor DJ, O'Sullivan MD, Hazan GJ. Variability of measurement of glenoid version on computed tomography scan. *J Shoulder Elbow Surg.* 1999;8(6):595–598.

46. Klein SM, Dunning P, Mulieri P, Pupello D, Downes K, Frankle MA. Effects of acquired glenoid bone defects on surgical technique and clinical outcomes in reverse shoulder arthroplasty. *J Bone Jt Surg Am.* 2010;92(5):1144–1154. https://doi.org/10.2106/JBJS.I.00778 [published Online First: Epub Date].

47. Throckmorton TW, Gulotta LV, Bonnarens FO, et al. Patient-specific targeting guides compared with traditional instrumentation for glenoid component placement in shoulder arthroplasty: a multi-surgeon study in 70 arthritic cadaver specimens. *J Shoulder Elbow Surg.* 2015;24(6):965–971. https://doi.org/10.1016/j.jse.2014.10.013 [published Online First: Epub Date].

48. Levy JC, Everding NG, Frankle MA, Keppler LJ. Accuracy of patient-specific guided glenoid baseplate positioning for reverse shoulder arthroplasty. *J Shoulder Elbow Surg.* 2014;23(10):1563–1567. https://doi.org/10.1016/j.jse.2014.01.051 [published Online First: Epub Date].

49. Walch G, Vezeridis PS, Boileau P, Deransart P, Chaoui J. Three-dimensional planning and use of patient-specific guides improve glenoid component position: an in vitro study. *J Shoulder Elbow Surg.* 2015;24(2):302–309. https://doi.org/10.1016/j.jse.2014.05.029 [published Online First: Epub Date].

50. Gauci MO, Boileau P, Baba M, Chaoui J, Walch G. Patient-specific glenoid guides provide accuracy and reproducibility in total shoulder arthroplasty. *Bone Jt J.* 2016;98-B(8):1080–1085. https://doi.org/10.1302/0301-620X.98B8.37257 [published Online First: Epub Date].

51. Dallalana RJ, McMahon RA, East B, Geraghty L. Accuracy of patient-specific instrumentation in anatomic and reverse total shoulder arthroplasty. *Int J Shoulder Surg.* 2016;10(2):59–66. https://doi.org/10.4103/0973-6042.180717 [published Online First: Epub Date].

52. Mulligan RP, Azar FM, Throckmorton TW. Generic targeting guides place revision glenoid components in more anatomic version than traditional techniques. *J Shoulder Elbow Surg.* 2017;26(5):786–791. https://doi.org/10.1016/j.jse.2016.09.002 [published Online First: Epub Date].

53. Lewis GS, Stevens NM, Armstrong AD. Testing of a novel pin array guide for accurate three-dimensional glenoid component positioning. *J Shoulder Elbow Surg.* 2015;24(12):1939–1947. https://doi.org/10.1016/j.jse.2015.06.022 [published Online First: Epub Date].

54. Sadoghi P, Vavken J, Leithner A, Vavken P. Benefit of intraoperative navigation on glenoid component positioning during total shoulder arthroplasty. *Arch Orthop Trauma Surg.* 2015;135(1):41–47. https://doi.org/10.1007/s00402-014-2126-1 [published Online First: Epub Date].

55. Edwards TB, Gartsman GM, O'Connor DP, Sarin VK. Safety and utility of computer-aided shoulder arthroplasty. *J Shoulder Elbow Surg.* 2008;17(3):503–508. https://doi.org/10.1016/j.jse.2007.10.005 [published Online First: Epub Date].

56. Kircher J, Wiedemann M, Magosch P, Lichtenberg S, Habermeyer P. Improved accuracy of glenoid positioning in total shoulder arthroplasty with intraoperative navigation: a prospective-randomized clinical study. *J Shoulder Elbow Surg.* 2009;18(4):515–520. https://doi.org/10.1016/j.jse.2009.03.014 [published Online First: Epub Date].

57. Dines DM, Gulotta L, Craig EV, Dines JS. Novel solution for massive glenoid defects in shoulder arthroplasty: a patient-specific glenoid vault reconstruction system. *Am J Orthop (Belle Mead NJ).* 2017;46(2):104–108.

58. Chammaa R, Uri O, Lambert S. Primary shoulder arthroplasty using a custom-made hip-inspired implant for the treatment of advanced glenohumeral arthritis in the presence of severe glenoid bone loss. *J Shoulder Elbow Surg.* 2017;26(1):101–107. https://doi.org/10.1016/j.jse.2016.05.027 [published Online First: Epub Date].

59. Miyake J, Shimada K, Oka K, et al. Arthroscopic debridement in the treatment of patients with osteoarthritis of the elbow, based on computer simulation. *Bone Jt J.* 2014;96-B(2):237–241. https://doi.org/10.1302/0301-620X.96B2.30714 [published Online First: Epub Date].

60. Nishiwaki M, Willing R, Johnson JA, King GJ, Athwal GS. Identifying the location and volume of bony impingement in elbow osteoarthritis by 3-dimensional computational modeling. *J Hand Surg Am.* 2013;38(7):1370–1376. https://doi.org/10.1016/j.jhsa.2013.03.035 [published Online First: Epub Date].

61. Willing RT, Nishiwaki M, Johnson JA, King GJ, Athwal GS. Evaluation of a computational model to predict elbow range of motion. *Comput Aided Surg.* 2014;19(4–6):57–63. https://doi.org/10.3109/10929088.2014.886083 [published Online First: Epub Date].

62. Yamamoto M, Murakami Y, Iwatsuki K, Kurimoto S, Hirata H. Feasibility of four-dimensional preoperative simulation for elbow debridement arthroplasty. *BMC Musculoskelet Disord.* 2016;17:144. https://doi.org/10.1186/s12891-016-0996-9 [published Online First: Epub Date].

CHAPTER 14

3D Printing in Hip and Knee Arthroplasty

MUHAMMAD NADEEM, MBBS • ERIC JACKSON, DO • SRIDHAR R. RACHALA, MD

3D-printed physical objects can be utilized for studying complex cases, teaching students and patients, rehearsing the procedures in risk-free settings, and pre-procedure designing of grafts and implants.[1-3] In this chapter, we will discuss some applications of 3D printing technologies in lower extremity total joint arthroplasty and how they may benefit the surgeon and patient.

ROLE OF 3D PRINTING IN LOWER EXTREMITY ARTHROPLASTY

Before using any new technology, a surgeon should analyze the following questions:

1. What is the problem that we are trying to fix?
2. What are the limitations of the current method of fixing this problem?
3. Does the innovation indeed address the problem better than existing options and improving patient outcomes?
4. What is the added cost of the innovation?

HIP

Restoration of the biomechanics of the hip (leg length and offset) is important not only for improved function of the hip but also to decrease the incidence of limp and dislocation.[4-9] In about 32% of the cases the femoral offset and the leg length are not restored simultaneously.[4] According to a study, limb length discrepancy (LLD) > 1 cm exists in about 62% of the patients who had uncemented total hip arthroplasty[10] resulting in lower clinical scores, patient dissatisfaction, and legal issues for operating surgeons. Navigation helps in fixing the offset precisely and protects from LLD; however, it adds to the cost and increases the operating time.[11] A 3D CT scan technique utilization during preoperative planning results in precise anatomy restoration.[12] In addition, results for the femoral offset and the leg length restoration are comparable with navigation.[11] Preoperative templating may be used to aid the surgeon

in their surgical preparation. It assists in giving the start point not only for prediction of implant size range but also for implant position. In lieu of anatomical variations, cases such as developmental dysplasia of hip where 2D radiographs do not show the acetabular morphology, 2D radiographs centered preoperative templating is usually not perfect.[13] Some surgeons would argue that placement of the acetabular component is the most important part of THA. Complications from malpositioning of the acetabular implant can lead to decreased range of motion, increased revision rate, increased dislocation, squeaking, edge-loading, and early wearing and loosening. Several systems have been introduced to control malpositioned hip implants and to get better implant alignment reproducibility including[14-24]:

- Computer-assisted navigation—image-assisted and imageless.
- Use of anatomic landmarks.
- Intraoperative X-ray.
- CT-based robotic assisted surgery.

These systems have increased precision and decreased outlier rates.[19-24] The navigation systems increase cost and operative time, so those are not used frequently despite the improved accuracy.[20,21] 3D preoperative planning based on CT image gives improved stability and high precision for hip reconstruction.[12]

3D RAPID PROTOTYPING

3D preoperative planning plays a vital role in increasing accuracy of anteversion restoration and lowering the outliers' percentage without affecting operative time (see Figs. 14.1 to 14.3A—C,[25]).[15] Stereolithography (STL) file format is used in STL CAD software for rapid prototyping. It is the industry standard and carries the actual size info. The model is triangulated and kept stored in STL file format after segmenting the specific sections. These files elaborate a raw amorphous triangulated surface by the unit normal and triangles vertices by means of the 3D Cartesian coordinate system. Afterward, STL files are transferred to the 3D printer. CT scan matching software and its designated nature assists to get 1:1 scale. A pelvis model, built based on 3D CT scan is used for preoperative simulated acetabular cup placing and reaming. The bone that lies under the osteophyte could be less dense. The overhanging osteophyte is taken off.[13]

Using a 3D-printed model allows the surgeon both tactile and visual inspection of bone loss in the setting of a complex reconstruction. It can give the surgeon clues as to column stability, medial wall stability, and whether the acetabular rim is intact or not. The tactile

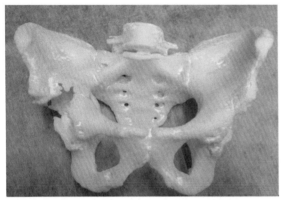

FIG. 14.1 3D-printed model of pelvis displaying the defects.

feel can aid a less experienced surgeon in planning the trajectory of screw placement especially when planning to place screws in a less utilized quadrant.

Implant manufacturers have utilized 3D printing in the hip reconstruction setting. In a complex hip that has pelvic discontinuity or significant bone loss a reasonable implant to use is a custom triflange acetabular component. ZimmerBiomet (Warsaw, Indiana) can produce a patient-specific triflange acetabular implants that are produced based on the patient's preoperative CT scan. The following steps include a 3D-printed acetabulum followed by the creation of a prototype implant. Lastly, the prototype is reviewed by the surgeon prior to final creation by the implant company. The process typically takes 4−6 weeks.

KNEE

End-stage osteoarthritis of the knee can be debilitating and affect the quality of life of the patient suffering from it. It can be managed surgically by total knee arthroplasty (TKA). The demand for TKA has increased in the last decade and is projected to increase substantially in the next decade with the aging baby boomers and increased incidence of obesity.[26] Despite the advances, one in five patients undergoing TKA can be dissatisfied with the result.[27] While the patient factors play a role in this, the role of altered knee kinematics, knee anatomy, and soft tissue balance cannot be discounted.[28,29]

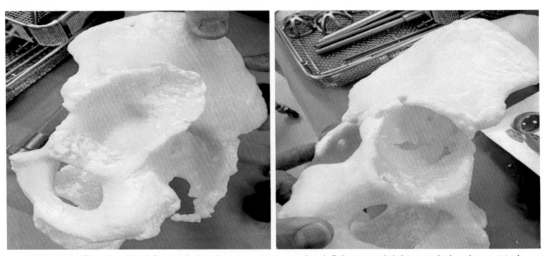

FIG. 14.2 Showing that left acetabulum has a posterosuperior deficiency and right acetabulum has central discontinuation due to bone loss.

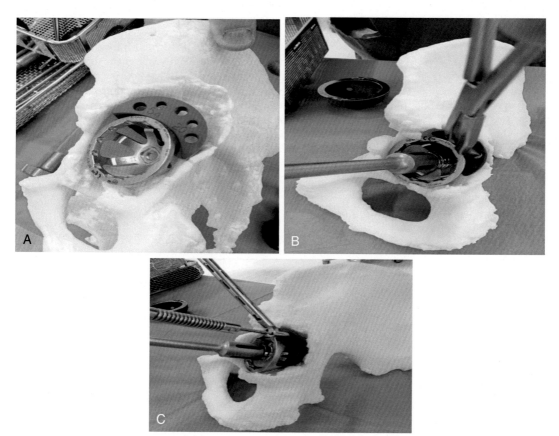

FIG. 14.3 (A–C) Showing preoperative templating, implant sizing, and surgical simulation.

The 3D printing technology has a role in knee replacement in three predominant areas:
1. Patient-specific instrumentation (PSI).
2. Custom implants prepared by using 3D-printed molds.
3. 3D-printed ingrowth surface on noncustom implants as an additive manufacturing process.

Patient-Specific Instrumentation

PSI involves generation of 3D-printed custom cutting blocks using preoperative CT data to improve the accuracy of component positioning and the extremity alignment. By linking a 3D printing system to preoperative CT data, PSI can be designed for bone cuts that are not only accurate but also unique to each patient (Kinematic alignment).[30,31] The plan is made preoperatively and based on the surgeon preference, the custom 3D-printed cutting blocks and jigs are created based on the CT data. Printed guides are sterilized at 121–126°C for 20–30 min.[32]

Intraoperatively there is no need for intramedullary alignment thereby potentially decreasing blood loss and fat embolization. Predefined template-specific rotation and orientation have been attained that result in improved rotational alignment. Also, prepackaged cutting blocks and trials mean decrease in number of instrument trays thereby decreasing the turnover time and improving efficiency.[33,34] It also decreases the load on the sterile processing department and decreases the inventory the hospital needs to hold. Because of the anticipated escalation in PSI applications, it may be a substitute for a conventional instrumentation technique and computer navigation and can lessen malalignment by accomplishing personalized cuts with an added benefit of bone conservation. The PSI system is 0.010 and 0.01 mm in precision. Patient-specific cutting guides have been used both in the total knee replacement setting and in the unicompartmental knee replacement setting.

Preoperative CT data ➡️ 3D printing system ➡️ PSI.

Advantages of PSI[35,36]:

- Improved bone cutting.
- Reduced negative effects impacted by surgeon experience.
- Reduced operative time and turnover time and inventory.
- Less blood loss.
- Invasiveness.
- Less operative decision making by preoperative planning.

PSI, however, adds cost to the procedure, as a CT scan is required preoperatively in addition to the cost of making the 3D-printed cutting blocks. This is partially offset by decreasing the turnover time and decreased number of trays to be processed by the sterile processing department. While there are many theoretical advantages to PSI, it has not yet been shown to unequivocally improve the patient outcomes.[33,37-39] The reason for that might have to do with the fact that multiple factors affect the patient outcomes (patient selection, surgeon's technical skill, and implant design). However, we believe that the high-volume centers might see the biggest benefits of this technology as the cost can be offset by improved efficiency with comparable outcomes.

Implants

3D printing technology has been utilized by implant manufactures to create a bone implant interface that more closely approaches the young's modulus of elasticity of cancellous bone. Stryker (Mahwah, New Jersey) uncemented triathalon tibial base plate utilizes 3D-printed tritantium substrate at the implant bone interface. The idea is that this will yield greater bone ingrowth and improve biologic fixation (see Figs. 14.4—14.6).[40]

Custom femoral implants have also been in use using this technology. Metal implants are casted in the custom molds created by 3D printing (Conformis).

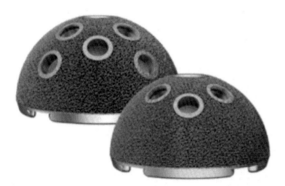

FIG. 14.4 3D printed Trident II Titanium acetabular cup for cementless fixation. (Image used after getting permission from Stryker.com.)

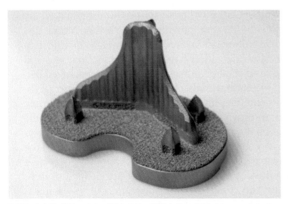

FIG. 14.5 3D printed Triathlon Tritanium tibial baseplate for cementless fixation. (Image used after getting permission from Stryker.com.)

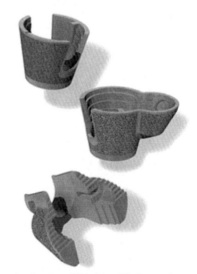

FIG. 14.6 3D printed Triathlon TS Cones for revision knee procedures. (Image used after getting permission from Stryker.com.)

CONCLUSION

3D printing is innovative new technology that is bound to have many applications in the future. It is currently limited by the type of materials that can be processed using the 3D printer and the turnover time for the process involving 3D-printed models, implants, and jigs. We believe the full potential of this technology is not yet realized in orthopedic surgery. It will have a bigger role in future to improve intraoperative efficiency, custom implants, and patient-specific positioning of the implants as these processes demonstrate improved outcomes. But, the benefits of this technology have to be carefully weighed against added cost to minimize the healthcare cost burden.

REFERENCES

1. Wurm G, Tomancok B, Pogady P, Holl K, Trenkler J. Cerebrovascular stereolithographic biomodeling for aneurysm surgery. Technical note. *J Neurosurg.* 2004;100(1): 139−145.
2. Zerr J, Chatzinoff Y, Chopra R, Estrera K, Chhabra A. Three-dimensional printing for preoperative planning of total hip arthroplasty revision: case report. *Skelet Radiol.* 2016; 45(10):1431−1435.
3. Nadeem M, Noor S. Coil embolization in 3D models. *J Vasc Surg.* 2017;65(6):99S.
4. Asayama I, Chamnongkich S, Simpson KJ, Kinsey TL, Mahoney OM. Reconstructed hip joint position and abductor muscle strength after total hip arthroplasty. *J Arthroplas.* 2005;20(4):414−420.
5. Bourne RB, Rorabeck CH. Soft tissue balancing: the hip. *J Arthroplas.* 2002;17(4 suppl 1):17−22.
6. Downing ND, Clark DI, Hutchinson JW, Colclough K, Howard PW. Hip abductor strength following total hip arthroplasty: a prospective comparison of the posterior and lateral approach in 100 patients. *Acta Orthop Scand.* 2001;72(3):215−220.
7. Kiyama T, Naito M, Shinoda T, Maeyama A. Hip abductor strengths after total hip arthroplasty via the lateral and posterolateral approaches. *J Arthroplast.* 2010;25(1): 76−80.
8. McGrory BJ, Morrey BF, Cahalan TD, An KN, Cabanela ME. Effect of femoral offset on range of motion and abductor muscle strength after total hip arthroplasty. *J Bone Joint Surg Br Vol.* 1995;77(6):865−869.
9. Flecher X, Pearce O, Parratte S, Aubaniac JM, Argenson JN. Custom cementless stem improves hip function in young patients at 15-year followup. *Clin Orthop Relat Res.* 2010; 468(3):747−755.
10. Konyves A, Bannister GC. The importance of leg length discrepancy after total hip arthroplasty. *J Bone Joint Surg Br Vol.* 2005;87(2):155−157.
11. Kitada M, Nakamura N, Iwana D, Kakimoto A, Nishii T, Sugano N. Evaluation of the accuracy of computed tomography-based navigation for femoral stem orientation and leg length discrepancy. *J Arthroplast.* 2011;26(5): 674−679.
12. Sariali E, Mouttet A, Pasquier G, Durante E, Catone Y. Accuracy of reconstruction of the hip using computerised three-dimensional pre-operative planning and a cementless modular neck. *J Bone Joint Surg Br Vol.* 2009;91(3):333−340.
13. Xu J, Li D, Ma RF, Barden B, Ding Y. Application of rapid prototyping pelvic model for patients with DDH to facilitate arthroplasty planning: a pilot study. *J Arthroplast.* 2015;30(11):1963−1970.
14. Parratte S, Argenson JN, Flecher X, Aubaniac JM. Computer-assisted surgery for acetabular cup positioning in total hip arthroplasty: comparative prospective randomized study. *Revue de Chir Orthop reparatrice de l'appareil moteur.* 2007;93(3):238−246.
15. Sariali E, Boukhelifa N, Catonne Y, Pascal Moussellard H. Comparison of three-dimensional planning-assisted and conventional acetabular cup positioning in total hip arthroplasty: a randomized controlled trial. *J Bone Joint Surg Am Vol.* 2016;98(2):108−116.
16. Kennedy JG, Rogers WB, Soffe KE, Sullivan RJ, Griffen DG, Sheehan LJ. Effect of acetabular component orientation on recurrent dislocation, pelvic osteolysis, polyethylene wear, and component migration. *J Arthroplast.* 1998;13(5): 530−534.
17. Murphy SB, Ecker TM. Evaluation of a new leg length measurement algorithm in hip arthroplasty. *Clin Orthop Relat Res.* 2007;463:85−89.
18. Archbold HA, Mockford B, Molloy D, McConway J, Ogonda L, Beverland D. The transverse acetabular ligament: an aid to orientation of the acetabular component during primary total hip replacement: a preliminary study of 1000 cases investigating postoperative stability. *J Bone Joint Surg Br Vol.* 2006;88(7):883−886.
19. Kalteis T, Sendtner E, Beverland D, et al. The role of the transverse acetabular ligament for acetabular component orientation in total hip replacement: an analysis of acetabular component position and range of movement using navigation software. *J Bone Joint Surg Br Vol.* 2011;93(8): 1021−1026.
20. Domb BG, El Bitar YF, Sadik AY, Stake CE, Botser IB. Comparison of robotic-assisted and conventional acetabular cup placement in THA: a matched-pair controlled study. *Clin Orthop Relat Res.* 2014;472(1):329−336.
21. Parratte S, Argenson JN. Validation and usefulness of a computer-assisted cup-positioning system in total hip arthroplasty. A prospective, randomized, controlled study. *J Bone Joint Surg Am Vol.* 2007;89(3):494−499.
22. Hube R, Birke A, Hein W, Klima S. CT-based and fluoroscopy-based navigation for cup implantation in total hip arthroplasty (THA). *Surg Technol Int.* 2003;11: 275−280.

23. Iwana D, Nakamura N, Miki H, Kitada M, Hananouchi T, Sugano N. Accuracy of angle and position of the cup using computed tomography-based navigation systems in total hip arthroplasty. *Comput Aided Surg.* 2013;18(5–6): 187–194.

24. Sugano N, Takao M, Sakai T, Nishii T, Miki H. Does CT-based navigation improve the long-term survival in ceramic-on-ceramic THA? *Clin Orthop Relat Res.* 2012; 470(11):3054–3059.

25. Hughes AJ, DeBuitleir C, Soden P, et al. 3D printing aids acetabular reconstruction in complex revision hip arthroplasty. *Adv Orthop.* 2017;2017:8925050.

26. Cavaignac E, Pailhe R, Laumond G, et al. Evaluation of the accuracy of patient-specific cutting blocks for total knee arthroplasty: a meta-analysis. *Int Orthop.* 2015;39(8): 1541–1552.

27. Mannan A, Smith TO. Favourable rotational alignment outcomes in PSI knee arthroplasty: a Level 1 systematic review and meta-analysis. *Knee.* 2016;23(2):186–190.

28. Hansen DC, Kusuma SK, Palmer RM, Harris KB. Robotic guidance does not improve component position or short-term outcome in medial unicompartmental knee arthroplasty. *J Arthroplast.* 2014;29(9):1784–1789.

29. Jiang J, Kang X, Lin Q, et al. Accuracy of patient-specific instrumentation compared with conventional instrumentation in total knee arthroplasty. *Orthopedics.* 2015;38(4): e305–e313.

30. Watters TS, Mather 3rd RC, Browne JA, Berend KR, Lombardi Jr AV, Bolognesi MP. Analysis of procedure-related costs and proposed benefits of using patient-specific approach in total knee arthroplasty. *J Surg Orthop Adv.* 2011;20(2):112–116.

31. Xiao J, Wang C, Zhu L, et al. Improved method for planning intramedullary guiding rod entry point in total knee arthroplasty. *Arch Orthop Trauma Surg.* 2014;134(5): 693–698.

32. Qiu B, Liu F, Tang B, et al. Clinical study of 3D imaging and 3D printing technique for patient-specific instrumentation in total knee arthroplasty. *J Knee Surg.* 2017;30(8): 822–828.

33. Lonner JH. Robotically assisted unicompartmental knee arthroplasty with a handheld image-free sculpting tool. *Orthop Clin N. Am.* 2016;47(1):29–40.

34. Jacofsky DJ, Allen M. Robotics in arthroplasty: a comprehensive review. *J Arthroplast.* 2016;31(10):2353–2363.

35. Leone WA, Elson LC, Anderson CR. A systematic literature review of three modalities in technologically assisted TKA. *Adv Orthop.* 2015;2015:719091.

36. Camarda L, D'Arienzo A, Morello S, Peri G, Valentino B, D'Arienzo M. Patient-specific instrumentation for total knee arthroplasty: a literature review. *Musculoskelet Surg.* 2015;99(1):11–18.

37. Banerjee S, Cherian JJ, Elmallah RK, Jauregui JJ, Pierce TP, Mont MA. Robotic-assisted knee arthroplasty. *Expert Rev Med Dev.* 2015;12(6):727–735.

38. Chua KH, Chen Y, Lingaraj K. Navigated total knee arthroplasty: is it error-free? *Knee Surg Sports Traumatol Arthrosc.* 2014;22(3):643–649.

39. Calliess T, Bauer K, Stukenborg-Colsman C, Windhagen H, Budde S, Ettinger M. PSI kinematic versus non-PSI mechanical alignment in total knee arthroplasty: a prospective, randomized study. *Knee Surg Sports Traumatol Arthrosc.* 2017;25(6):1743–1748.

40. Stryker. Hip and Knee Joint.

FURTHER READING

1. Kido T, Kurata A, Higashino H, et al. Cardiac imaging using 256-detector row four-dimensional CT: preliminary clinical report. *Radiat Med.* 2007;25(1):38–44.

2. Meaney JF, Goyen M. Recent advances in contrast-enhanced magnetic resonance angiography. *Eur Radiol.* 2007; 17(suppl 2):B2–B6.

3. Tack P, Victor J, Gemmel P, Annemans L. 3D-printing techniques in a medical setting: a systematic literature review. *Biomed Eng Online.* 2016;15(1):115.

4. Doi K. Diagnostic imaging over the last 50 years: research and development in medical imaging science and technology. *Phys Med Biol.* 2006;51(13):R5–R27.

5. Kirchgeorg MA, Prokop M. Increasing spiral CT benefits with postprocessing applications. *Eur J Radiol.* 1998;28(1): 39–54.

6. Von Tengg-Kobligk H, Weber TF, Rengier F, et al. Imaging modalities for the thoracic aorta. *J Cardiovasc Surg.* 2008; 49(4):429–447.

7. McGurk M, Amis AA, Potamianos P, Goodger NM. Rapid prototyping techniques for anatomical modelling in medicine. *Ann R Coll Surg Engl.* 1997;79(3):169–174.

8. Mulford JS, Babazadeh S, Mackay N. Three-dimensional printing in orthopaedic surgery: review of current and future applications. *ANZ J Surg.* 2016;86(9):648–653.

9. Eltorai AE, Nguyen E, Daniels AH. Three-dimensional printing in orthopedic surgery. *Orthopedics.* 2015;38(11):684–687.

10. Rengier F, Mehndiratta A, von Tengg-Kobligk H, et al. 3D printing based on imaging data: review of medical applications. *Int J Comput Assist Radiol Surg.* 2010;5(4): 335–341.

11. Hahn HK, Millar WS, Klinghammer O, Durkin MS, Tulipano PK, Peitgen HO. A reliable and efficient method for cerebral ventricular volumetry in pediatric neuroimaging. *Methods Inf Med.* 2004;43(4):376–382.

12. Fuller SM, Butz DR, Vevang CB, Makhlouf MV. Application of 3-dimensional printing in hand surgery for production of a novel bone reduction clamp. *J Hand Surg.* 2014;39(9): 1840–1845.

13. Salmi M, Paloheimo KS, Tuomi J, Wolff J, Makitie A. Accuracy of medical models made by additive manufacturing (rapid manufacturing). *J Cranio-Maxillo-Facial Surg.* 2013; 41(7):603–609.

14. Engineers ASOM. Top 10 Materials for 3D Printing. https://www.asme.org/engineering-topics/articles/manufacturing-processing/top-10-materials-3d-printing.

15. D'Urso PS, Thompson RG, Atkinson RL, et al. Cerebrovascular biomodelling: a technical note. *Surg Neurol.* 1999; 52(5):490–500.

16. Izatt MT, Thorpe PL, Thompson RG, et al. The use of physical biomodelling in complex spinal surgery. *Eur Spine J.* 2007;16(9):1507–1518.
17. D'Urso PS, Earwaker WJ, Barker TM, et al. Custom cranioplasty using stereolithography and acrylic. *Br J Plast Surg.* 2000;53(3):200–204.
18. Starosolski ZA, Kan JH, Rosenfeld SD, Krishnamurthy R, Annapragada A. Application of 3-D printing (rapid prototyping) for creating physical models of pediatric orthopedic disorders. *Pediatr Radiol.* 2014;44(2):216–221.
19. Conn KS, Clarke MT, Hallett JP. A simple guide to determine the magnification of radiographs and to improve the accuracy of preoperative templating. *J Bone Joint Surg Br Vol.* 2002;84(2):269–272.
20. Huppertz A, Radmer S, Asbach P, et al. Computed tomography for preoperative planning in minimal-invasive total hip arthroplasty: radiation exposure and cost analysis. *Eur J Radiol.* 2011;78(3):406–413.
21. Sharkey PF, Hozack WJ, Rothman RH, Shastri S, Jacoby SM. Insall Award paper. Why are total knee arthroplasties failing today? *Clin Orthop Relat Res.* 2002;(404):7–13.
22. Roche M. Robotic-assisted unicompartmental knee arthroplasty: the MAKO experience. *Clin Sports Med.* 2014;33(1):123–132.
23. Liow MH, Chin PL, Tay KJ, Chia SL, Lo NN, Yeo SJ. Early experiences with robot-assisted total knee arthroplasty using the DigiMatch ROBODOC(R) surgical system. *Singap Med J.* 2014;55(10):529–534.
24. Calliess T, Ettinger M, Windhagen H. Computer-assisted systems in total knee arthroplasty. Useful aid or only additional costs. *Der Orthopade.* 2014;43(6):529–533.
25. Shang P, Zhang L, Hou Z, et al. Morphometric measurement of the patella on 3D model reconstructed from CT scan images for the southern Chinese population. *Chin Med J.* 2014;127(1):96–101.

CHAPTER 15

3D Printing in Orthopedic Oncology

AMIR STERNHEIM, MD • YAIR GORTZAK, MD • YEHUDA KOLANDER, MD •
SOLOMON DADIA, MD

INTRODUCTION

Basic Concepts in Oncologic Surgery

Orthopedic oncology focuses on the treatment of primary sarcomas, which are mesenchymal tumors arising from bone and connective tissues. The majority of bone sarcomas are comprised of three different tumors: osteosarcoma, Ewing's sarcoma, and chondrosarcoma. The former two commonly affect patients between the ages of 5 and 25 years and account for up to 15% of all malignancies in that age group.[1-3] Chondrosarcomas commonly affect patients 50 years of age and older and account for less than 1% of all malignancies in that age group.[4,5] The annual incidence of primary bone sarcomas varies from 10 to 26 per million worldwide.[6] Patients present with localized pain and swelling and the development of a limp when a lower limb is involved. Osteosarcomas usually arise around the knee, i.e., the distal femur and proximal tibia, followed by the proximal humerus, whereas Ewing's sarcoma is more likely to be found in the diaphysis of long bones, especially the femur, as well as in the pelvis. These tumors have a tendency to spread systemically through the bloodstream, usually to the lungs and less often to other bones. They spread either directly as skip lesions or as distant metastasis, and approximately 20% of the patients have evidence of disseminated disease at presentation.

The diagnosis of Ewing's sarcoma and osteosarcoma dictates a chemotherapy regimen of approximately 6–12 months.[7-9] These lesions are treated with (neo) adjuvant chemotherapy and surgery. Proper staging for assessment of the local and systemic extent of disease is crucial and entails a local magnetic resonance imaging (MRI) scan with gadolinium and whole body imaging with a bone scan and a chest computerized tomogram (CT) or a positron emission tomogram CT (PET-CT). A biopsy will provide the pathologic diagnosis as well as the grade of the tumor and will guide the oncologist in recommending the appropriate chemotherapy protocol for a given patient. Surgical resection is an integral part of the treatment and must be planned carefully in order to ensure a wide resection of the tumor.

Imaging is carried out at the time of diagnosis and again toward the end of the preoperative chemotherapy administration in order to evaluate the extent of the tumor and response to chemotherapy. Tumor size can decrease dramatically with treatment, especially the soft tissue component in Ewing's sarcoma.

The goal of treatment is to eradicate both local and systemic tumor cells. This can be achieved by a combined modality treatment, which includes systemic chemotherapy and local surgical resection for osteosarcoma, while radiation therapy can play a significant role in addition to chemotherapy and surgery in Ewing's sarcoma. In contrast, chondrosarcomas are resistant to chemotherapy and are therefore treated by surgery alone.[4] High-grade chondrosarcomas have a worse prognosis compared with osteosarcomas and Ewing's sarcomas. The cure rates of osteosarcomas and Ewing's sarcomas are around 65%–70% for localized disease of the appendicular skeleton.[9]

The goal of surgery in bone sarcomas is a negative margin resection. This entails resection of the whole tumor mass with a surrounding margin of healthy tissue.[10] A negative margin resection is determined by frozen pathologic evaluation of the medullary canal (bone marrow) taken during surgery and pathologic evaluation of the whole resected specimen. There is an ongoing debate regarding the definition of a wide negative margin. Smaller margins have been shown to be adequate as long as all the tumor has been resected and the risk of local recurrence depends mainly on histologic grade of the tumor and whether the tumor was resected en bloc.[11-13] MRI findings, specifically, the amount of edema around the tumor on T2 MRI

3D Printing in Orthopaedic Surgery. https://doi.org/10.1016/B978-0-323-58118-9.00015-4

sequence and gadolinium enhancement, can help predict tumor response to treatment and planning the surgical procedure necessary to render the patient disease free. Local recurrence of a bone sarcoma is influenced by the grade of the disease, size of the initial tumor, initial response to chemotherapy, and the tumor's anatomic location. Pelvic tumors have a higher rate of recurrence.[14,15] The most significant factor influencing risk of recurrence is the margin status.[16] Positive margins on initial resection portend a high rate of recurrence, whereas negative margin resections are associated with low rates of local recurrence. Acceptable local recurrence rates among high-volume sarcoma centers are less than 10%, thus local recurrence rates may be considered a good indication of the appropriateness of the surgical treatment.

Wide margins are intended to account for all sarcoma cells in the periphery of the tumor, and those cells have been shown to exist in the peritumoral edema as well. In addition, those margins account for all the imaging and surgical inaccuracies of the surgical procedure. Imaging inaccuracies include the inability to locate the exact point where the tumor ends. A T1 MRI imaging series will show marrow replacement in bone. Gross tumor is thereby well displayed, but all the microscopic tumor cells that are often prevalent in the edema surrounding tumor are not always accounted for. A region with edema reportedly contains tumor cells up to several centimeters away from a gross tumor in soft tissue sarcomas and is probably similar to some extent in bone sarcomas.[17] Gadolinium-enhanced imaging can help differentiate between viable cancer cells, which have a high gadolinium uptake, and necrotic tissue and edema, which have much lower gadolinium uptake. The compiled data obtained from MRI T1, T2, and gadolinium-enhanced series make it possible to define a safe resection margin which does not reach the tumor and allows for resection of the tumor with a healthy soft tissue cuff. Another source of significant inaccuracies involves the accurate execution of the surgical plan. Bone cuts are measured and planned from the MRI imaging findings. The cuts are first measured away from the tumor (this is the "planned" margin), and the distance from this line of cutting is then measured from the adjacent joint. These measurements are also susceptible to some inaccuracy, as the exact anatomic point from which the measurement is taken on imaging is never the exact same point of measurement on the patient in surgery. Additionally, the measurement on the MRI is on a two-dimensional (2D) image (coronal/sagittal), whereas the measurement in surgery in the may not be on the same 2D. Throughout this chapter

we will explore whether 3D planning and 3D printing can improve accuracy and enable smaller resection margins while maintaining negative margin resection.

CT and MRI Imaging

MRI is the preferred modality of imaging of bone sarcomas. It is superior to CT by virtue of its ability to show the extent of tumor within the medullary space, where T1 weighted images will clearly demonstrate marrow replacement with tumor.[18,19] MRI is also superior to CT with regard to the evaluation of soft tissue extension of tumor outside the involved bone.[20] In order to preserve function, it is paramount to delineate the relation between that extension of the tumor and normal and critical anatomic structures, such as arteries, veins, and nerves. Acquiring an MRI is time-consuming, however. Typical scans that include axial, sagittal, and coronal cuts in T1, T2, and gadolinium series may take up to 30–45 min each and necessitate patient compliance as well as sedation in the case of young patients. The scan field must include the tumor and a surrounding region. Several cuts, which include the entire bone of interest, are also acquired to rule out skip metastasis in the same bone. There are several disadvantages to MRI scans. Each of the three modalities and each of the three cuts (i.e., axial, sagittal, and coronal) are acquired separately and cannot be reconstructed volumetrically from pixels to voxels to form a 3D image. Additionally, MRI cuts are often 1 mm in slice thickness acquired every 4 mm, limiting the level of accuracy. This can be improved with scans performed using the neurosurgical protocol of 1 mm cuts every 1 mm, although that is currently not the standard and is even more time consuming.

CT scans have the advantage of high resolution (1 mm cut every 1 mm step). Being volumetric, pixels can be constructed into 3D voxels, and scans can be acquired in short lengths of time.[18,21] The main disadvantage of CT scans, as opposed to MRI scans, is poorer accuracy in depicting soft tissue and bone medullary involvement, thus precluding its ability to act as a stand-alone imaging modality for bone tumor surgery.

The technique of fusion of CT and MRI scans superimposes the images of one modality over the other thus combining the fine details seen only on MRI scans with the higher resolution CT data set.[21] Image fusion is based on accurately matching anatomic landmarks on the involved bone of both imaging modalities in all three axes (X,Y,Z). It should be noted that as MRI scans are not volumetric, only one MRI series at a time can be fused to the CT scan.

Segmentation

Segmentation is the delineation of structures (e.g., tumor, anatomic parts) on the CT or MRI scan by defining their contours. Segmentation can be done manually (slice-by-slice), automatically, or, as is most commonly done, with a combination of manual and automatic techniques. Segmentation is carried out on dedicated software platforms as well as on several different imaging modalities and on different cuts and series. The various segmented structures can then be fused to the highest resolution scan, often the CT scan.

The bone from which the tumor arises and all relevant adjacent bones should be segmented for definition. There are multiple segmentation software packages available. The newer generations have an improved user interface which makes segmentation accessible to the surgeon within an acceptable timeframe of approximately 20 min. The tumor is segmented on the MRI scan as it is superior to CT with regard to the extent of the tumor inside bone (as noted on MRI by bone marrow replacement on T1) as well as the extent of soft tissue involvement. Only one MRI series is generally used for this purpose, and the additional MRI series may be used for cross-check validation. It is preferable that the MRI series with the largest amount of cuts be used as it often contains the largest volume. It is up to the surgeon's personal preference which of the three modalities (MRI T1, T2, or gadolinium) to use for segmentation. The step that follows is the fusion of the CT-based bone segmentation and the MRI-based tumor segmentation. During fusion, one image data set is superimposed on the other image data set. Registering the MRI data set to the CT data set is done by identifying identical anatomic landmarks on the CT and MRI images before fusion.

Each step of image acquisition, segmentation, and fusion has some level of inaccuracy but probably within only 2–3 mm.[22] Larger errors can occur when a process includes several steps, therefore the final assessment should always be compared with the initial image data set.

CHALLENGES IN ONCOLOGY SURGERY

Precision surgery aims to improve surgical accuracy through improving our understanding and ability to extract information from the findings demonstrated on imaging scans, as well as enhancing the definition (segmentation) of the tumor and important anatomic structures.[21] This is the basis for greater specificity in the surgical plan and greatest accuracy in its execution. Precision surgery through 3D planning and printing is a structured, multistep process that enables this improvement of accuracy in each of the steps, yielding significant overall improvement. Each step needs to be carried out in a structured and precise manner, and each must be measured and monitored.

Planning an Adequate Margin is Based Mostly on the Findings of MRI Imaging

The grade and histologic subtype of the tumor are also taken into account. Higher grade and chemoresistant tumor subtypes require a wider resection margin.[13–16] On MRI series, T1 imaging clearly shows the exact extent of macroscopic tumor.[20] T2 imaging clarifies the edema surrounding the gross tumor which has the potential to contain residual microscopic disease.[17] Gadolinium avidity shows areas of viable tumor with increased uptake and areas of necrotic tumor with decreased uptake. A tumor occasionally responds to chemotherapy by decreasing in size. There is also a lesser extent of bone and soft tissue involvement, as well as reduced edema. Planning the resection cuts to account for all these factors is crucial (Fig. 15.1). The authors believe the plan should always account for a worst case scenario where the edema surrounding the tumor contains microscopic disease and where those tumor cells have not responded well to chemotherapy and are still viable, thereby posing a risk of local recurrence. Thus, the lines representing the planned bone cuts need to be outside this range.

The necessity for the planned cut lines to be distanced away from the tumor accounts for various inaccuracies that impact the surgical process.[23] Tool error is a major culprit: it derives from the oscillating saw because of vibrations, the thickness of the saw blade, the length of the blade, and the blade's ability to bend. Saw vibrations and the coarseness of the tool cause it to jump about, specifically, on initial contact with bone. This is exacerbated with freehand use. The use of cutting jigs limits most of these tool errors. The thickness of the saw blade influences the thickness of the cut in bone. A 1 mm thick saw blade will make a 2 mm cut in bone. When the saw blade is longer and thinner, it has a greater tendency to bend, thus making it harder to control the exact direction it will take when it enters bone. In our experience, these different tool characteristics account for about 5 mm of inaccuracy in cutting. The resection plan should account for this factor by expanding the planned cuts 5 mm away from the tumor compared with the original plan.

During surgery, once the bone cuts that are made to resect the bone segment containing the tumor are

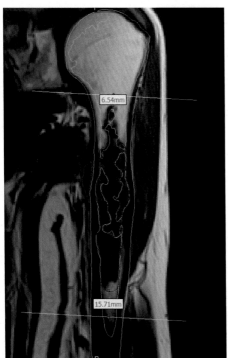

FIG. 15.1 **Plans:** Pre-op plan for resection of a chondrosarcoma of the proximal humerus. The completed plan is validated on a coronal T1 MRI image. It includes tumor which is outlined in red and humerus which is contoured in white. The planned bone cuts for a segmental resection of the tumor and the diaphysis of the humerus. Measurements mark the distance from the proximal tip of the greater tuberosity to the bone cut. Tumor is initially segmented on the MRI scan, the image is then fused with the CT scan where the humerus has been segmented. The bone cuts are then planned away from tumor to achieve a wide resection. The complete plan is then transferred back to the MRI scan for validation.

completed, marrow samples from the remaining bone are sent for pathologic analysis to validate that no tumor is microscopically apparent beyond the bone cuts. Macroscopic assessment of the different cut ends yields added information, as surgeons are experienced in identifying normal tissue compared to tissue with tumor content.

The pathologic assessment of the resection specimen includes longitudinal cuts, decalcification, and macroscopic assessment. A grid is then drawn on each longitudinal cut, and samples are taken from the margins and around the bone cuts.

Each of these steps in planning and analysis carries some level of inaccuracy. These have historically been accounted for with the 2 cm resection margin in bone. Improving accuracy may help in decreasing these margins to 1 cm or less without increasing the risk of a positive margin and a local recurrence.[18,20]

Deciding Upon the Surgical Approach and Soft Tissue Exposure.

The surgical approach is dictated by the location of tumor, the extent of soft tissue involvement, and the critical neurovascular structures which lay in close proximity. All of these elements should be visualized during surgery for a safe resection. The anatomic location dictates the approach. In the humerus, the approach to the arm is often deltopectoral, which can be extended to the anterolateral arm. In the distal femur, the most common approach is the medial, as the femoral vessels run off the medial aspect of the thigh before turning to the posterior popliteal region behind the knee. The second factor influencing the approach is the location and extent of tumor, especially the extent of soft tissue involvement. In the distal femur, when the soft tissue component of the tumor is more significant on the lateral aspect, a lateral surgical approach is indicated so that the tumor and its extent can be better visualized. The artery and vein are initially visualized behind the knee joint and they are dissected free in a proximal direction. The goal of the surgical approach is to optimize the safety of the soft tissue exposure where critical anatomic structures (arteries, veins, and nerves) are located, identified, and then dissected away from the tumor and the bone. The goal of the soft tissue exposure is to provide safe bone cuts for resecting the tumor without unnecessarily compromising important neurovascular structures. All of these factors influence the surgical planning process as they dictate the direction in which the bone cuts will be made and the bone surface that will be exposed and visualized for the placement of the cutting tool and cutting jig.

SURGICAL RECONSTRUCTION CHALLENGES

The preservation of limb function is the most important secondary goal of surgery, the primary goal being complete resection of the tumor.[24,25] Multiple factors impact functional outcome, including neurologic and vascular status, edema in the limb, joint stability, the amount of muscle resected, and limb length discrepancy that may develop in the pediatric growing population. Accuracy in the reconstruction of the defect created by resection of tumor is critical.[26] Preservation of the native knee joint is a common challenge as most primary bone tumors arise in the distal femur or the proximal tibia. Joint resections in tumor surgery are reconstructed with implants that are hinged joints with limited rotation and longevity which only incompletely replicate native motion. Those implants enable mobility but significantly limit function. Joint preservation together with that of the cruciate and collateral ligaments will result in significantly improved function and a closer to natural feel. Limb length and alignment are no less important in achieving good functional outcomes. Bone tumors originating around the distal femur and proximal tibia often arise in the metaphysis. The distance between the tumor and the knee joint is often only a few centimeters. The ability to improve accuracy in preoperative planning and in the actual surgery using 3D planning imaging platforms and 3D printed tools may impact our ability to spare the native joint in bone tumor resections and thus improve function without compromising the oncologic outcome.

3D Models

Three-dimensional computerized and printed models improve the surgeon's understanding of the surgical challenge at hand (Fig. 15.2). They enable preoperative trial runs of several surgical options and can serve as a tool for dry-run simulations. Although this is currently not common practice in surgery, different professional fields, such as aviation and automotive and construction industries, routinely use models and simulations to improve safety in real-life situations. Making tactical decisions on whether to make pelvic cuts inside-out or outside-in, which rely on soft tissue exposure and having an acceptable working angle for making a cut, can be tested and discussed on the model by the surgical team before finalizing the surgical plan.

The process of producing a 3D model starts with a CT scan of the field of interest, which includes the surgical field of interest, and it should have a 1 mm cut every 1 mm step. This yields a voxel size of 1 mm square which will define the level of accuracy of the plan. Next, a 3D box is used to focus the field of interest for the

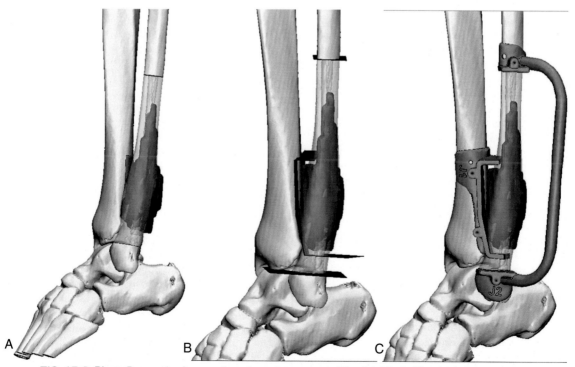

FIG. 15.2 **Plans:** Pre-op plan for resection of an osteosarcoma of the distal fibula. The plan is for a segmental resection sparing the lateral malleolus. Tumor is segmented from an MRI scan and bones are segmented from the CT scan. A fused 3D image shown **(A)**. The resection planes are placed away from tumor for a wide resection **(B)** protecting the lateral malleolus in order to preserve ankle motion and stability. Cutting jigs are then planned to account for the bone cuts and the footprint on bone which will guide their accurate placement **(C)**. The jigs are planned for a lateral approach, one for the fibula and a second for the posterior cortex of the tibia given the intimate proximity of tumor to it.

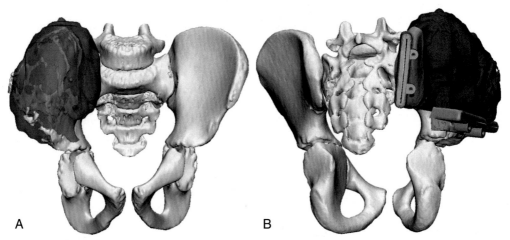

FIG. 15.3 **Plans:** Pelvic Ewing with a large soft tissue component which is best visualized and segmented on an MRI. Bone anatomy segmented from CT. 3D computer image of tumor and bone anatomy **(A)**. Resection planes and bone footprint are incorporated into the design of the jigs. These are planed for a supra-acetabular cut and a posterior cut through the sacroiliac joint both planned from the outside inwards **(B)**.

model. It should include the involved body part within the surgical field as well as the anatomic landmarks nearby. A scale of 1:1 enables the model to be used to test the printed surgical tools, which should also fit the surgical instruments. The larger the model, the harder it is to reproduce it on an average commercial printer, most of which can accommodate a 30 cm^3 model.

Finally, smoothness and opacity are defined. Smoothness relates to the surfaces of bone and tumor. The rougher the surface, the more it is identical to the imaging data set and therefore more accurate. A smoother finish is achieved by averaging the high and low points on the surface. This produces an image with a better look and feel. Opacity relates to the ability to see though an object. It is important in order to visualize the extent of tumor inside a bone that is not apparent on the bone surface. These steps define the process of reconstructing a 3D image of the critical structural anatomy of the body part involved and the ability to visualize the extent of the tumor under discussion.

The choice of printing materials should vary, depending mostly on the expectations of the model. A basic white model can be printed from relatively inexpensive fused deposition modeling material. Models can be printed from materials which are heat stable or which can withstand chlorhexidine sterilization when there is a need for the surgeon to have access to the model during surgery. Bone models can be printed

from transparent material in order to visualize the extent of tumor within the bone (Fig. 15.8).

The surgical plan is defined by a set of planar bone cuts that should enable the surgeon to resect the bone tumor with adequate margins (Fig. 15.6). Each one of these planes can be located around the tumor to achieve sufficient resection. One or more cut planes are necessary for an end of bone resection. Two or more cut planes are necessary to achieve a segmental (intercalary) resection. Three or more planes may be necessary for a geometric resection which spares bone continuity. Whether it is on a computer or a printed model, this surgical plan helps the surgeon to assess their ability to perform the desired resection and enable preparation for the reconstruction of the defect created by the resection (Fig. 15.7). There are several different plans that take into account the direction of the surgical approach, the amount of exposure needed, the critical structures surrounding the involved bone, and the ability to access and make the bone cuts with the different cutting tools, such as an osteotome, Gigli saw, or an oscillating saw. The cut plane lines are marked on the bone surface as lines that indicate where the bone cuts will pass.

This printed model contains the surgical plan. There is value in having the model at hand in the operating theatre during surgery where it can be oriented in the same position as the patient and help with correct orientation. Printed surgical tools can be tested out on the model to validate their accuracy and improve their positioning during surgery. Distance measurements

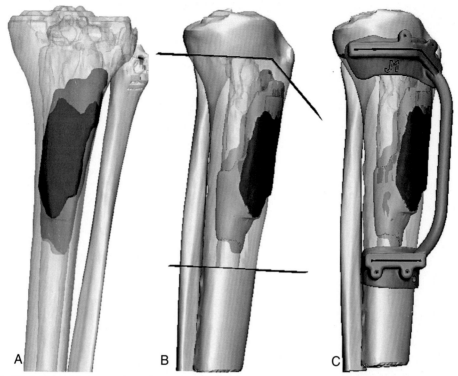

FIG. 15.4 **Plans:** Proximal tibial Ewing sarcoma in close proximity to the tibial tuberosity insertion of the extensor mechanism. 3D computer model shows tumor contoured in red **(A)**. Bone cuts are planned for a segmental resection sparing the tibial tuberosity **(B)**. A cutting jig is planned for an anteromedial surgical approach. The handle doubles as a soft tissue retractor **(C)**.

between the joint surface and the bone cuts can be made along the bone surface. These measurements have the potential of being more accurate than cut measurements taken from sagittal or coronal 2D image cuts, provided the model is scaled one to one.

Models can contain detachable parts to accommodate the surgical plan and plan for reconstruction options when needed (Fig. 15.6). The detachable soft tissue components of the tumor will expose the model bone surface that will remain after tumor resection. Internal fixation plates can be tested and prebent if necessary prior to surgery in order to achieve an optimal fit (Fig. 15.5). In segmental resections where only a short bone segment remains, the choice of plate and planning of screw placement will save time and avoid intraoperative compromises during reconstruction.

Surgical simulators and dry-run models are uncommon in surgery and are mostly used during the training of residents in surgical skills laboratories. They are seldom used by staff surgeons. In recent years, 3D

modeling and 3D printed models are being used by surgeons to plan and prepare more complex and challenging cases. Surgical safety may be improved with running through the surgical plan on a printed model and actually performing the surgical cuts on the model prior to performing the actual surgery. This practice is common in various industrial fields, as well as in aviation and the military. New printing materials that have recently become available can accurately simulate the consistency of bone and provide the surgeon the look and feel of drilling and cutting through bone while accommodating an oscillating saw, thus enabling trial runs of bone tumor resections on a surgical model simulator.

3D printing can also be used to enhance surgery for metastatic bone disease, where the goal is to improve a patient's quality of life. For example, in cases of metastatic bone lesions of the pelvis which cause pain due to mechanical hip instability and possible pelvic discontinuity, reconstruction after resection of the

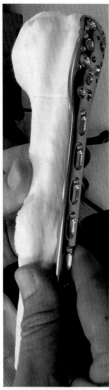

FIG. 15.5 3D Models (Photos): Using models to plan and precontour a plate chondrosarcoma of the humerus, diaphysial tumor, the surgical plan included intercalary resection and reconstruction with an allograft and a plate. The model shows the resection cuts and enables pre-op planning of the optimal plate used to fix the reconstruction with regard to size and contour.

involved bone can be achieved by inserting Steinmann pins through the iliac crest and advancing them into the anterior and posterior acetabular columns (Fig. 15.14). This provides a scaffold for bone cement to bridge the bone defect created by the metastasis. Preparing a model that includes the bone defect based on the patient's imaging studies will allow surgeons to determine the number of Steinmann pins required for reconstruction and, with the use of drill guides prepared beforehand, will enable them to navigate the pins accurately to their desired position. This will minimize the risk of damage to internal organs and blood vessels due to misplaced hardware and enhance the patient's safety. Furthermore, the trials on surgical guides during simulation will shorten the time needed to perform the actual surgical procedure.

3D-PRINTED SURGICAL TOOLS

Three-dimensional printing is a simple and accurate method for simulating surgical tools that enable the surgeon to carry out the prepared surgical plan based on preoperative imaging studies before actually implementing it.[27,28] Executing the surgical plan accurately is not a simple task. Bone cuts and drill holes have an entry point into bone, a pitch, and a roll. The ability to accurately contend with all three elements simultaneously has been shown to be significantly more accurate with guidance tools, such as navigation systems, compared with freehand cutting.[23]

Cutting jigs have long been the standard practice for performing accurate bone cuts in total knee arthroplasty. The cutting jigs optimize implant positioning and thus enhance implant longevity and patient function. They have recently been used in the reconstruction phase of the surgical defect created during a sarcoma resection.[29,30]

Each patient with bone sarcoma poses a distinct surgical challenge, as each tumor is unique in size and has its own 3D geometry. This precludes the use of the standard cutting jigs used in arthroplasty surgery and stresses the need for personalized tools. Custom planned and printed personalized cutting jigs meet this need for ensuring a safe oncologic margin and an improved functional outcome.

The types of 3D printed tools used in orthopedic oncology include cutting jigs, drilling guides, and ablation guides. These tools need to be fashioned from biocompatible materials that have been proven to be safe when in contact with human tissue and which can be sterilized for surgery without being deformed or breaking. Several such materials are available commercially.

General Design

Three-dimensional printed guides and cutting jigs align a cutting or drilling tool to a specific location in bone and are therefore made of two parts, one that aligns the tool and the other that aligns the jig to the bone. The footprint is the part which aligns the guide to the target bone. The footprint is designed in such a way that it will conform perfectly to the bone surface at only one specific location. A good choice of footprint has a nonuniform surface, contains clear and specific anatomic landmarks, and contains areas where bone is easily exposed. For example, footprints in the pelvic region cannot rely solely on iliac bone, which is uniform but should rely on the greater sciatic notch and iliac crest for pelvic resections. Footprints along the tibia should rely on the curved surfaces of the proximal tibia.

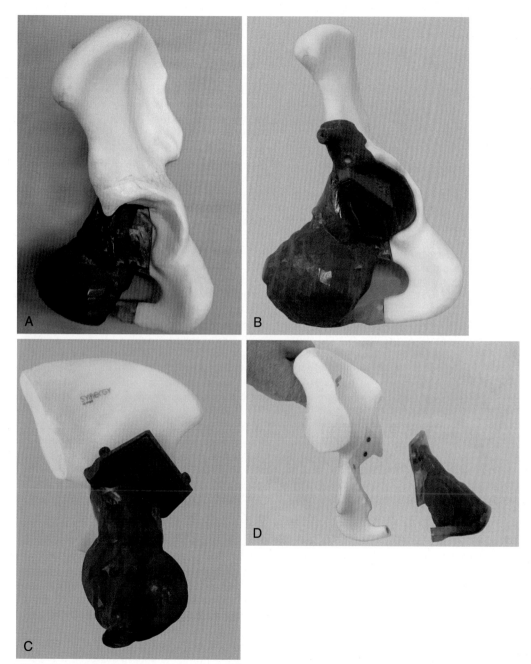

FIG. 15.6 **3D Models (Photos):** A pelvic model of a 16-year-old patient with a pelvic osteosarcoma involving the pubic rami and the medial wall of the acetabulum. The hemipelvic model **(A)** shows tumor in red. The bone away from tumor is white and the bone surrounding tumor which is planned to be resected as margins is transparent, which enables tumor extent within the bone to be visualized. Cutting jigs are planned and tested on the model **(B** and **C)** and include an intra-acetabular cutting jig and a second jig planed for the inner table of the ilium. The ability to dry-run test the jig on the model is important for surgical preparation. Finally the resected part is planned and printed as a separate part and magnets fold it together to the pelvic model. This gives the option to simulate the anatomy before and after resection of the tumor **(D)**.

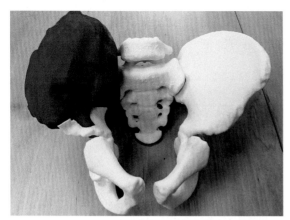

FIG. 15.7 **3D Models (Photos):** A pelvic Ewing sarcoma of the Ilium with a large soft tissue component. 3D printed pelvic model shows tumor in red and bone in white. The model enables volumetric visualization and a trial potion for accurate placement of the cutting jigs ahead of surgery.

The tibial tuberosity with its insertion of the patellar tendon is also not a good choice because of soft tissue coverage that must not be detached unless absolutely necessary. The larger the footprint on a nonuniform surface, the more accurate the fit, but this will call for wider exposure and the detaching of soft tissue insertions during surgery. The mid-diaphysis of long bones, such as the femur, tibia, and humerus are specific locations where footprints need to be made larger because of the relative paucity of anatomic features. Fixation points to bone are part of the footprint and they are placed on the periphery of the jig. The jig is usually fixed to the bone with a number of K-wires, once the cutting jig has been correctly placed. Fixation is especially important as the vibration of the cutting tool may displace the jig and hamper accuracy.

Cutting jigs are guides for oscillating saws and osteotomes (Figs. 15.2–15.4, 15.9–15.12). They should be planned ahead for a specific blade. The cutting slit through which the blade is inserted should be 0.1–0.2 mm wider than the thickness of the blade and wider than the range of motion of the oscillating saw in order to avoid excessively strong vibrations. We recommend the height and thickness of the walls of the cutting jig be approximately 1 cm high and 3 mm thick for stability. The length of the cutting slit in the jig should extend beyond the length of the cut in bone. The correct location of the cutting jig on bone can be tested by measurement to the closest joint line and with fluoroscopic imaging which visualizes the cutting slit on bone. In addition, the depth of the cut can

be measured preoperatively and thus help avoid unnecessary bone cuts.

For bulk allograft reconstructions, a second identical cutting jig can be used to cut the allograft to fit the size of the resected segment, which is then used for reconstruction. Handle location is important as it should not interfere with the saw blade and tool during cutting and should not obstruct the surgical field. This is best achieved by planning it to be sufficiently distant (3–5 cm) from the bone. Cutting jigs used for segmental cuts often use two footprints, one for each cutting slot, and a handle which connects these two parts. Handle and cutting slot positions must be carefully planned. They must take into account the local anatomy, the surgical dissection, and the relation to soft tissue. For example, a cutting guide based on the acetabulum should take into account that the femoral head needs to be displaced after dislocation, which is not an easy task, in order to position the jig. The handle can be planned in such a fashion that it will aid in the retraction of the soft tissue flap and thus improve exposure.

Ablation guides can be used to guide ablative therapy probes, such as cryosurgery probes and radiofrequency probes. Benign aggressive bone tumors and metastatic lesions that are not treated by a wide margin resection, such as giant cell tumor of bone, are responsive to ablation therapies. These have been used as adjuvants to curettage and high-speed burring in order to reduce local recurrence. The ablation probes have a fixed radius of tumor destruction. Preoperative planning based on the patient's tumor characteristics as seen on 3D imaging facilitate cryo-probe positioning and help determine the optimal number of probes necessary to ensure optimal tumor destruction. A custom guiding tool can be designed to guide the probes based on anatomic landmarks of the individual patient. The probes are inserted under direct vision when there is a bone window or else under fluoroscopy. Each probe is inserted to a preplanned and measured depth. Guide holes should be 0.1–0.2 mm larger in diameter than the probe diameter.

Drill guides are used to guide drill holes that are planned for a specific trajectory. Drill guides can be used in the drilling of sites of avascular necrosis of the femoral head through a trochanteric entry point for decompression (Fig. 15.13). They can also be used to guide Steinmann pins inserted through the iliac crest to support the acetabular region in metastatic bone disease or after partial iliac resections (Fig. 15.14). These guide holes should be planned 0.1–0.2 mm larger in diameter compared with the drill diameter.

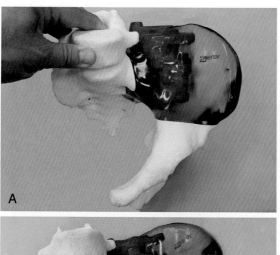
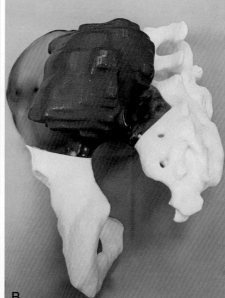
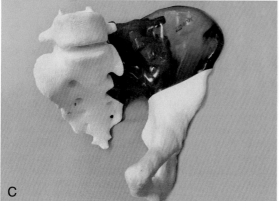

FIG. 15.8 **3D Models (Photos):** A posterior pelvic tumor involving the posterior ilium and sacrum. The tumor has a large soft tissue component, posteriorly. The tumor, in red, has been segmented off the MRI. The bone surrounding tumor is transparent in order to visualize the extent of tumor inside bone. Resection plains are planned between transparent and white bone **(A)**. View of the pelvic model from front to back showing tumor reaches the sacro-iliac joint in the front **(B)**. A view of the pelvic model from the back showing a large soft tissue component surrounding the sacroiliac joint and limiting access for a posterior bone cut **(C)**. A superior view of the model showing the tumor mass in the posterior ilium reaching the sacroiliac joint. The model helps visualize the needed bone cuts, as well as the surgical approach and exposure which is needed given the large soft tissue mass in this challenging location.

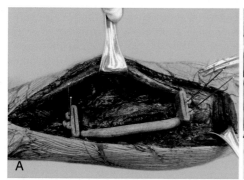
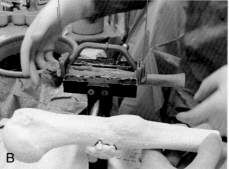

FIG. 15.9 **Guides:** Cutting jig used for segmental resection of a chondrosarcoma of the humerus **(A)**. An identical jig is used to cut an allograft for the reconstruction of the defect **(B)**.

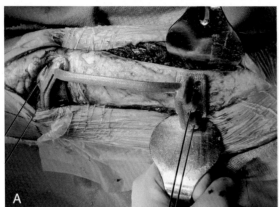
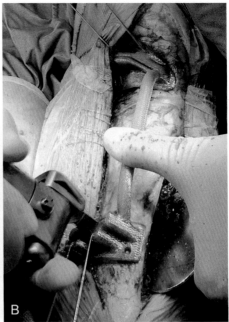

FIG. 15.10 **Guides:** Cutting jig planned for an anteromedial approach to the proximal tibia for resection of a Ewing bone sarcoma. (A) The proximal cut is planned to spare the insertion of the patellar tendon. A segmental resection of the proximal tibia is planned. The jig has two proximal and two distal fixation points which are away from the bone cuts and the tumor. The jig handle doubles as a soft tissue retractor. The footprint of the jig that needs to conform to the bone surface is planned for the medial side of the tibia that does not have much soft tissue coverage except for the Pes Anserine. (B) An oscillating saw is used to make the cuts through the slots of the cutting jigs.

3D-PRINTED CUSTOM IMPLANTS

Three-dimensional custom implants printed in titanium metal have the value of exact fit for reconstructing segmental bone defects after bone tumor resections.[31] These custom implants are offered as a service by the major implant companies. The basic plan is similar to the resection plan. The length of the implant is similar to the distance between the two bone cuts made for resection. Three basic types of implants are available for long bones: a cage and nail type implant, a single piece cage and stem implant, and an interlocking 2-piece cage and stem implant. Pelvic implants are designed to reconstruct the pelvic bone defects after type I iliac bone resection or after type I + II acetabular resections. They are fixed with multiple screws designed for fixation to the remaining surrounding bone. A cemented polyethylene liner and a hip replacement complete the reconstruction when needed. The challenge in the use of custom implants is achieving a perfect fit. It is difficult to compensate for any

miscalculation, especially if the implant is too small or too short. Planning is therefore a major subject of focus, and designing two implant sizes so that one will have the exact resection dimensions while the other is 3–5 mm longer is a good backup plan.

A custom implant can replace a bulk allograft (Fig. 15.15) or a segmental prosthesis in segmental defects in long bones. It has the added value of being exactly sized to the planned resection. Large cage constructs are designed with a lattice structure and can carry large amounts of morcellized iliac crest autografts. As they are prepared from the resection plan, they can offer an exact fit at the bone/implant junctions. An intramedullary nail serving as a load-sharing device can complement this construct. The inner diameter of the cage should be designed to accommodate the nail size with an additional 2 mm in diameter. The bone should also be reamed by at least 2 mm above the nail size in order to avoid distraction of the distal bone segment when the nail is

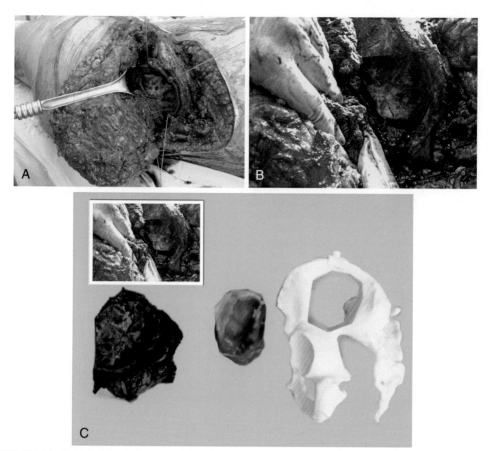

FIG. 15.11 **Guides:** An osteosarcoma of the posterior ilium with a large inner table soft tissue component. The cutting jig is planned for the outer table of the ilium, the bone cuts are planned for a geometric resection thus preserving a bone bridge between ilium and sacrum **(A)**. The image shows the cutting jig positioned on the exposed iliac bone **(B)**. The bone cuts have been completed and tumor is removed through the inner pelvis **(C)**. The model of the pelvis is shown on the right, the model to the tumor (in red) and the planned resection specimen including the margins is shown in the middle. The resected part which includes tumor and surrounding margin is shown on left to emphasize the similarity between the resection plan and the actual outcome.

inserted. The planning of a cage and a nail construct must account for the whole length of the bone, with special focus on the nail entry point into the bone. The entry point significantly impacts nail positioning, which can cause a tilt in the cage bone construct if there is a miscalculation.

One-piece cage stem implants have value in segmental resections which leave short bone segments adjacent to the joint. These short segments cannot always be stabilized with a nail because of the metaphyseal flair. The one-piece construct has a short interlocking stem facing the adjacent joint, and so

insertion needs to be planned ahead in the tibia with osteotomy of the fibula to enable distraction and hyperextension of the lower leg.

Soft tissue coverage of the implant is crucial to avoid infection in cases of wound dehiscence. This has long been the case for tibial implants that are augmented with a gastrocnemius pedicle flap and skin graft. Proximal tibia resections with patellar tendon reattachment to the implant have a special need for gastrocnemius flap augmentation in order to augment the blood supply to the patellar tendon at its reattachment to the implant.

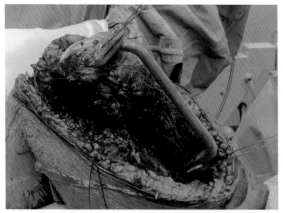

FIG. 15.12 **Guides**: A distal femur osteosarcoma that does not cross the physis. It has therefore been planned for a joint sparing segmental resection. An intraoperative image of the femur and the tumor. A medial approach has been used and the vessels have been dissected away from tumor off the posterior aspect of the femur. The cutting jig is placed flush on the distal femur and the distal cut is made through the cutting slot and the physis. Two jig fixation holes on both the distal and proximal aspect aid in fixation to bone and avoiding movement. Cutting slots have walls which are between 1 and 1.5 cm high to guide the saw blade.

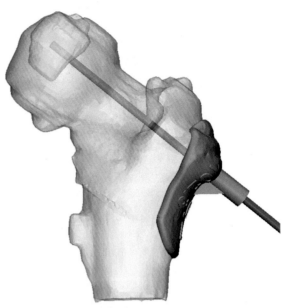

FIG. 15.13 **Guides**: Drill guide, planned from an MRI scan for decompression of avascular necrosis of the femoral head viewed only on MRI scan but not seen on CT scan. The guide footprint was based off of the greater trochanter and drilling depth was measured in the plan. A guide wire was then drilled using the guide and a cannulated drill was used for decompression.

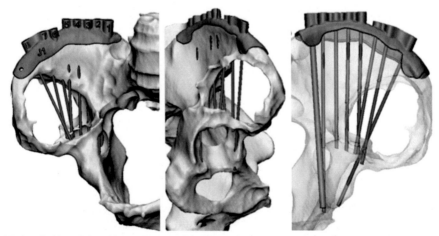

FIG. 15.14 **Guides**: Drill guide—a 67-year-old patient with metastatic bone disease involving the ilium and supra-acetabular region causing mechanical hip joint pain. Reconstruction of the lytic bone defect in the supra-acetalular region is mandatory to support a total hip replacement. Stability is achieved with metal pins which begin in healthy solid bone and continue into the bone defect. A multihole drill guide tool is designed to fit on the iliac crest. Each drill hole guides a pin to an exact preplanned position around the acetabulum. This tool aids in accurate pin placement and shortens the time needed for this part of the procedure. As each pin is inserted once without trial and error in and out motion, they are more stable.

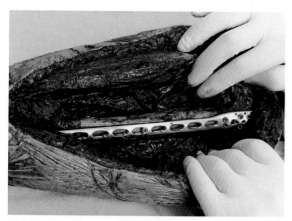

FIG. 15.15 **Allograft Reconstruction:** Segmental resection of a chondrosarcoma of the humerus reconstructed with an allograft and a plate. The segmental resection of the tumor and the allograft were both done with an identical cutting jig which ensures an exact fit. The fixation plate was planned and measured ahead of surgery, thus decreasing surgical time.

CONCLUSION

The goal in orthopedic oncology surgery is wide resection of the primary tumor as this influences the risk of a local recurrence. Tumors which arise and grow in bone cannot always be fully viewed and palpated in surgery, making complete resection challenging. 3D reconstruction using CT imaging adds an additional dimension of understanding of the surgical challenge. Although most surgeons are comfortable with 2D imaging, the surgical challenge is 3D, and so should be preparation for the case. Fusion between CT and MRI can add valuable data to that understanding as the soft tissue and marrow extent of the tumor is more prominent on MRI. A surgical plan based on the 3D model reconstructed from the imaging is a tool to plan an optimal resection that best accounts for a wide resection of the tumor, while sparing adjacent joints and preserving bone continuity where possible to improve long-term function. It accounts for the surgical approach and exposure necessary to safely carry out the resection plan. 3D printed models of the tumor, bone, and surgical plan can be used to visualize and better understand the surgical challenge. They are useful in communicating the plan to the surgical team. They can serve as simulators for dry-run practice ahead of the surgical case. The models are also useful for measuring and prebending plates that will be used in the reconstruction. Custom printed surgical guides, such as cutting jigs and aiming guides, are a way to accurately carry out the surgical plan. These printed guides have a footprint that accommodates to the bone surface in one specific location. The cutting slots guide the saw or osteotome to the correct entry plane into bone while controlling for the pitch and roll of the tool. Custom printed metal implants are useful for reconstructing segmental bone defects. They can be planned and printed from the surgical plan to reconstruct the defect with an exact fit and allow for initial and long-term stability. These tools should allow for improved understanding, planning, surgical resection of bone tumors, and accurate reconstruction, with the potential to improve oncologic and functional outcomes.

REFERENCES

1. Moore DD, Haydon RC. Ewing's sarcoma of bone. *Cancer Treat Res.* 2014;162:93–115.
2. Franchi A. Epidemiology and classification of bone tumors. *Clin Cases Miner Bone.* 2012;9(2):92–95.
3. Stiller CA. International patterns of cancer incidence in adolescents. *Cancer Treat Rev.* 2007;33(7):631–645.
4. Riedel RF, Larrier N, Dodd L, Kirsch D, Martinez S, Brigman BE. The clinical management of chondrosarcoma. *Curr Treat Options Oncol.* 2009;10(1–2):94–106.
5. Gelderblom H, Hogendoorn PC, Dijkstra SD, et al. The clinical approach towards chondrosarcoma. *Oncol.* 2008;13(3):320–329.
6. Ottaviani G, Jaffe N. The epidemiology of osteosarcoma. *Cancer Treat Res.* 2009;152:3–13.
7. Reed DR, Hayashi M, Wagner L, et al. Treatment pathway of bone sarcoma in children, adolescents, and young adults. *Cancer.* 2017;123(12):2206–2218.
8. Harrison DJ, Schwartz CL. Osteogenic sarcoma: systemic chemotherapy options for localized disease. *Curr Treat Options Oncol.* 2017;18(4):24.
9. Ou JY, Spraker-Perlman H, Dietz AC, Smits-Seemann RR, Kaul S, Kirchhoff AC. Conditional survival of pediatric, adolescent, and young adult soft tissue sarcoma and bone tumor patients. *Cancer Epidemiol.* 2017;50(Pt A):150–157.
10. Kawaguchi N, Ahmed AR, Matsumoto S, Manabe J, Matsushita Y. The concept of curative margin in surgery for bone and soft tissue sarcoma. *Clin Orthop Relat Res.* 2004;(419):165–172.
11. Li J, Shi L, Chen GJ. Image navigation assisted joint-saving surgery for treatment of bone sarcoma around knee in skeletally immature patients. *Surg Oncol.* 2014;23(3):132–139.
12. Andreou D, Bielack SS, Carrle D, et al. The influence of tumor- and treatment-related factors on the development of local recurrence in osteosarcoma after adequate surgery. An analysis of 1355 patients treated on neoadjuvant cooperative osteosarcoma study group protocols. *Ann Oncol.* 2011;22(5):1228–1235.

13. Loh AH, Wu H, Bahrami A, et al. Influence of bony resection margins and surgicopathological factors on outcomes in limb-sparing surgery for extremity osteosarcoma. *Pediatr Blood Cancer.* 2015;62(2):246–251.

14. He F, Zhang W, Shen Y, et al. Effects of resection margins on local recurrence of osteosarcoma in extremity and pelvis: systematic review and meta-analysis. *Int J Surg.* 2016;36(Pt A):283–292.

15. Jeys LM, Thorne CJ, Parry M, Gaston CL, Sumathi VP, Grimer JR. A novel system for the surgical staging of primary high-grade osteosarcoma: the Birmingham classification. *Clin Orthop Relat Res.* 2017;475(3): 842–850.

16. Bacci G, Forni C, Longhi A, et al. Local recurrence and local control of non-metastatic osteosarcoma of the extremities: a 27-year experience in a single institution. *J Surg Oncol.* 2007;96(2):118–123.

17. White LM, Wunder JS, Bell RS, et al. Histologic assessment of peritumoral edema in soft tissue sarcoma. *Int J Radiat Oncol Biol Phys.* 2005;61(5):1439–1445.

18. Caracciolo JT, Letson GD. Radiologic approach to bone and soft tissue sarcomas. *Surg Clin N Am.* 2016;96(5): 963–976.

19. Saifuddin A. The accuracy of imaging in the local staging of appendicular osteosarcoma. *Skelet Radiol.* 2002;31(4): 191–201.

20. Ahmad S, Stevenson J, Mangham C, Cribb G, Cool P. Accuracy of magnetic resonance imaging in planning the osseous resection margins of bony tumours in the proximal femur: based on coronal T1-weighted versus STIR images. *Skelet Radiol.* 2014;43(12):1679–1686.

21. Ritacco LE, Milano FE, Farfalli GL, Ayerza MA, Muscolo DL, Aponte-Tinao LA. Accuracy of 3-D planning and navigation in bone tumor resection. *Orthopedics.* 2013;36(7):e942–e950.

22. van Eijnatten M, van Dijk R, Dobbe J, Streekstra G, Koivisto J, Wolff J. CT image segmentation methods for bone used in medical additive manufacturing. *Med Eng Phys.* 2018;51(Suppl. C):6–16.

23. Sternheim A, Daly M, Qiu J, et al. Navigated pelvic osteotomy and tumor resection: a study assessing the accuracy and reproducibility of resection planes in Sawbones and cadavers. *J Bone Joint Surg Am.* 2015;97(1):40–46.

24. Wong KC, Kumta SM, Antonio GE, Tse LF. Image fusion for computer-assisted bone tumor surgery. *Clin Orthop Relat Res.* 2008;466(10):2533–2541.

25. Jeys LM, Kulkarni A, Grimer RJ, Carter SR, Tillman RM, Abudu A. Endoprosthetic reconstruction for the treatment of musculoskeletal tumors of the appendicular skeleton and pelvis. *J Bone Joint Surg Am.* 2008;90(6):1265–1271.

26. Kunz P, Bernd L. Methods of biological reconstruction for bone sarcoma: indications and limits. *Recent results Cancer.* 2009;179:113–140.

27. Levin AS, Arkader A, Morris CD. Reconstruction following tumor resections in skeletally immature patients. *J Am Acad Orthop Surg.* 2017;25(3):204–213.

28. Wong KC, Sze KY, Wong IO, Wong CM, Kumta SM. Patient-specific instrument can achieve same accuracy with less resection time than navigation assistance in periacetabular pelvic tumor surgery: a cadaveric study. *Int J Comput Assist Radiol Surg.* 2016;11(2):307–316.

29. Khan FA, Lipman JD, Pearle AD, Boland PJ, Healey JH. Surgical technique: computer-generated custom jigs improve accuracy of wide resection of bone tumors. *Clin Orthop Relat Res.* 2013;471(6):2007–2016.

30. Gouin F, Paul L, Odri GA, Cartiaux O. Computer-assisted planning and patient-specific instruments for bone tumor resection within the pelvis: a series of 11 patients. *Sarcoma.* 2014;2014:842709.

31. Jentzsch T, Vlachopoulos L, Furnstahl P, Muller DA, Fuchs B. Tumor resection at the pelvis using three-dimensional planning and patient-specific instruments: a case series. *World J Surg Oncol.* 2016;14(1):249.

FURTHER READING

1. Wong KC, Kumta SM, Geel NV, Demol J. One-step reconstruction with a 3D-printed, biomechanically evaluated custom implant after complex pelvic tumor resection. *Comput Aided Surg.* 2015;20(1):14–23.

CHAPTER 16

Setting Up Your Own Home 3D Printing "Plant"

BRUNO BORRALHO GOBBATO, MD

INTRODUCTION

Orthopedic 3D Printing From the Home and Office

3D printing is revolutionizing manufacturing processes in industry and medicine. Because the practice of orthopedics centers around visualizing structural musculoskeletal anatomy, it lends itself well to 3D print modeling.

Today there are many ways to have anatomic models or guides built that may aid surgical execution. Many companies are emerging to provide this service, while other clinics are investing in their own service equipment. Nobody knows for sure how 3D printing will take root among practitioners. While we do not have the definitive answer, our choice was not to wait to depend on anyone or any institutions but to set up our own "Maker Lab" and learn the process of creating orthopedic 3D printed models ourselves. We think a case can be made for you to consider 3D printing your own models from your home or office as well.

There are many advantages to learning how to 3D print in your own home.

Where 3D printing at home/office costs around four cents per cubic centimeter, it is not uncommon to see a price of 50 cents to $1 per cubic centimeter from online services. That represents a $10\times$ increase in price over printing it yourself.

The main words we use with this technology is freedom and creativity. Having a printer at home gives you the chance to play with almost everything. You can test how many models you want. For example, it is possible to print the whole anatomy (a scapula) but also many small copies of the main part (glenoid) for testing different implants or corrective surgeries.

Creating guides and even instruments such as special retractors is one of the most challenging but rewarding tasks. Here is where our creativity and medical knowledge emerge. Sometimes you actually perform most of the surgery in your office and use the guide or instrument just to replicate that effort.

A disadvantage for self-printing is everything that "surrounds" the actual 3D printing. This includes preparing the model, leveling the machine, making sure your filament is stored properly, and other factors. For the most part, once you have gone through your initial learning process for 3D printing, the process becomes much faster and easier.

This chapter will briefly introduce a few of the technologies integral to the 3D printing process. The main thrust, however, will be to convey some of the essential considerations of setting up a 3D printing operation at your home or office. The information that will follow was distilled from many hours of the author's own tinkering and experience garnered from trial and error and should serve to guide the novice down he rewarding path of 3D printing.

The term 3D printing covers a host of processes and technologies that offer a full spectrum of capabilities for the production of models, anatomy parts, guides, and instruments in different materials.[1]

Essentially, what all of the processes and technologies have in common is the manner in which production is carried out—layer by layer in an additive process—which is in contrast to traditional methods of production involving subtractive methods or molding/casting processes. Applications of 3D printing are emerging almost by the day, and, as this technology continues to penetrate more widely and deeply across the medical industry, this is only set to increase. We

3D Printing in Orthopaedic Surgery. https://doi.org/10.1016/B978-0-323-58118-9.00016-6

195

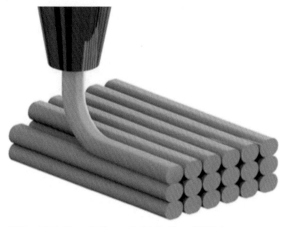

FIG. 16.1 Fused filament fabrication (FFF) is a uses a continuous filament of a thermoplastic material through a moving, heated printer extruder head layer-by-layer. https://eu.wikipedia.org/wiki/3D_inprimaketa.

are only just beginning to see the true potential of 3D printing in medicine.

Simply put, 3D printing is a method of creating a solid physical object from a digital 3D model. The reason it is called 3D "printing" is because the assembly process is similar to the way you would print ink on paper. Most popular 3D printers are "extrusion printers," (meaning they spray their material out of maneuverable nozzles) where base material—usually thermoplastic filament—are laid down in layers that eventually create the finished product. 3D printing is an "additive" process, which means that the object is created by adding layers from bottom up, with each layer being printed on top of the last one over and over until the job is done.[2] (Fig. 16.1).

The earliest 3D printing technologies first emerged in the late 1980s, at which time they were called rapid prototyping (RP) technologies. This is because the processes were originally conceived as a fast and more cost-effective method for creating prototypes for product development within industry. As an interesting aside, Dr. Kodama, in Japan, filed the very first patent application for RP technology in May 1980. Unfortunately for Dr. Kodama, the full patent specification was subsequently not filed before the 1-year deadline after the application. In real terms, however, the origins of 3D printing can be traced back to 1986, when the first patent was issued for stereolithography apparatus (SLA). This patent belonged to Charles (Chuck) Hull, who first invented his SLA machine in 1983. Hull went on to cofound 3D Systems Corporation—one of the largest and most prolific organizations operating in the 3D printing sector today.

3D Printing Technology

The starting point for any 3D printing process is a 3D digital model, which can be created using a variety of 3D software, from a 3D model extracted from a CT scan, MRI, or even scanned with a 3D scanner. The model is then "sliced" into layers, thereby converting the design into a file readable by the 3D printer—the opposite process that the CT scans do. The material processed by the 3D printer is then layered according to the design and the process. There are a number of different types of 3D printing technologies, which process different materials in different ways to create the final object. Functional plastics, metals, ceramics, and sand are, now, all routinely used for medical and production applications. Research is also being conducted for 3D printing biomaterials and different types of food. Generally speaking though, at the entry level of the market, materials are much more limited. Plastic is currently the only widely used material—usually acrylonitrile butadiene styrene (ABS) or polylactic acid (PLA), but there are a growing number of alternatives, including nylon.

The different types of 3D printers each employ a different technology that processes different materials in different ways. It is important to understand that one of the most basic limitations of 3D printing—in terms of materials and applications—is that there no one solution fits all. For example, some 3D printers process powdered materials (nylon, plastic, ceramic, metal), which utilize a light/heat source to sinter/melt/fuse layers of the powder together in the defined shape. Others process polymer resin materials and again utilize a light/laser to solidify the resin in ultra-thin layers. Jetting of fine droplets is another 3D printing process, reminiscent of 2D inkjet printing, but with superior materials to ink and a binder to fix the layers. Perhaps the most common and easily recognized process is deposition, and this is the process employed by the majority of entry-level 3D printers. These are the machines we recommend for every doctor to start your own 3D printing office.

This process extrudes plastics, commonly PLA or ABS, in filament form through a heated extruder to form layers and create the predetermined shape. Because parts can be printed directly, it is possible to produce very detailed and intricate objects, often with functionality built in and negating the need for assembly. We are able to create almost any anatomic part using rigid or flexible materials. Another important point to stress is none of the 3D printing processes come as plug and play options. There are many steps prior to pressing print and more once the part comes off the printer—these are often overlooked.

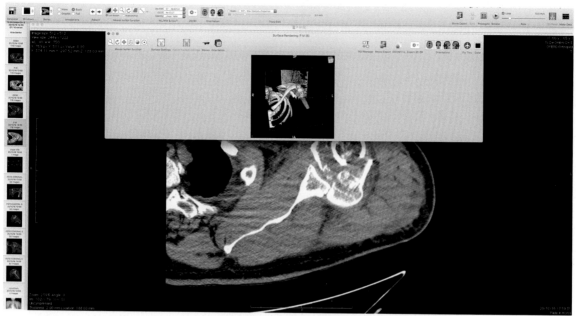

FIG. 16.2 Creating a 3D file from a regular CT-Scan using Horos Software.

Apart from the realities of preparing the anatomy for 3D printing (Fig. 16.2), which can be demanding, file preparation and conversion can also prove time-consuming and complicated, particularly for parts that demand intricate supports during the build process. However, there are continual updates and upgrades of software for these functions and the situation is improving. Furthermore, once off the printer, many anatomy models will need to undergo finishing operations such as support removal, sanding, lacquer, paint, or other types of traditional finishing touches, which all typically need to be done by hand and require skill, time, and patience (Fig. 16.3).

The following section will briefly outline some of the basic technologies and materials used in 3D printing with the intended purpose of guiding you toward our preferred methods and materials for orthopedic applications. After this section we will guide you through various hardware and software options for orthopedic applications.

PRINTERS
Stereolithography

The 3D printing process called stereolithography is generally considered to be the pioneer of all other 3D printing processes. SL is a laser-based process that works

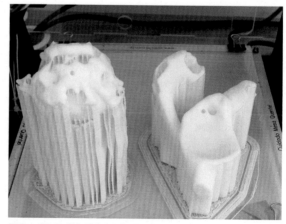

FIG. 16.3 3D Printer bed of a proximal humerus and glenoid with support material.

with photopolymer resins that react with the laser and cure to form a solid in a very precise way to produce very accurate parts. It is a complex process, but simply put use of a vat of liquid photopolymer resin that is cured by a UV laser. The laser solidifies that resin layer by layer in order to create the whole object. Once the layer is completed, the platform within the vat drops down by a fraction (in the Z axis) and the subsequent

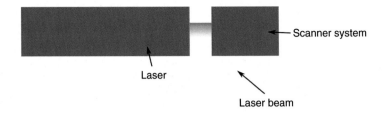

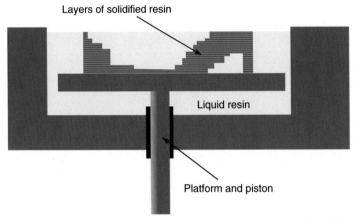

FIG. 16.4 SL 3D Printer with laser or UV light that cure the resign layer-by-layer. https://commons.wikimedia. org/wiki/File:Stereolithography_apparatus_vector.svg.

layer is traced out by the laser. This continues until the entire object is completed and the platform can be raised out of the vat for removal. Because of the nature of the SL process, it requires support structures for some parts, specifically those with overhangs or undercuts. These structures need to be manually removed. In terms of other postprocessing steps, many objects 3D printed using SL need to be cleaned and cured (Fig. 16.4).

Digital Light Processing

Digital light processing (DLP) is a similar process to SL in that it is a 3D printing process that works with photopolymers. The major difference is the light source. DLP uses a more conventional light source, such as an arc lamp. DLP produces highly accurate parts with excellent resolution, but its similarities also include the same requirements for support structures and postcuring. These machines are affordable and are used principally for creating cutting guides for odontology and bucomaxilofacial surgeries. It has a very good resolution (10–50 μm), but the size of the printed part for regular use is normally limited to 10–15 cm in all axes.

Selective Laser Sintering

Selective laser sintering (SLS) is one of the most commonly used 3D printing technologies. During the

SLS printing process, tiny particles of ceramic, glass, or plastic such as nylon are fused together by a high-power laser. The heat from the laser fuses together these particles to form 3D objects. This technology is the most used for medical applications for creating anatomy models and surgery guides. Generally, it uses nylon (polyamide) powder that is inert to the body. But these printers are expensive for end consumers (Fig. 16.5).

Multi-Jet Modeling

The principle of working of a 3D printer utilizing multi-jet modeling is starkly similar to that of an ink jet printer. This process is sometimes also referred to as thermojet. It is a type of a RP process that can create waxlike plastic models. Owing to the fact that this technology does not have the same kind of limitations as SLA, it is able to produce exceptionally detailed objects with thickness as fine as 16 μm. This process is used to create those anatomic models with many colors and different transparencies. These machines are very expensive.

Fused Deposition Modeling

3D printing utilizing the extrusion of thermoplastic material is easily the most common—and recognizable—3DP process. The most popular name for the process

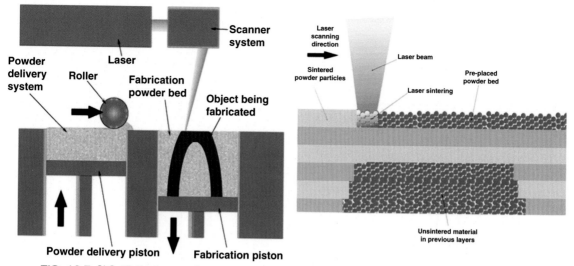

FIG. 16.5 SLS 3D Printer uses laser to melt a powder material. https://commons.wikimedia.org/wiki/File: Selective_laser_melting_system_schematic.jpg.

is fused deposition modeling (FDM), due to its longevity; however, this is a trade name, registered by Stratasys, the company that originally developed it. Stratasys' FDM technology has been around since the early 1990s and today is an industrial-grade 3D printing process. This method also works by creating an object layer by layer. However, there are some differences in the way the materials are used by this technology.

The process works by melting plastic filament that is deposited, via a heated extruder, a layer at a time, onto a build platform according to the 3D data supplied to the printer. Each layer hardens as it is deposited and bonds to the previous layer. The benefits offered by FDM make it suitable for use in offices, as it is a clean and easy-to-use method. We recommend this as the technology of choice for every doctor that wants to produce his or her own models at the office (Fig. 16.6).

MATERIALS

The materials available for 3D printing have come a long way since the early days of the technology. There are now a wide variety of different material types that are supplied in different states (powder, filament, pellets, granules, resin, etc). Specific materials are now generally developed for specific platforms performing dedicated applications (an example would be the dental and medical sector) with material properties that more precisely suit the application. However, there are now way too many proprietary materials from the many different 3D printer vendors to cover them all

here. Instead, this book will look at the most popular types of material in a more generic way.[3]

Acrylonitrile Butadiene Styrene

ABS is a commonly used plastic material that melts at about 220°C, then quickly reforms into a tough, glossy, impact-resistant material. It is made from crude oil and is nontoxic; it can be easily dyed and retains color well. Legos are made of ABS for this reason: it is easy to shape but tough to break. However, ABS does release some unpleasant (and possibly poisonous) chemicals when heated or burned (Fig. 16.7).

These properties make ABS very suitable for 3D printing. You do need a large heater to reach that 220°C melting point, but ABS flows easily when heated and sets quickly to form the print. You will need a 3D printer with a **heated print bed** that can reach about 100°C, as ABS becomes sticky at this temperature and will adhere to a glass print bed.

A print using ABS will be very tough, similar to a Lego piece. The print will also be water and chemical resistant.

Pros: Tough, impact-resistant material; commonly used; nontoxic and water resistant.

Cons: High melting point makes it harder to liquefy; gives off unpleasant fumes; not suitable for outdoor use.

Cost: $20 to $50 per kg.

Compatible with: Printers with extruders that heat to 220°C and have a heated print bed.

Author Tip: The natural ABS color is very similar to bone color. It is my personal choice for anatomy

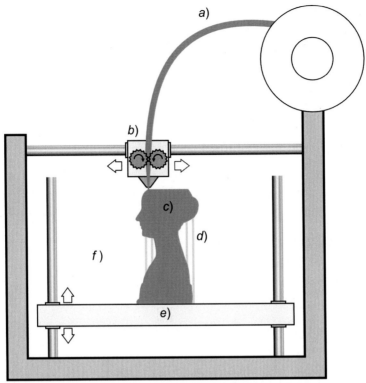

FIG. 16.6 A desktop FFF Printer with a) filament, b) extruder, c) object, d) support material, e) printer bed, f) printer
https://commons.wikimedia.org/wiki/File:Schematic_representation_of_Fused_Filament_Fabrication_01.png.

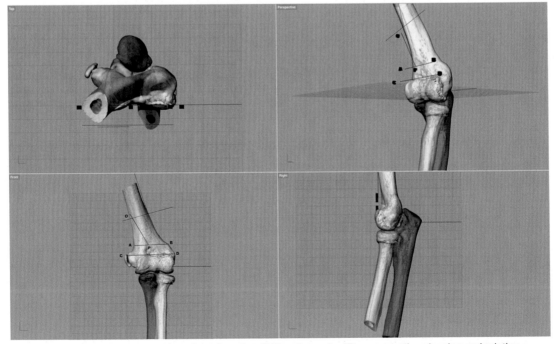

FIG. 16.7 A 3D representation of an elbow in a CAD software for 3D pre-operative planning and printing.

models to be used for planning surgeries with no contact to the patient. It can handle autoclave sterilization with some care.

Polylactic Acid

PLA is a relatively new polymer plastic, made from biologic materials such as cornstarch or sugarcane. It is similar to the material used in biodegradable plastic packaging, which melts at between 180 and 200°C, depending on other materials that are added for color and texture. PLA then quickly cools to form a tough, resilient material with a matte, opaque quality, but it is not as tolerant of heat as ABS is. PLA begins to deform at temperatures above 60°C. There is a slight smell when it is heated, rather like microwave popcorn.

PLA is generally the preferred option for low-cost 3D printers because it is easier to print with than ABS, as it sticks to other surfaces and itself better. It will stick well to the print base using white glue or blue painter's tape, which means that a printer with a heated print bed is not needed. The material is also biodegradable; like other corn- or sugar-based materials, it is slowly consumed by many common bacteria. It will last a long time in normal conditions, though. It is only when buried that it breaks down.

Pros: Easier to print with than ABS; biodegradable.

Cons: Prints degrade over time; rougher texture than ABS.

Cost: $20 to $50 per kg.

Compatible with: All FDM 3D printers.

Author Tip: The PLA is the easiest material to start printing. PLA is used in many medical products such as bioabsorbable anchors and sutures, but it is not exactly the same.

Polyvinyl Alcohol

Polyvinyl alcohol (PVA) is one of a new class of 3D printing materials that are used to make supports. A synthetic polymer, PVA, is used in biodegradable products, such as fishing lures and medical devices that need to work, but then dissolve away. It melts at about 200°C and can release some nasty chemicals if heated to higher temperatures. Another interesting property: it is water soluble.

This is why PVA is often used in 3D printing. It can be melted for printing by a standard 3D printer extruder to form parts that support other objects, and it sticks to a heated, glass print bed well. Once the printing is complete, if the material is immersed in water, the PVA parts will dissolve, leaving the rest of the print behind. This makes it easier to print complex models that require supports, or even models that include moving parts. If you

do use water to dissolve PVA, you will need to properly dispose of the water, as dissolved PVA can clog drains.

Pros: Water soluble; good for supports; fairly easy to print.

Cons: Can release toxic vapors if overheated; expensive; requires safe disposal.

Cost: More than $100 per kg.

Compatible with: Standard FDM printers with multiple extruders.

Author Tip: If you are planning to use a multiextruder machine, PVA will be very important when creating anatomy. To date, the author does not have a multiextruder machine to give a personal comment, but it is very important to consider.

Nylon (Polyamide)

The name nylon can be used for any one of a number of synthetic polymers originally created as replacements for silk. Nylon is a tough material that has a very high tensile strength, meaning that it can hold a lot of weight without breaking. It melts at about 250°C and is nontoxic.

Nylon's use as a 3D printing material is relatively new, but the material is becoming popular because the prints it produces are very tough and resistant to damage. However, nylon does require high temperatures to print: 250°C is hotter than many extruders can manage. And it is harder to get it to stick to the print bed than with ABS or PLA. Generally, nylon requires both a heated print bed and white glue to stick while printing.

Pros: Tough; medical approved.

Cons: Requires high temperatures to print.

Cost: $18−70 per kg.

Author Tip: Nylon is the most widely material used in the medical industry. It is autoclavable and the choice for medical guides. Most printers can print, but it is for experts!

Flexible

Most 3D printing materials strive for rigidity, creating prints that are strong. That is not always what you need, though, and flexible filaments produce prints that are stretchable and flexible. These rubberlike materials can be used to make things such as wearable parts that need to flex with your body.

However, this flexibility also poses a problem. FDM 3D printers work by pushing the filament into the heated extruder, where it melts. You cannot do that as easily if the material is flexible, so most printers will require modification to use these flexible filaments.

Pros: Produces squishy, flexible prints.

Cons: Requires modification of the printer or extruder.

Cost: $50 to $120 per kg.

Compatible with: Any FDM printer with a replaceable extruder.

Where Can You Buy the Material?

The printing material (or filament) that is required for the 3D printer can be from a wide range of sources. A kilogram of 1.75 mm ABS filament reel costs around $30 on Amazon, which is where we recommend you buy your filament. Search around to find the best deal and the lowest shipping cost for your location.

GETTING STARTED WITH 3D PRINTING

Getting started with 3D printing can be challenging. With so many new things to learn, novices can find it extremely hard to figure out where they should begin. There are many questions that need to be answered before you actually take the plunge and enter the world of 3D printing.

The first question you may want to ask yourself is whether you actually need a 3D printer of your own. Even though desktop 3D printers can now be purchased at an affordable price, there are a great number of online resources that can print models and deliver them to you without all of the steps of creating your own 3D print shop. So if you only need to get something printed occasionally, then it might be best to simply send the anatomic model to one of these services, and avoid all the hassle completely. But let us assume that you are ready to take on the challenge and actually build a 3D print yourself. What are the next steps?

Modeling: The Preprinting Phase
Where can you get 3D models?

You can transform any CT scan into a 3D. STL file that is suitable for printing or design your own models, like guides, or you can find many models on a website called the Thingiverse. Any CT scan can be turned into a 3D file. There is no need to be a specific 3D CT. However, there are some protocols that make the models better and more accurate.

All slices must have the same field of view and the same slice spacing; if possible, use a high-resolution algorithm usually described as Bone. Use only axial images, no other reconstructions or reformations in different planes (sagittal or coronal). The slices thickness should be 0.1–1.5 mm (ideal 1.0) and the number of slices 40–1500 (ideal 200–400).

Now that you have your CT examination, the first step is to open the DICOM files with a DICOM viewer.

This software will allow you to open and transform the CT into a 3D file. There are many on the market. Some very expensive but others are totally free (InVesalius and Horos). After opening the examination in this software, choose the axial view and select the threshold that "paints" only the bone part. A good number is 170–300. Now that the bone pixels are selected, create the 3D model and save into a 3D STL file.

Prior to printing, you will likely need to do more preprocessing. For example, if you are interested in a scapula model, the shoulder examination will have the ribs, sternum, clavicle, humerus, and spine. You should open this complete anatomic file and separate the exact parts for printing by removing the bony anatomy that you do not want to print. This task is done with Meshmixer or Meshlab (Adobe) (Fig. 16.9).

How can you make your own models?

There was a time when computer-aided design (CAD) software was designed by engineers, for engineers. That is not the case anymore. The software has become much more user-friendly for the average individual. In order to learn the basics of CAD designing software, check out Autodesk's 123D Design and Inventor Fusion. Both of these programs are free for limited licenses. You can use the free versions of these software tools to design models for printing (Fig. 16.6 and 16.7).

Can you simply scan real objects and print them?

A lot of people wonder whether it is possible to "simply scan and print" objects. It is possible, and there are a few companies that create dedicated 3D scanning equipment; however, the scanned models generally require a lot of tweaking before they can be used to print objects. This idea is undoubtedly ingenious, but it will take a little time to mature; at present you are still better to create the files individually and then print from there.

How should you go about printing models?

If you have downloaded models from websites or created models at home, chances are that they will already be in STL format. This format is halfway to becoming a printable file.

For the printer to be able to manage the design files, they have to be sliced—which means that it has to be transformed into the exact layer-by-layer description of the object, including the temperature, the speed, and wall thickness controls. The resulting file is called a G-Code file that can be interpreted by the printer.

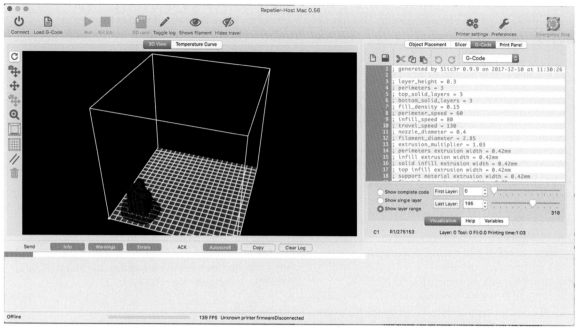

FIG. 16.8 A Slicer software transforms the 3D object into code (G-Code) for the printer.

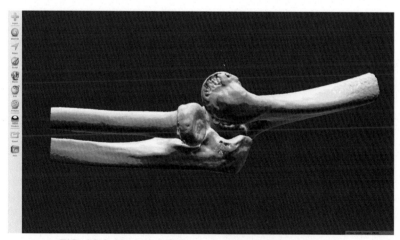

FIG. 16.9 Meshmixer Software for adjusting files for printing.

You can choose from a number of slicing applications in the market, including free ones such as ReplicatorG, Cura, and KISSlicer. Most printers have their own software or versions (Fig. 16.8).

3D Printers: Hardware

Buying a 3D printer of your own can be one of the most exciting purchases you will ever make. But it will not be an easy decision because there are many brands and machine types. You will need to choose between buying a preassembled machine and getting one that you have to build yourself. Both routes come with their own set of advantages and disadvantages. If you are blessed with do-it-yourself skills and a fair bit of technical knowledge, you may find the latter option more appealing. Building your own 3D printer will also cost you less money but certainly more time. You will need at least 2 days of work to build it from a kit to run perfectly. The cost of 3D printers has gone down significantly over the past few years. However, at this time you should still expect to spend around $1000–1500 to get a decent desktop 3D printer (Fig. 16.10).

Essential Hardware

Here we will review some of the components and inner workings of the most common 3D printing machine, the FDM printer. Knowledge of the hardware of a 3D printer is essential if you want to make the most of this technology. It will help you make good decisions when purchasing these machines. It will also help you if you ever have to troubleshoot a problem (and if you are doing this at home, at some point you will have a problem).

How a 3D Printer Works: The Anatomy of a 3D Printer

A printer consists of a frame and features three axes:
X-axis (left-to-right movement)
Y-axis (front-to-back movement)
Z-axis (up-and-down movement)

A part called an extruder is installed on the X-axis and its function is to feed the material that is used to create an object. The lowest part of the extruder itself is called the extruder head—this is the part where the filament is

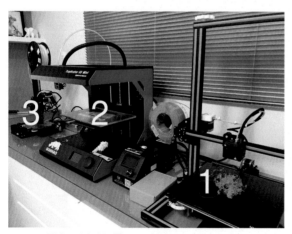

FIG. 16.10 Three desktop printers at author's office.

melted and "extruded" from a tiny hole that has a diameter of no more than a millimeter (Fig. 16.12).

Extruder

The extruder is often considered to be the component from where the plastic filament extrudes. However, this is not entirely true; the extruder is a part that is responsible for pulling and feeding the filament to a part called the hot end.

Hot End

The hot end in a 3D printer is comprised of a heater, a temperature sensor, and an extrusion tip through which the filament is fed. Just as their name implies, they can get extremely hot and should never be handled directly. There are holes in the nozzle that range in size: between 0.2 and 0.8 mm (most common is 0.4).

The smaller the nozzle of the hot end, the finer the print will be; however, the time taken to print the object will also be greater (Fig. 16.13).

Print Bed

The print bed is the area where the objects are created layer by layer by the printer. Based on the type of filament you are using, the print bed itself may be heated. Some filaments such as ABS require a heated bed. The print bed size will determine the X and Y dimensions of your model.

How to Choose a 3D Printer

Choosing a 3D printer is like choosing your car. As there is no definitive car model for every person in the world, with all the technologies and prices, we must choose wisely. We suggest choosing the features you think are most important and buy a machine with good technical support.

It is virtually impossible to calculate how many models and machines there are in the world as many are made by individuals from the ground up. Just as an example, I personally already had (and have) three machines bought from some friends that were totally designed and constructed from scratch by them! A lot of savvy technology enthusiasts attempt to make their

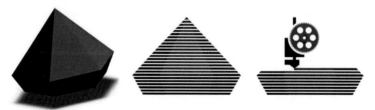

FIG. 16.11 Representation of a layer-by-layer object. http://hotmess3d.com/en/about-3d-printing.

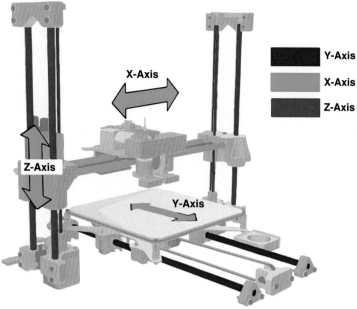

FIG. 16.12 The axis of a desktop 3D printer. https://revolution3dprinters.zendesk.com/hc/en-us/articles/225108188-X-Y-Z-Axis-Movement-Control.

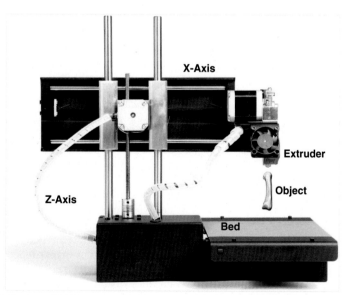

FIG. 16.13 Desktop 3D Printer anatomy. https://pt.slideshare.net/nettrice/biomimicry-3d-printing.

own 3D printer from scratch. This requires some exceptional mechanical and programming skills to begin with, so if you have the skills and patience, then by all means, take this route to the 3D printing arena. I personally created my own machine using bars and connectors from External Fixators and Ilizarov parts (Fig. 16.14).

Overall you need to identify your skill level as well as your needs so that you can pinpoint the exact outcomes that you expect from your 3D printer. This is the first step on the way to purchase a 3D printer.

Kits—Another option is a 3D printer kit. These kits come with all the necessary parts required to set up a

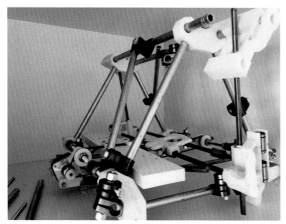

FIG. 16.14 Experimental 3D printer made out 3D-Printed Parts and Orthopedic External Fixators bars.

printer. They do, however, require a fair bit of mechanical and programming knowledge on your part. This is a great way to get to know your machine from inside out so if you ever have to troubleshoot problems, you will have a good idea of where to look. It generally takes 1–2 days to have a kit ready for printing.

Assembled Machine—The easiest and fastest method of getting your hands on a 3D printer is to get an assembled one. Most 3D printing companies now offer ready-made desktop 3D printers. When you purchase a printer, many of them are delivered to you ready to use (even the calibration has been done). This method does cost a little more than the abovementioned two routes, but you save yourself a lot of time and potential hassle.

3D Printers: What to Look for When Comparing Printers

A comparison of 3D printers must be carried out before choosing one that suits your needs. Here are some of the factors that you need to look for when comparing 3D printers:

Price
Build platform size
Filament type
Reviews
Customer service

Price

Price is a major factor that needs to be considered. How much are you willing to spend? There are numerous types of 3D printers available, and their cost varies according to their capabilities.

For instance, FDM printers are comparatively the cheapest desktop printers that you can get. Decent ones start from as low as $1000. The filament that they use

is also quite cheap. Keep in mind that if you are new to 3D printing, you will mess up a few projects (this means wastage of filament) before you get the basic idea. Be prepared to spend the first 10–20 h with your printer in a state of frustration, as you battle to get decent quality prints. This is why you should consider getting a printer that is not only within your budget but also supports a wide variety of affordable filaments.

Build Platform Size

The build platform is the area also known as the print surface. The greater the size of the print area, the larger the size of objects and models that you will be able to print. But "with great power comes great responsibility." Bigger models increase the time needed to print and the chance of failure.

Filament Type

The desktop printers currently available can generally print using two filaments: ABS and PLA. We discussed the different properties of these two materials in great detail previously. Most of the printers will come with interchangeable filament spools, allowing you to use any compatible reel of filaments. A kilogram of ABS or PLA plastic filament typically costs between $30 and $50 depending on its quality.

Keep in mind that the main cost incurred during 3D printing does not lie with the expenses of materials; it is actually the time the printer takes to create a model. Electricity, and your own time, all add up!

Reviews

It is important to read the reviews of the 3D printers that interest you before you actually buy one. A detailed review can help reveal the intricacies of the printer, including any good and bad points that you need to consider.

Customer Support

Because you are likely to make a few mistakes as you are just getting started and technology is complex, it is vital that the company you purchase your printer from provides superb customer support. You can learn about support quality by reading reviews and from their previous customers in discussion forums. The majority of companies that create and sell 3D printers offers exceptional customer support because they want to encourage the expansion and use of 3D printing technology among the masses.

Print Speed

The term print speed may mean different things, but generally it is how far it can move. This seems an important feature because of the printing time, but in a practical job, the print speed has little effect.

Resolution

The resolution of a machine is how thin it can produce a layer. Generally, FMD machines work with 0.1 and 0.2 mm resolution. The higher the resolution of the machine, the more detailed the printed object can be.

How to Transform Your CT Imaging Into a 3D Printed File

These are the tools for manipulating and creating. Not all are necessary, but probably in some part of the job you will need one of these. We are going to suggest in this chapter only software programs that are available **free**. It will be easy to find them on the Internet.

1. Transforming the CT (or MRI) to a 3D file

    When printing anatomy models, this must be the first step. Here we are going to get the anatomic part from your patient's examination and transform it into a 3D file that can be edited, cropped, modified, and printed.

    First, we must have the DICOM files from your patient's CT scan. Normally, these files are inside the CD-ROM or can be downloaded from your cloud server. Open one of these software below and select the examination you want. The software will open all the images. Select the axial examination. Both bone and the soft tissue window will work. I prefer the second. Now is the time to select the pixel density. Every tissue has a specific value. For bone, we suggest a number between 170 and 300. Now that the bone tissue is selected, just create the file and export as a .STL file.

    a. Horos (Mac)
    b. InVesalius (Windows and Mac)
    c. Osirix (Mac)
    d. 3D Slicer

2. Adjusting software—cleaning and preparing the models

    When you transform a CT scan into a 3D file, all the anatomy is represented in that file. But, most of the time, you are only interested in some part. These software are used to separate the models, clean some parts, and even reduce the resolution for better working.

    I suggest starting with Meshmixer. Open the .STL file you have created with the segmentation software. Now, it is time to clean the parts of the anatomy you do not want. Use the selection tool to select and delete. Use the analysis tool and inspector to verify errors that are common and could ruin your print.

    a. Meshlab
    b. Meshmixer

3. CAD software—creating guides, implants, planning surgeries

    Most doctors will not need to work with this kind of software if you are planning just to print anatomy. If you want to design your own instrument, modify, create implants, and plan surgeries using any material or implant, you should have a basic knowledge of CAD.

    a. 3D Builder: It is a Windows 10 software already installed in every new machine
    b. Autodesk 123
    c. Tinkercad

4. Slicing and printer control software

    The models that you design go through one further process on their way to becoming an anatomic model. This process is called slicing.

    Slicing divides the model into several printable layers and plots the toolpaths for them. The control software then sends these "instructions" to the printer which then creates an object layer by layer.

    3D printers are generally controlled through an onboard control screen or by a computer through a USB connection. This user interface enables the control software (which can be the slicer software itself) to send the computer code (instructions) to the printer and controls the major parameters such as the speed, flow, and the temperature required for each layer(Fig. 16.11).

    Every printer has a "preferred" slicing software that is suggested on the manual, but the Slicers software can be used in almost every 3D printer in the world. So you can choose what fits better for you.

    a. Slic3r
    b. Cura
    c. KISSlicer

CONCLUSION

There are a lot of steps to transform your patient's examination into a 3D-printed anatomy model. It can be a time-consuming process. But by the end of this process, you will be an expert in that anatomy, pathology, and all the steps needed to correct it.

While there is a lot to learn, creating your own 3D printed anatomic models and guides in your own home or office can be rewarding and enlightening. We anticipate as more individuals employ 3D printing in the future, the steps and learning curves will continue to improve.

REFERENCES

1. *The Free Beginner's Guide.* 3dprintingindustry Website; 2017. https://3dprintingindustry.com/3d-printing-basics-free-beginners-guide.
2. Henry A. *How to Get Started With 3D Printing (Without Spending a Fortune).* Lifehacker Website; 2017. Updated September 18, 2013. https://lifehacker.com/how-to-get-started-with-3d-printing-without-spending-a-1340345210.
3. Baguley R. *3D Printing Materials: the Pros and Cons of Each Type.* Tom's Guide Website; 2017. Updated February 02, 2017. https://www.tomsguide.com/us/3d-printing-materials,news-24392.html.

FURTHER READING

1. Kloski LWKN. *Getting Started With 3d Printing: a Hands-on Guide to the Hardware, Software, and Services Behind the New Manufacturing Revolution.* Oreilly & Associates Inc.; 2016.
2. Multiple Authors. *Reprap Forum. RepRap Forums*; 2017. http://forums.reprap.org/.
3. Coburn J, Lee J, Patkar M. *Ultimate beginner's guide to 3D printing.* MakeUseOf; 2017. Published February 20, 2017. http://www.makeuseof.com/tag/beginners-guide-3d-printing/.

Index

A

Ablation guides, 188
Ablation probes, 188
Ablative therapy probes, 188
ABS. *See* Acrylonitrile butadiene styrene (ABS)
ACEA. *See* Anterior center edge angle (ACEA)
Acellular biomaterials, 10
Acetabular fracture classifications, 56–57
Acetabulum, 123–126, 129
  AVN/perthes with hip dysplasia, 129–131, 131f–134f
  hip dysplasia, 123–126, 126f–128f
  SCFE, 126–129, 128f–130f
Acrylonitrile butadiene styrene (ABS), 7, 21–22, 57, 105–106, 196, 199–201
Addidas/carbon shoes, 76f
Additive manufacturing (AM), 1, 3–4, 6, 6f, 17, 46, 49, 55, 65, 105–106
  assumptions underpinning medical regulation, 46–47
  basics, 49–50
  FDA
    guidance, 47–48
    regulation of 3D printing, 45–46
    review process, 47
  innovation, 44–45
  in medical applications, 50–52
  3D printing, 45–48
  3D printing–economic considerations, 41–43
  total joint implants, 52
Adult-acquired posterior tibial deficiency, 99–101
Advanced biomaterials medical 3D printing, 11–12
Advanced biomedical 3D printing, 5
Advanced hydrogels, 10
Advanced image visualization techniques, 31
Advanced Regenerative Manufacturing Institute (ARMI), 5
ALARA principle. *See* As low as reasonably achievable principle (ALARA principle)
Allograft reconstruction, 193f
Alloys, 10
AM. *See* Additive manufacturing (AM)
America Makes. *See* National Additive Manufacturing Innovation Institute (NAMII)
American Society of Testing and Materials (ASTM), 19, 49
Anatomic TSA, 152–153
Anatomy education, 56
Anterior center edge angle (ACEA), 123–124, 125f
Apis Cor 3D printing, 18
Archeology, 3D printing in, 19
ARMI. *See* Advanced Regenerative Manufacturing Institute (ARMI)
Art, 3D printing in, 19
As low as reasonably achievable principle (ALARA principle), 34
ASTM. *See* American Society of Testing and Materials (ASTM)
ASTM International, 51, 51f
Automobile, 3D printing in, 19
Avascular necrosis (AVN), 129–131
Aviation, 19
AVN/perthes with hip dysplasia, 129–131, 131f, 133f–134f
  comparison of planned and executed osteotomies, 131

B

Baseplate, 153
  fixation, 153
Beamhardening, 34
Benign aggressive bone tumors, 188
Binder jetting (BJ), 19, 19t, 24–25
Biocompatibility, 81
Bioinks, 12–14, 13f
Bioprinting, 8, 10, 12–14
BJ. *See* Binder jetting (BJ)
Blender, 36t
Blooming, 34
Bone
  cuts, 180
  grafting, 152
  models, 184
  sarcomas, 179–180
Both-bone malunion, 88
Build platform size, 206
Bulk allograft reconstructions, 188

C

CAD. *See* Computer-aided design (CAD)
CAM. *See* computer-aided manufacturing (CAM)
Carcinomatous kidneys, 56
Cardiothoracic surgery, 49
Cardiovascular surgery, 55
CATIA, 26
Center for Devices and Radiological Health (CDRH), 78
Center of rotation (COR), 153
Ceramics, 10
Cervical spine, 57, 58f–59f
  patient-specific implant guides, 110–111
  patient-specific implants, 114
Chondrosarcoma, 179
Clavicle fracture models, 90
CLIP. *See* Continuous liquid interface polymerization (CLIP)
CMF. *See* Craniomaxillofacial (CMF)
Combination energy-material deposition technologies, 8–9
Combined modality treatment, 179
Commercial orthopedic applications 3D printing
  in medicine, 65–81
  in orthopedic applications, 65–74
Complex spinal deformities associated with myelomeningocele, 137–143
Computational semitransparent models of elbow, 166f
Computed tomography scan (CT scan), 31, 51, 66–67, 137–139, 179–180
  CT–guided navigation, 105
Computer modeling software, 123
Computer-aided design (CAD), 36, 106–108, 164–165, 202, 207
computer-aided manufacturing (CAM), 164–165
  deformity, 127–129
Computer-aided tomography, 4
Computer-generated datasets, 95
Computerized navigation system, 112–113
ConforMIS iUni/iDuo product, 68f
Congenital kyphosis, 139–143
  following neonatal kyphectomy, 143
Congenital scoliosis, 137–139, 141–143
Construction, 3D printing in, 18
Consumer market, 3D printed products impacting, 75
Continuous liquid interface polymerization (CLIP), 7

Note: Page numbers followed by "f" indicate figures, "t" indicate tables.

Conventional manufacturing techniques, 114
Conventional surgical instruments, 105
Conventional volar plates, 86
COR. *See* Center of rotation (COR)
Corrective osteotomy/fixation planning and templating, 72–73, 73f
Cortices, 99
Cost, 29
Cranio-maxillo-facial surgery, 49
Craniofacial surgery, 55
Craniomaxillofacial (CMF), 4
Cryosurgery probes, 188
CT and MR images to 3D printed models
  educational websites and resources, 38t
  service bureaus for outsourcing 3D printing, 39t
  steps in workflow creating medical 3D model
    ideation, 31–33
    image acquisition, 33–34
    image segmentation, 34–36
    mesh model creation, smoothing, and preparing for print process, 36
    postprint processing/polishing, 37
    printing, 36–37
    segmentation software examples, 35t
    tips, tricks, and traps, 37–38
    validation and quality control, 37
    workflow for printing patient-specific models, 32f
CT scan. *See* Computed tomography scan (CT scan)
Cubitus valgus, 88
Cubitus varus, 88
Cura, 203
Custom 3D printed guides use
  DRUJ instability after pediatric forearm malunion, 146
  indications/contraindications, 143
  for pediatric upper extremity osteotomies, 143–146
  planning and surgical technique, 143–146
Custom and patient-specific arthroplasty implants, 50–52
Custom devices, 80
Custom femoral implants, 174
Custom implants, 190
Custom talar prosthesis, 95
Cutting jigs, 186, 188

D

DDH. *See* Developmental dysplasia of the hip (DDH)
DED. *See* Directed energy deposition (DED)
Deformity, 106
  CAM, 127–129
  correction, 95

Deltopectoral arm, 182
Department of Defense (DoD), 5
Department of Veteran Affairs (VA), 5
Developmental dysplasia of the hip (DDH), 124
"Diagnostic" imaging, 33
Digital guide, 72
Digital Imaging and Communications in Medicine (DICOM), 31, 95–97, 106–108
Digital light processing (DLP), 20–21, 198
Digital materials, 75
Direct ink writing (DIW), 7
Direct laser melting (DLM), 6
Direct metal laser sintering (DMLS), 23, 49, 66
Directed energy deposition (DED), 19, 19t, 24
Disease morphology, 56–57
Dislocation, 188
Distal humerus correctional osteotomy, 88
Distal humerus fracture fixation with 3D-printed plate, 86–87, 87f
Distal radioulnar joint (DRUJ), 143
  instability after pediatric forearm malunion, 146
Distal radius fracture fixation with 3D-printed plates, 86
Distal radius malunion, 89–90
DIW. *See* Direct ink writing (DIW)
DJO Matchpoint system, 159
DLM. *See* Direct laser melting (DLM)
DLP. *See* Digital light processing (DLP)
DMLS. *See* Direct metal laser sintering (DMLS)
DoD. *See* Department of Defense (DoD)
Drill guides, 105, 188, 192f
DRUJ. *See* Distal radioulnar joint (DRUJ)
Dry-run models, 185
Dynamic pathoanatomy, 60
Dysplastic pedicles, 106

E

EBB. *See* Extrusion-based bioprinting (EBB)
EBM. *See* Electron beam melting (EBM)
Education, 3D printing for, 55–58
  anatomy education, 56
  patient education, 56
  surgical simulation, 57–58
  teaching pathoanatomy, 56–57
Elbow arthritis, 3D planning application in, 165–166
Elbow fracture model, 90
Electron beam melting (EBM), 23–24, 49–50, 66
Energy-based technologies, 6–7
Ewing's sarcoma, 179
Extraperiosteal approach, 143

Extruder, 204
Extrusion 3D printing, 8
Extrusion-based bioprinting (EBB), 22

F

FDA. *See* US Food and Drug Administration (FDA)
FDCA. *See* Federal Food, Drug, and Cosmetic Act (FDCA)
FDM. *See* Fused deposition modeling (FDM)
Federal Food, Drug, and Cosmetic Act (FDCA), 76–77, 80
Femoral head extrusion index (FHEI), 123–124, 125f
FFF. *See* Fused filament fabrication (FFF)
FHEI. *See* Femoral head extrusion index (FHEI)
Filament type, 206
Fixation, 186–188
Flexible prints, 201–202
Flexion valgus internal rotation osteotomy, 126–127
Fluoroscopic images, 123
Food, 3D printing in, 18, 18f
Food and Drug Administration Modernization Act (1997), 78
Foodini, 18, 18f
Foot and ankle surgery, 61, 95. *See also* Oncologic surgery; Spine surgery
  deformity correction, 95
  innovation, 104
  jigs, 97
  3D printing considerations, 99–103
  3D-printed implants, 98–99
  Footprint, 186–188
Foundational 3D printing technologies, 2–3
Free market, 44–45
  economics, 43
  framework, 41
Fused deposition modeling (FDM), 3–4, 7, 10, 17, 19, 198–199
Fused filament fabrication (FFF), 19

G

G-Code file, 202
Gadolinium-enhanced imaging, 180
Gigli saw, 184
Glenohumeral arthritis, 162
Glenoid pathology, 3D planning in assessment of, 155–159
Glenosphere, 153
Good Manufacturing Practice (GMP), 78
Gross tumor, 180

H

Hallux valgus, 95
Hands-on simulation of surgery/osteotomies, 67–68
HB. *See* Hyperelastic "bone" (HB)

HDE route. *See* Humanitarian Device Exempt route (HDE route)
High-grade chondrosarcomas, 179
High-impact polystyrene (HIPS), 23, 106
High-resolution technique, 37
Hip
  3D printing in, 171
  dysplasia, 123–126, 126f–128f
    PAO to normalizing LCEA, 125f
  preservation surgery, 123
HIPS. *See* High-impact polystyrene (HIPS)
Hochman infiltrated 3D printed temporal bone, 57
Hot end, 204
HOYA Yuniku eyeglasses, 76f
Human civilization, 1
Humanitarian Device Exempt route (HDE route), 78
Humanitarian use devices, 79
Hydroxyapatite, 115–118
Hyperelastic "bone" (HB), 11–12

I
IDE. *See* Investigation Device Exemption (IDE)
Iliac bone, 186–188
Image acquisition, 33–34
Imaging, 179
Implants, 174
  manufacturers, 172
  principles in implant placement
    anatomic TSA, 152–153
    application of 3D planning in elbow arthritis, 165–166
    patient-specific guides, 159–164
    reverse TSA, 153–154
    3D planning in assessment of glenoid pathology, 155–159
    3D printed implants in shoulder arthoplasty, 164–165
    two-dimensional *vs.* three-dimensional CT imaging, 154–155
    virtual implant templating, 155–159
In-hospital 3D printing, 75
In-out-in technique, 111
Inkjet binding, 8
Inkjet printing. *See* Material jetting (MJ)
Inkjetting/polyjetting, 7
Instruments, 3D printed, 91, 91f
Intelligent Reusable Instrument (IRI), 161f, 162, 163f
Internal pelvectomy for management of tumors, 60
International Standards Organization (ISO), 51, 51f
Intertrochanteric osteotomy (ITO), 124, 126
Intraoperative fluoroscopy, 124
Intraoperative navigation system, 164

Intraoperative reference, 68
InVesalius software, 35t
Investigation Device Exemption (IDE), 78–79
IRI. *See* Intelligent Reusable Instrument (IRI)
ISO. *See* International Standards Organization (ISO)
ITO. *See* Intertrochanteric osteotomy (ITO)

J
Jigs, 97, 99f, 186–188
Joint preservation, 60–61

K
K-wires, 186–188
KISSlicer, 203
Knee, 172–174
  implants, 174
  PSI, 173–174

L
Lambskin latex-free condom, 57
Laminated object manufacturing (LOM), 8–9
Laminoplasty plates, 57
Large pelvic resection, 69f
Laser metal/wire deposition processes, 8
Laser sintering (LS), 23
Lateral center edge angle (LCEA), 123–124, 125f
Lateral mass screws, 110
LCEA. *See* Lateral center edge angle (LCEA)
LCPs. *See* Locking compression plates (LCPs)
Light-based polymerization, 7
Limb function preservation, 182–183
Limb length discrepancy (LLD), 171
Liquid photopolymer, 20
Live cells, 10
LLD. *See* Limb length discrepancy (LLD)
Local healthcare system, 44
Locking compression plates (LCPs), 86, 87f
LOM. *See* Laminated object manufacturing (LOM)
Lower extremity arthroplasty, 3D printing in, 171
LS. *See* Laser sintering (LS)
Lumbar spine, 57
  patient-specific implant guides, 112–113
  patient-specific implants, 114

M
Magnetic resonance imaging (MRI), 4, 31, 67–68, 179–180
"Maker Lab", 195
"Maker movement", 2–3

Material deposition–based technologies, 7–9
  combination energy-material deposition technologies, 8–9
Material extrusion, 19, 19t, 21–23
  Stratasys Mojo, 22f
  Stratasys uPrint SE, 22f
Material jetting (MJ), 19, 19t, 25
  Stratasys Objet30 Prime, 25f
Material-named ages, 1
Materialise's *Mimics*, 9–10
3-Matic, 36t
Mayo elbow performance score (MEPS), 86–87
MDI. *See* Meter dose inhaler (MDI)
Medacta company, 106
Medial approach, 182
Medical 3D model, steps in workflow creating, 31–38
Medical 3D printing, 8, 11–14, 12f
Medical applications, 66
  AM in, 50–52
    of custom and patient-specific arthroplasty implants, 50–52
    total knee baseplate, 50f
Medical devices, FDA regulation of, 76–79
Medical imaging modalities, 31
Medical regulation, assumptions, 46–47
Medical-image-based anatomic modeling, 67–68
Medicine
  corrective osteotomy/fixation planning and templating, 72–73
  custom devices *vs.* patient-matched devices, 80
  expanded access/compassionate use, 80
  FDA
    guidance on 3D printing, 80
    regulation of medical devices, 76–79
  future directions, 81
  humanitarian use devices, 79
  in-hospital 3D printing, 75
  mainstream knowledge of 3DP, 75
  materials expansion, 75
  patient-matched
    fixation plates, 71
    implants, 68–69
    oncologic reconstruction components, 70
    primary total joint components, 69
    revision total joint components, 69
  practice, 79
  presurgical anatomic modeling, 67–68
  technological advancements, 80–81
  3D printing, 65–81, 67f
    for off-the-shelf implants, 73–74
    products impacting consumer market, 75

Medicine (*Continued*)
total joint arthroplasty planning and templating, 71–72
Melting processes, 7, 24
MEPS. *See* Mayo elbow performance score (MEPS)
Mesh manipulation/cleaning software, 36t
Mesh model for print process, 36
MeshLab, 95–97
Meshmixer, 36t, 207
Metal(s), 10
implants, 174
Metaphyseal prominence, 126–127
Metastatic lesions, 188
Meter dose inhaler (MDI), 43
3MF. *See* 3D Manufacturing Format (3MF)
Mid-diaphysis of long bones, 186–188
Mimics inPrint software, 35t
MJ. *See* Material jetting (MJ)
Monteggia malunion, 88–89
Moore's Law, 18
MRI. *See* Magnetic resonance imaging (MRI)
Multi-jet modeling, 198
Myelomeningocele, complex spinal deformities associating with, 137–143
congenital kyphosis, 139–141
following neonatal kyphectomy, 143
and scoliosis, 141–143
neuromuscular and congenital scoliosis, 137–139
neuromuscular scoliosis and pelvic anomaly, 141

N

Naftulin, 55–56
Nail positioning, 190–191
National Additive Manufacturing Innovation Institute (NAMII), 4–5
National Institutes of Health (NIH), 5
National Network for Manufacturing Innovation (NNMI), 4–5
Native knee joint preservation, 182–183
Negative margin resection, 179–180
Neonatal kyphectomy, congenital kyphosis, 143
Neuromuscular scoliosis, 137–139, 141
NIH. *See* National Institutes of Health (NIH)
NNMI. *See* National Network for Manufacturing Innovation (NNMI)
Nonuniform rational basis spline (NURBS), 37
Non–weight-bearing 3D print of patient, 99–101
NURBS. *See* Nonuniform rational basis spline (NURBS)
Nylon, 201

O

Off-the-shelf
implants, 73–74, 73f
3D-printed bone wedge, 99
Oncologic surgery
challenges in, 181–182
planning adequate margin, 181–182
surgical approach and soft tissue exposure, 182
concepts in, 179–180
One-piece cage stem implants, 191
Opacity, 184
Open reduction and internal fixation (ORIF), 85
Operating room (OR), 110
ORIF. *See* Open reduction and internal fixation (ORIF)
Orthopedic(s)
imaging, 99
oncology, 60, 179
challenges in oncology surgery, 181–182
concepts in oncologic surgery, 179–180
CT and MRI imaging, 180
segmentation, 181
surgical reconstruction challenges, 182–186
3D-printed custom implants, 190–191
3D-printed surgical tools, 186–188
orthopedics–upper extremity arthroplasty
principles in implant placement, 152–166
surgery, 49
3D models for surgical planning, 58–61
education, 55–58
systematic reviews, 55
3D
osteotomy guides for upper extremity malunion correction, 87–90
printing from home and office, 195–196
printing in orthopedic applications, 65–74, 67f
3D-printed guides and plates for primary fracture fixation, 85–87
3D-printed instruments, implants, and prostheses, 91
3D-printed model, 90–91
Oscillating saw, 184
Osirix MD/Osirix Lite software, 35t
Osteosarcoma, 179
Osteotome, 184
Osteotomy, 58–59, 69f
comparison of planned and executed, 131, 134f
techniques, 143

P

PACS. *See* Picture archiving and communication system (PACS)
PAO. *See* Periacetabular osteotomy (PAO)
Patellar tendon, 186–188
Pathoanatomic diseases, 57–58
Patient education, 56
Patient-matched
devices, 80
fixation plates, 70f, 71
implants, 68–69
oncologic reconstruction components, 70
primary total joint components, 69
revision total joint components, 69
Patient-specific arthroplasty implants, 50–52
Patient-specific devices (PMDs), 80
Patient-specific drill guides of varying design, 106
Patient-specific implants, 113–119
cervical spine, 114
future direction, 119
instructions for creating and printing surgeon-designed implants, 115t
legal and regulatory considerations, 118–119
lumbar spine, 114
patient-specific implant guides, 106–113
cervical spine, 110–111
future direction, 113
lumbar spine, 112–113
thoracic spine, 111
surface coating, 114–118
thoracic spine, 114
Patient-specific instrumentation (PSI), 151, 173–174
Zimmer PSI for trabecular metal reverse glenoid system, 160f
Patient-specific porous coatings, 106
PBF. *See* Powder bed fusion (PBF)
PCL. *See* Polycaprolactone (PCL)
Pediatric hip
AVN/perthes with hip dysplasia, 129–131, 131f–134f
dysplasia, 123–126, 126f–128f
SCFE, 126–129, 128f–130f
Pediatric orthopedic surgery, 61
Pediatric spine and extremity
complex spinal deformities associating with myelomeningocele, 137–143
current clinical literature, 146–149
custom 3D printed guides use for pediatric upper extremity osteotomies, 143–146
PEEK. *See* Poly ether ketone (PEEK)
PEKK. *See* Polyetherketoneketone (PEKK)
Pelvic anomaly, 141
Pelvic CT scan, 123
Pelvic implants, 190

Pelvic tumors, 179–180
"Perfect-fit" jig or guide, 97
Periacetabular osteotomy (PAO), 123–126, 125f
Peripherally projecting osteophytes, 155
PET-CT. See Positron emission tomogram CT (PET-CT)
Phalanges, 101
Phantom-based quality analysis, 37
Physical guide, 72
Picture archiving and communication system (PACS), 34
PLA. See Polylactic acid (PLA)
Plasterized cadaveric specimens, 56
Plastics, 106
Ployetherimide, 106
PMA pathway. See Pre-Market Approval pathway (PMA pathway)
PMDs. See Patient-specific devices (PMDs)
Point-of-care manufacturing, 75
Poly ether ketone (PEEK), 52
Polyamide, 201
Polycaprolactone (PCL), 7
Polyetherketoneketone (PEKK), 7, 74, 74f, 106
Polyethylene glycol, 12–14
Polylactic acid (PLA), 7, 21–22, 105–106, 196, 201
Polymer, 10
Polyvinyl alcohol (PVA), 106, 201
Positron emission tomogram CT (PET-CT), 179
Postoperative coronal CT scan, 110–111, 111f
Postoperative CT scan, 114, 116f
Postprint processing/polishing, 36t, 37
Powder bed fusion (PBF), 19, 19t, 23
Powder bed–based selective sintering, 7
PPE. See Proper personal protective equipment (PPE)
Pre-Market Approval pathway (PMA pathway), 78
Prebending plates, 90
Preoperative planning and education, 3D printing for, 119–121
Preprinting phase, 202–203
Preprocessing of 3D printing workflow, 26–27
preparing CAD model, 26
STL conversion, 26–27
uploading part to printer, 27
Presurgical anatomic modeling, 67–68, 67–69, 69f
Presurgical visualization, 67
Primary fracture fixation, 3D-printed guides and plates for
distal humerus fracture fixation, 86–87
distal radius fracture fixation, 86
scaphoid fracture, 85–86

Primary fracture fixation, plates for, 85–87, 86f
Primary sarcomas, 179
Print bed, 204
Print speed, 206–207
Print surface. See Build platform size
Printed surgical tools, 183–184
Printer(s), 197–199
control software, 207
DLP, 198
FDM, 198–199
multi-jet modeling, 198
SL, 197–198
SLS, 198
Printing, 36–37
Proper personal protective equipment (PPE), 24
Prophecy navigation guide, 97
Proto Additive Manufacturing, 2–3
Prototype phase, 66
Proximal humerus fracture model, 90
Proximal tibial osteotomy, 60–61
PSI. See Patient-specific instrumentation (PSI)
PVA. See Polyvinyl alcohol (PVA)

Q
Quality control, 37
Quality System Regulation (QSR), 78

R
Radial head fracture model, 90–91
Radiation therapy, 179
Radiofrequency probes, 188
Radiographs, 124
Radiological Society of North America (RSNA), 75
Rafts, 109
Randomized control trial, 86–87
Rapid prototyping technologies (RP technologies), 3–4, 10, 17, 196
Refined mesh model, 36–37
Regulation principles, 45
Renal carcinoma, 56
ReplicatorG, 203
RepRap Project, 4, 17–19
Resin bath–based lithographic process, 7
Reverse shoulder arthroplasty (RSA), 151
Reverse TSA, 153–154
Robotics, 72
RP technologies. See Rapid prototyping technologies (RP technologies)
RSA. See Reverse shoulder arthroplasty (RSA)
RSNA. See Radiological Society of North America (RSNA)
Rule of thumb, 33

S
Safe Medical Device Act (1990), 78
Scaffolding, 106–109

Scaphoid fracture, 85–86
SCFE. See Slipped capital femoral epiphysis (SCFE)
Sciaky's Electron Beam Additive Manufacturing process, 24
Screw guide templates (SGTs), 106, 109, 109f
three-step, 112f
unilateral three-step, 110f
Screw positioning, 111
Second-generation 3D printing, 5
"Secondary curing" process, 7
Segmentation, 181
software programs, 34, 35t
Selective heat sintering (SHS), 23
Selective laser melting (SLM), 23–24, 49, 106, 115–118
Selective laser sintering (SLS), 3–4, 23, 55, 198
Serratus anterior resection, 60
SGTs. See Screw guide templates (SGTs)
Sheet lamination (SL), 19, 19t, 25–26
Shoulder arthroplasty, 3D printed implants in, 164–165
SHS. See Selective heat sintering (SHS)
Silberstein 3D printed models, 56
Simple biologic tissues, 10
Simplify3D, 106–108
SL. See Sheet lamination (SL); Stereolithography (STL)
SLA. See Stereolithography apparatus (SLA)
Slicing, 207
Slipped capital femoral epiphysis (SCFE), 123, 126–129, 128f–130f
SLM. See Selective laser melting (SLM)
SLS. See Selective laser sintering (SLS)
Smoothness, 184
Soft tissue
coverage of implant, 191
exposure, 182
Softer kernel, 33–34
Southwick/Imhauser-type osteotomy, 126–127
SPECT-CT scans, 104
Spine, 59–60
Spine surgery, 105. See also Foot and ankle surgery
instructions for creating and printing 3D Model of patient's spine, 120t
patient-specific implant guides, 106–113
patient-specific implants, 113–119
pedicle screw drill guide, 107t–108t
3D printing for preoperative planning and education, 119–121
Sports medicine, 60
Standard Tessellation Language, 36
Steinmann pins, 185–186, 188
Stereolithography (STL), 20, 171–172, 197–198
conversion, 26–27
files, 106–108

Stereolithography apparatus (SLA), 3, 17, 65, 66f, 196
Sterile X-ray bags, 121
Sterilization, 72
STL. *See* Stereolithography (STL)
Stratasys Mojo, 22f
Stratasys Objet30 Prime, 25f
Stratasys uPrint SE, 22f
Stryker uncemented triathalon tibial base plate, 174
Subchondral bone support, 152
Supracondylar malunion, 88
Surface coating, patient-specific implants, 114—118
Surgeons, 89
Surgical approach, 182
Surgical plan, 184
Surgical reconstruction challenges, 182—186
    3D models, 183—186, 186f
Surgical resection, 179
Surgical simulation, 57—58
Surgical simulators, 185

T

Technical Considerations for Additive Manufactured Medical Devices, 118—119
Thermojet. *See* Multi-jet modeling
Thermoplastic composites, 10
Thingiverse, 202
Thoracic pedicle screws, 110—111
Thoracic spine
    patient-specific implant guides, 111
    patient-specific implants, 114
Three-dimension (3D)
    computer modeling, 124, 131
    CT imaging, 154—155
    digital model, 196
    imaging, 143
    modeling and printing, 123
    models, 183—186, 186f—189f
        foot and ankle surgery, 61
        joint preservation, 60—61
        orthopedic oncology, 60
        pediatric orthopedic surgery, 61
        spine, 59—60
        sports medicine, 60
        for surgical planning, 58—61
        total joint arthroplasty, 61
        trauma, 60
    osteotomy guides for upper extremity malunion correction, 87—90
    painting, 8, 11—12
    preoperative planning, 171—172
    rapid prototyping, 171—172
    scanning, 27—28
    Slicer software, 35t
    software, 17
    templating using OrthoVis preoperative planning software, 156f—157f
    3D-printed prosthesis, 91
    visualization, 31

Three-dimensional printers (3D printers), 196
    build platform size, 206
    comparison, 206
    customer support, 206
    filament type, 206
    hardware, 203—204
    kits, 205—206
    price, 206
    print speed, 206—207
    resolution, 207
    reviews, 206
    selection, 204—206
    works, 204
Three-dimensional printing (3D printing), 1—5, 17—18, 41, 45—48, 52, 85, 90—91, 95, 105, 114, 137, 172, 186, 196
    additive manufacturing, 3—4
    advantages, 28
    applications, 18—19
        archeology, 19
        art, 19
        automobile, 19
        aviation, 19
        construction, 18
        food, 18, 18f
        medical applications, 19
    clavicle fracture models and prebending plates, 90
    components, processes, materials, and classifications, 6
        technologies and processes, 6, 6f
    computational capabilities increase and industrial 3D printing matures, 4
    custom implants, 190—191
    drill guides, 111
    elbow fracture model, 90
    energy-based technologies, 6—7
    FDA regulation of, 45—46
    general distinction between subtractive and AM processes, 2f
    hardware, software, and material, 9—11, 9f
    implants, 98—99
    implants in shoulder arthoplasty, 164—165
    limitations, 29
    material deposition—based technologies, 7—9
    medical, 11—14, 12f
        future, 14
    new materials
        and advanced biomedical, 5
        and technologies and second-generation, 5
    physical objects, 171
    plant, 202—207
        CT imaging into 3D printed file, 207
        essential hardware, 204
        extruder, 204
        hot end, 204

Three-dimensional printing (3D printing) (*Continued*)
    materials, 199—202
    orthopedic 3D printing from home and office, 195—196
    preprinting phase, 202—203
    print bed, 204
    printers, 197—199
    technology, 196—197
    for preoperative planning and education, 119—121
    proto additive manufacturing, 3
    proximal humerus fracture model, 90
    radial head fracture model, 90—91
    rapid expansion and increased awareness of, 4—5
    surgical tools, 186—188
        general design, 186—188
    3D printing—economic considerations, 41—43
    types, 19—26
        BJ, 24—25
        directed energy deposition, 24
        DLP, 20—21
        LS, 23
        material extrusion, 21—23
        melting, 24
        MJ, 25
        PBF, 23
        SL, 25—26
        stereolithography, 20
        vat photopolymerization, 20
    workflow SL, 26—27
        postprocessing, 27
        preprocessing, 26—27
        processing, 27
3D grapheme (3DG), 11—12
3D Manufacturing Format (3MF), 37
3D-printed model. *See* Three-dimensional printing (3D printing)
Ti64. *See* Titanium-6 aluminum-4 vanadium (Ti64)
Titanium alloy powder, 86
Titanium plasma spray (TPS), 114—118
Titanium-6 aluminum-4 vanadium (Ti64), 7
TKA. *See* Total knee arthroplasty (TKA)
Tool error, 181
Total joint arthroplasty, 61
    planning and templating, 71—72
Total joint implants, 52
Total knee arthroplasty (TKA), 70f, 72, 172
Total shoulder arthroplasty (TSA), 151
Traditional manufacturing techniques, 17
Traditional medical 3D printing, 11
Transpedicular transdiscal screw trajectory (TPTD screw trajectory), 112—113, 112f

Trauma, 60
TSA. *See* Total shoulder arthroplasty
(TSA)
Two-dimension (2D), 180
CT imaging, 154–155
Two-photon polymerization, 7

U
Ultra-high molecular weight
polyethylene (UHMWPE), 69
Upper extremity malunion correction,
87–90, 89f
both-bone malunion, 88
distal humerus correctional
osteotomy, 88
distal radius malunion, 89–90
Monteggia malunion, 88–89
supracondylar malunion, cubitus
varus, and cubitus valgus, 88

US Food and Drug Administration
(FDA), 5, 44–45, 73, 118–119
guidance
in december 2017, 47–48
on 3D printing, 80
regulation
of medical devices, 65f, 76–79, 79t
of 3D printing, 45–46
review process, 47

V
VA. *See* Department of Veteran Affairs
(VA)
Vat photopolymerization, 19–20, 19t
Vault model, 158
Viable cancer cells, 180
Virtual implant templating, 3D
planning in assessment of,
155–159

Virtual Reality Modeling Language
(VRML), 37
Voxels, 20

W
4WEB Medical company, 98–99
3D-printed implantable cage, 101f
Weight-bearing effect, 99
White glue or blue painter's tape, 201

Z
ZEdit software, 37
Zimmer Trabecular Metal Reverse
Shoulder System, 153–154
ZimmerBiomet, 172
ZPrint software, 37